Contemporary Endocrinology

Series editor

Leonid Poretsky, Friedman Transgender Health and Wellness Program,
Division of Endocrinology, Lenox Hill Hospital, Donald and Barbara Zucker
School of Medicine at Hofstra/Northwell, New York, NY, USA

More information about this series at http://www.springer.com/series/7680

Leonid Poretsky · Wylie C. Hembree
Editors

Transgender Medicine

A Multidisciplinary Approach

Humana Press

Editors
Leonid Poretsky
Friedman Transgender Health and Wellness Program, Division of Endocrinology
Lenox Hill Hospital, Donald and Barbara Zucker School of Medicine at Hofstra/Northwell
New York, NY, USA

Wylie C. Hembree
Columbia University
New York, NY, USA

ISSN 2523-3785 ISSN 2523-3793 (electronic)
Contemporary Endocrinology
ISBN 978-3-030-05682-7 ISBN 978-3-030-05683-4 (eBook)
https://doi.org/10.1007/978-3-030-05683-4

Library of Congress Control Number: 2018963998

This Humana Press imprint is published by the registered company Springer Nature Switzerland AG
The registered company address is: Gewerbestrasse 11, 6330 Cham, Switzerland

Series Editor Foreword

Transgender medicine, like transgender rights, is a new frontier. Endocrinologists, however, have been inhabiting this frontier for decades because of the patients' need for hormonal therapy. For this reason, I thought it would be appropriate to publish *Transgender Medicine: A Multidisciplinary Approach* in the *Contemporary Endocrinology* series.

Needless to say, comprehensive care of a transgender individual requires much more than hormonal therapy—primary care physicians, mental health professionals, pediatricians, plastic surgeons, specialists in reproductive health, and other medical specialists all have important roles to play. Further, because transgender patients' needs often extend beyond medicine, social workers, legal professionals, and spiritual counselors also may have to be involved. Hence, the interdisciplinary nature of this book.

I am thankful to an outstanding group of accomplished experts passionately devoted to this field who enthusiastically contributed their time and effort to this volume. I realize that there is no publication that can match our transgender patients' perseverance, determination, and courage in their pursuit of a fulfilling and happy life. I hope that this text will make a contribution to the development of the knowledge base sorely needed to help transgender individuals achieve their life goals.

New York, NY, USA Leonid Poretsky, MD

Preface

Medical and social care of transgender persons require complicated, multidisciplinary efforts with complex strategies and many unknowns. The biology of gender identity, gender dysphoria, and gender incongruence is still incompletely understood. The best medical practice options are often based upon retrospective or empirical studies rather than upon controlled, randomized, double-blind trials common to most other areas of medicine.

Even hormone therapy for transgender individuals is commonly based upon the strategies used for estrogen replacement in menopausal women or testosterone in hypogonadal men—treatment modalities whose goals differ from those of gender affirming hormone therapy in transgender individuals. As a result, treatment may lack consistent standards of care required to ensure an acceptable transition in hormone levels using the best available therapeutic options. To make things even more complex, in addition to hormone therapy, transgender persons have a multitude of coincident needs—medical, surgical, educational, social, and legal—all of which must be addressed.

In planning this volume, we attempted to address as many of these needs as possible. We have engaged a multidisciplinary group of experts and asked them to provide recommendations and advice based upon the best available evidence. Clearly, the important and compelling field of transgender medicine will continue to evolve and the next edition of this text (if and when it comes) may look very different. So, in the meantime, we hope that the reader will find this text a useful guide for safe and efficient care of transgender persons.

We are grateful to all contributors who embraced this project with immense enthusiasm and to our students who keep asking good questions and demanding evidence-based answers. Most importantly, we are indebted to those transgender persons from whom we continue to learn daily and with whom we are proud to share their accomplishments.

New York, NY, USA

Leonid Poretsky, MD
Wylie C. Hembree, MD

Preface

Contents

Contributors

Ladan Ahmadi, MD Department of Internal Medicine, Lenox Hill Hospital, Northwell Health, New York, NY, USA

Brittany J. Allen, MD Department of Pediatrics, University of Wisconsin School of Medicine and Public Health, Madison, WI, USA

Adrian Araya, MD Department of Pediatrics, Mott Children's Hospital, Michigan Medicine, Ann Arbor, MI, USA

Stephanie Baum, MD Department of OBGYN and Reproductive Endocrinology and Infertility, Lenox Hill Hospital, Northwell Health, New York, NY, USA

Boback M. Berookhim, MD Department of Urology, Lenox Hill Hospital, Northwell Health, New York, NY, USA

Kelly J. Chan, BA Boston Medical Center and Boston University School of Medicine, Boston, MA, USA

Deeangelys Colón, BA Department of Endocrinology, Lenox Hill Hospital, Northwell Health, New York, NY, USA

Dennis Dacarett-Galeano, BA Icahn School of Medicine at Mount Sinai, New York, NY, USA

Aaron Devor, Phd University of Victoria, Victoria, BC, Canada

Nancy Neveloff Dubler, AB, LL.B Division of Medical Ethics, Department of Population Health, NYU School of Medicine, New York, NY, USA;
NYC Health + Hospitals, New York, USA

Mark Fisher, MD Department of Plastic and Reconstructive Surgery, Zucker School of Medicine at Hofstra/Northwell, Hempstead, NY, USA

Sarah L. Fishman, MD, Phd Division of Endocrinology, Lenox Hill Hospital, Northwell Health, New York, NY, USA

Kelly McBride Folkers, MA Division of Medical Ethics, Department of Population Health, NYU School of Medicine, New York, NY, USA

Samantha Goldstein, DO Department of Internal Medicine, Lenox Hill Hospital, Northwell Health, New York, NY, USA

Zil Goldstein, MSN Department of Medical Education, The Mount Sinai Health System, New York, NY, USA

Oksana Hamidi, DO Department of Endocrinology and Metabolism, UT Southwestern Medical Center, Dallas, TX, USA

Wylie C. Hembree, MD Division of Endocrinology, Columbia University College of Physicians and Surgeons, New York, NY, USA

Jo Hirschmann, BCC, ACPE Department of Spiritual Care and Education, Mount Sinai Beth Israel, New York, NY, USA

Aron Janssen, MD Department of Child and Adolescent Psychiatry, Hassenfeld Children's Hospital at NYU Langone, New York, NY, USA

Noelle Marie Javier, MD Department of Geriatrics and Palliative Medicine, Icahn School of Medicine at Mount Sinai, New York, NY, USA

Susan Jelinek, BCC Department of Pastoral Care, Cincinnati Children's Hospital Medical Center, Cincinnati, OH, USA

Sean Lare, LCSW-C Sean Lare Counseling and Consulting, Columbia, MD, USA

Noah E. Lewis, Esq. Transcend Legal, Jackson Heights, NY, USA

Todd B. Nippoldt, MD Department of Endocrinology, Diabetes and Nutrition, Mayo Clinic, Rochester, MN, USA

Angelica Nocerino, MD Department of Internal Medicine, Lenox Hill Hospital, Northwell Health, New York, NY, USA

Maria Paliou, MD Division of Endocrinology, Lenox Hill Hospital, Northwell Health, New York, NY, USA

Adam D. Perry, MD Department of Plastic and Reconstructive Surgery, Zucker School of Medicine at Hofstra/Northwell, Hempstead, NY, USA

Richard R. Pleak, MD Division of Child and Adolescent Psychiatry, Donald and Barbara Zucker School of Medicine at Hofstra/Northwell, Glen Oaks, NY, USA

Leonid Poretsky, MD Friedman Transgender Health and Wellness Program, Division of Endocrinology, Lenox Hill Hospital, Donald and Barbara Zucker School of Medicine at Hofstra/Northwell, New York, NY, USA

Tonia Poteat, Phd, MPH, PA-C Department of Social Medicine, University of North Carolina, Chapel Hill, NC, USA

Daniel Puneky, MD Department of Internal Medicine, Lenox Hill Hospital, Northwell Health, New York, NY, USA

Katherine Rachlin, Phd Clinical Psychologist in Private Practice, New York, NY, USA

Asa Radix, MD, MPH Department of Medicine, Callen-Lorde Community Health Center, New York, NY, USA

Tamar Reisman, MD Division of Endocrinology, Diabetes and Bone Disease, Department of Internal Medicine, Icahn School of Medicine at Mount Sinai, New York, NY, USA

Donna B. Riley, Phd, LCSW-R School of Social Welfare, Stony Brook University, Stony Brook, NY, USA

Joshua D. Safer, MD, FACP Center for Transgender Medicine and Surgery, Mount Sinai Health System and Icahn School of Medicine, New York, NY, USA

Jean Sawyer, Phd Department of Communication Sciences and Disorders, Illinois State University (This is a university and not a hospital), Normal, IL, USA

Warren M. Seigel, MD, MBA, FAAP, FSAHM Division of Adolescent Medicine, Bioethics Consultation Service, Department of Pediatrics, NYC Health + Hospitals/Coney Island, Brooklyn, NY, USA

Shervin Shadianloo, MD Division of Child and Adolescent Psychiatry, Zucker Hillside Hospital, Glen Oaks, NY, USA

Daniel Evan Shumer, MD, MPH Department of Pediatrics, Mott Children's Hospital, Michigan Medicine, Ann Arbor, MI, USA

Tomer Singer, MD Department of OBGYN and Reproductive Endocrinology and Infertility, Lenox Hill Hospital, Northwell Health, New York, NY, USA

Mark Smith, MD Department of Plastic and Reconstructive Surgery, Zucker School of Medicine at Hofstra/Northwell, Hempstead, NY, USA

Leon Telis, MD Department of Urology, Lenox Hill Hospital, Northwell Health, New York, NY, USA

Emilee Walker-Cornetta, BCC Department of Pastoral Care and Education, New York-Presbyterian Hospital, Columbia University Irving Medical Center, New York, NY, USA

Chapter 1
History and Prevalence of Gender Dysphoria

Tonia Poteat, Katherine Rachlin, Sean Lare, Aron Janssen and Aaron Devor

Introduction

When asked to write about the history and prevalence of gender dysphoria, we carefully considered what that might include. We recognize that the transgender population is vastly diverse throughout the world. The evolution of transgender medicine is intricately connected to cultural attitudes regarding gender, to the evolution of language, to patient identities and narratives, diagnoses, and standards of care, as well as the ways transgender people are identified and counted. A discussion of the history and prevalence includes acknowledgement of all the people impacted by these systems, and how the strong voices and experiences of this population have contributed to the evolution of these systems.

The language used to describe transgender people is evolving. For the purposes of this chapter, we use the words trans, non-binary, and gender diverse to mean

T. Poteat (✉)
Department of Social Medicine, University of North Carolina, Chapel Hill, NC, USA
e-mail: tonia_poteat@med.unc.edu

K. Rachlin
Clinical Psychologist in Private Practice, New York, NY, USA
e-mail: kitrachlin@gmail.com

S. Lare
Sean Lare Counseling and Consulting, Columbia, MD, USA
e-mail: counseling@seanlare.com

A. Janssen
Department of Child and Adolescent Psychiatry, Hassenfeld Children's Hospital at NYU Langone, New York, NY, USA
e-mail: Aron.Janssen@nyumc.org

A. Devor
University of Victoria, Victoria, BC, Canada
e-mail: ahdevor@uvic.ca

L. Poretsky and W. C. Hembree (eds.), *Transgender Medicine*, Contemporary Endocrinology, https://doi.org/10.1007/978-3-030-05683-4_1

people whose gender identities do not match or align with their sex assigned at birth. We use these terms in an attempt to be inclusive of all gender identities, though we recognize that over time, trends in language will change. It is important to use the terms most affirming to each person when working with individual people. Of course, as a chapter that includes discussions of historical perspectives, we may use other terms when citing or quoting another source. When we use capitalization for Gender Dysphoria, we are referring to the diagnosis as defined in the *Diagnostic and Statistical Manual (DSM) 5*; when "Standards of Care" is capitalized, we are referring to the World Professional Association of Transgender Health's (WPATH) Standards of Care (SOC).

Trans and non-binary people throughout time have had rich, complex, and varied narratives about their lived experience that have not always aligned with either the diagnostic criteria laid forth or with the expectations of medical and mental health providers. Over the Past 50 years, in order to access gender-affirming care, trans and non-binary people have been required to undergo evaluations and receive a diagnosis associated with gender diversity. (As we will describe, the diagnostic label and criteria have changed over time). People who did not meet the diagnostic criteria would not get gender-affirming care; therefore, they would sometimes tailor their narratives to fit the diagnosis, even if the description did not accurately or fully reflect their experience. When this happened, providers remained uninformed about the real and varied experiences of their gender diverse patients [16]. The increasing outspokenness and visibility of trans and non-binary people have allowed for clinical decisions, diagnostic categories, and treatment protocols to evolve and to better serve these groups.

We hope to increase readers' understanding of the history and complexity of this topic and how we got to where we are at the time of this printing, particularly in the treatment of gender dysphoria. The purpose of this chapter is to briefly describe the long history of gender diversity; to address difficulties in estimating the number of gender diverse people worldwide and the challenges for researchers and medical and mental health professionals who wish to define and count this population; to look at the history and utility of Gender Dysphoria as a diagnosis in the *DSM-5* and the *International Classification of Diseases (ICD)*; and to provide some historical perspective on the evolution of standards of care over time.

We recognize that the field of transgender medicine is evolving and will continue to do so after this book is printed. Growing advocacy by, and visibility of, transgender people will also rightfully continue to influence this field and future work. That said, it is important to understand how we got here, how the history of diagnoses has influenced where we are, and how we move forward in the care and management of gender dysphoria. The chapter is divided into four sections: A Short History of Gender Diversity, Being Counted, A Brief Review of Diagnostic Changes over Time, and An Evolution of Guidelines. Each section ends with thoughts on future directions and the need for further work.

A Short History of Gender Diversity

The medicalization of gender diversity is a relatively new historical phenomenon. The word transgender and the concepts that it attempts to convey, are quite new in historical terms, really only becoming widely used in the 1990s. The terms trans, non-binary, and Two-Spirit are even newer, coming into common usage in the early 2000s. Earlier in the twentieth century, the words transvestite and transsexual were more commonly used in Western societies to describe people who cross-dressed periodically, or who pursued complete hormonal and surgical transitions.[1] Prior to the beginning of the twentieth century, however, there were no words in English or European languages specifically to describe what we now think of as trans or non-binary people. Nor were there hormonal treatments or gender affirmation surgeries. Thus, those in Western societies who wished to change gender expression could either present as gender-nonconforming or affect a social transition to the other binary gender and hope to remain undetected. However, evidence of people in the West who were gender diverse is as old as are our historical records.

While it would be anachronistic and/or colonialist to apply today's Western diagnostic or social categories to people of other times and places, it is possible to recognize that people who share some features with those who today might call themselves transgender, transsexual, trans, non-binary, or any of a wide range of related identity terms, have always been part of humanity. The historical evidence of earlier gender diversity that is available must be understood to be far from verifiable in the specifics, but the existence of gender diversity cannot be in doubt.

Often, the evidence comes to us through very incomplete reports made by observers rather than from the people themselves. Such reports can tell us something about people's actions; they can tell us less about their motivations and identities. In all cases, the reports are likely to be difficult to interpret in relation to today's sensibilities. In particular, throughout most of human history, and still quite common today, physical sex, social expressions of identities, and erotic inclinations and behaviors, have all been thought of as a single manifestation of more or less the same underlying factor. In some contexts, such dispositions were thought of as stemming from one's soul, in others, from one's biology. Thus, gender diversity in other times and places might have been interpreted as what today would be understood as differences of sex development, or as homosexuality, or having a soul in the wrong type of body, or as stemming from some combination of these and other factors.

One of the oldest historical records of gender diversity comes to us from a female-bodied pharaoh named Hatshepsut who ruled Ancient Egypt 1478–1458 BCE and was depicted as a king with a beard, standing in a masculine pose [22]. This scant evidence might indicate an individual who today would seek out transgender medicine. From the Roman period, historical records tell of Emperor

[1]The term transsexual has fallen out of favor with some due to its association with medicalization. However, there are individuals who embrace transsexual as an identity.

Elagabalus who ruled 218–222 CE. The little that we know about him includes that he was known for his sensuous beauty, his use of cosmetics, and his feminine clothing and mannerisms. Similar to many gender diverse people who seek gender-affirming medical treatment today, he wanted to be known as a female, and he sought a surgeon who could give him female genitalia [65, 93].

Many Indigenous peoples around the world have long had the language to describe gender diversity as it has been understood in their cultures. In many cases, these societies and cultures recognized and embraced three or more gender identities and such people were often seen as special healers or spiritual guides. As the influence of Western culture and medicine spreads, some of the language and attitudes of the West have begun to supplant, or coexist, with more traditional approaches. For example, the Hijra of modern-day India, who trace their lineage back 2000 years, typically start life with male genitalia and later undergo ritual castration, and sometimes penectomy, using traditional methods. They are then understood to be neither male nor female, but, rather, some of both. They dress in women's clothing, do not usually attempt to be seen as women, and exhibit a form of femininity that is both a parody of proper Indian womanhood and a bowdlerization of it [66]. Today, some Hijra also identify as transgender or transsexual and seek hormonal treatments and hospital-based surgical procedures [79].

Over 150 traditional Indigenous cultures of North America had culturally accepted roles for people who were recognized as different from women and men on the basis of their temperament, work roles, clothing, personal habits, spirituality, or sexuality. Today, the English term Two-Spirit functions as an umbrella term that includes lesbian, gay, bisexual, trans, non-binary, intersex, queer, and questioning people. Some Two-Spirit people identify more with specific aspects of gender or sexuality within the Two-Spirit umbrella, and other people prefer to simply identify as Two-Spirit [37, 74].

There are also numerous European historical figures who exhibited traits that, in today's world, might cause them to identify, or lead others to consider them to be trans. The story of Jean D'Arc is well known. Born in 1412 in France, at the age of 17 she had a vision from God that she was to dress in men's clothing and help lead France in the battle against England. Although she prevailed against the English, ultimately, she was burned at the stake, refusing until her death to dress in women's clothes and accept women's traditional gender role [82]. Spaniard Catalina de Erauso, the Lieutenant Nun, born in 1585, exhibited behavior that today might indicate a trans identity. Lacking any alternative for gender expression other than subterfuge, at the age of 15, de Erauso escaped from the convent where she had been deposited as a child and began to live as a young man. De Erauso became a sailor and traveled extensively. By 1626, de Erauso's story had become legendary and the Pope gave de Erauso a choice between living as a woman in a convent, or a man in the secular world. De Erauso chose to embrace manhood for the remainder of his life [25]. The Chevalier/Chevalière d'Éon, born in 1728 in France, demonstrated a gender expression similar to some of today's non-binary people. For the first 49 years of life, d'Éon lived as a man who served as a military Captain and as a spy. However, aspects of d'Eon's gender expression led many people at the time to believe that d'Éon was really a woman who dressed as a man in order to prove that women could do anything that men could do. Believing d'Eon to be a woman, in 1777, the King of France ordered d'Éon to only wear women's clothing from that time on—which d'Eon willingly did. Upon d'Eon's death in 1810, d'Éon's body was examined by several doctors who reported that d'Èon had male genitalia [56].

While people in earlier centuries might have wished that they could transform their bodies to align them with their gender identities, medicine did not begin to provide the means to do so until the first half of the twentieth century. Toward the end of the nineteenth century, medical professionals started to recognize that some people desired to live as a gender different from the one they were assigned at birth. Krafft-Ebing described a case of a young male who felt "as if I were a real woman," and referred to this case as an example of "effemination," which he classified as one of the most diseased forms of homosexuality [57]. In 1910, Magnus Hirschfeld, who established the Institute for Sex Research in Berlin in 1919, published one of the first professional books challenging the view that trans people were necessarily homosexual, *Transvestites: The Erotic Drive to Cross Dress* [47]. In 1930, some of the first experiments with gender-affirming surgeries were conducted on two trans women at Hirschfeld's Institute.

Michael Dillon was probably the first trans man to undergo a medical transition including hormonal treatments and genital surgeries. Born in 1915, Dillon displayed classic childhood and young adult signs of being trans. In 1939, at age 24, Dillon procured testosterone pills, the effects of which enabled him to live socially as a man. Dillon later had his breasts removed and then underwent a 4-year-long series of genital surgeries to create a penis. In 1958, a journalist exposed Dillon as trans, making him one of the earliest trans celebrities. Dillon died in 1962 as a Buddhist monk in India at age 47 [49].

Starting in the 1950s, a number of Americans came to prominence and influenced social and professional perceptions of who might be included under the trans umbrella. Christine Jorgensen (1926–1989) was the first transsexual person to achieve international fame when the story of her gender transition made front-page headlines in the *New York Daily News* on December 1, 1952. Four months later, the *Los Angeles Times* declared her the "most talked about" person in the world. At that time, trans people often had no words to describe how they felt and thought that they were the only ones in the world with their feelings. The news about Jorgensen's gender transition was transformative. It informed the public about the existence of trans people and offered hope to trans people that transition may be possible for them. For many service providers, members of the general public, and trans people themselves, Jorgensen's heteronormative appearance became the standard template for transsexual gender expression [31]. It was not until 1966 that the first major publication appeared that recommended gender-affirming treatments for transsexual people. Harry Benjamin, who had studied with Magnus Hirschfeld, published *The Transsexual Phenomenon*, setting a new direction for the treatment of gender diverse people. Some trans people used this book as a guide for pursuing treatment from a growing number of sympathetic physicians.

Virginia Prince (1912–2009) had a long career as a trans speaker, publisher, editor, and author. In 1960, she founded a very influential magazine, *Transvestia,* was its editor for 20 years, and used it effectively as a mouthpiece to spread her views on gender within trans circles. Prince also attended professional conferences and communicated extensively with leading gender experts of her day, influencing their views on gender diversity. Prince was an early, assertive, proponent of the separation of sex and gender, and of the primacy of gender identity in determining persons' social and legal rights and statuses. She proudly maintained that she was a woman irrespective of her retention of the penis with which she had been born. She coined the word transgenderist to describe how she lived full-time as a woman without the benefit of surgery and identified as neither a transsexual nor a transvestite. During the early 1960s, Prince started a group called "The Hose and Heels Club", which later evolved into the much larger Foundation for Full Personality Expression (FPE), and then into the even-larger Society for the Second Self (Tri-Ess), which still exists today with chapters across the United States. In the 1960s, Prince was arrested and convicted for sending sexually explicit letters to a heterosexual male cross-dresser through the US Mail. Her probation requirements included that she not cross-dress. However, her lawyer negotiated permission for her to cross-dress if she did it for educational purposes. Thus began Virginia Prince's successful public speaking career advocating for acceptance of heterosexual male cross-dressers. At age 55, Virginia Prince began to live full-time as a woman, which she continued to do until her death at age 96 [32].

Lou Sullivan (1951–1991) was another trans person, who was instrumental in advancing professional thought. Sullivan was androphilic (attracted to men) at the time when the professional opinion was that anyone who claimed to be a trans man and androphilic was not a true transsexual and should be denied hormonal and surgical treatment. Sullivan was a driving force in convincing professionals to provide gender-affirming treatment to gay and bisexual trans men. He wrote and spoke out for years, until he had amassed a group of other androphilic men and garnered the attention of influential professionals who joined him in his advocacy. Shortly before his death from AIDS in 1991, Sullivan commented that he took a certain pleasure in sharing his HIV status with some of the gender clinics that had rejected him because they thought that he could not live as a gay man because "…it looks like I'm gonna die like one" [80].

As trans people began to access the Internet in the 1990s, they built online communities for social support, knowledge exchange, and with strength in numbers necessary to influence medical and social policy. Similarly, social understandings of gender diversity have been expanding. For example, the number of individuals who assert non-binary identities is increasing [63, 73]. Gender non-binary people may eschew the term trans because they feel it implies movement from one point on a gender binary to another, an implication that does not accurately reflect them. Terms that non-binary people may prefer include: genderqueer (political non-binary identity); bi-gender (being both a man and a woman); pangender (being all genders, including more than two); agender, null gender, neutrois (having no gender); and gender creative or gender fluid (continuing to explore and change gender identity and expression). Current standards and practices of care are generally geared to assisting trans people to achieve binary forms of gender expression and embodiment. The needs of non-binary people may represent the next major challenge for professionals working in the field of transgender medicine.

Being Counted

"If you're not counted, you don't count" is an old adage that speaks to the importance of data as a tool to advocate for the needs of marginalized groups. Researchers determine who "counts" by first defining the population. They often use diagnostic criteria or clinical guidelines for this purpose, and individuals who do not fit within these parameters may not be counted as part of the population. Enduring challenges to gathering data on the numbers of gender diverse people include how to ascertain trans and gender diverse identities, identify "representative" samples, and overcome stigma-related barriers to disclosure. The dynamic and evolving nature of gender identity presents additional challenges for counting the numbers of gender diverse people and highlights the inherently reductionist nature of quantitative research [41, 58]. Nonetheless, being counted in health research is necessary to advance understanding of the diverse health needs of trans and non-binary people and to respond to that diversity in clinical care [77]. How researchers determine who "counts" as trans is impacted by, and has an impact on diagnostic criteria, clinical guidelines, and the lives of gender diverse people themselves.

The movement from pathologization toward understanding gender diversity as a normal variation of human existence is reflected in the evolution in ways researchers have attempted to define and describe the numbers of trans people in a given population [64]. Definitions are important, as they determine who is included or excluded from the population of interest and are often used to determine who receives care. For many years, the medical literature focused on counting trans people who sought gender-affirming medical interventions to transition from their assigned sex at birth to another gender [94]. Other studies included individuals who met DSM diagnostic criteria for "Gender Identity Disorder" or "Gender Dysphoria" or who had received an International Classification of Diseases (ICD) code for "transsexualism" [9]. This practice implicitly, or explicitly, excludes gender diverse people who do not seek gender transition services in a medical setting or at all.

Historical reports of population sizes of 1 in 4000 to 1 in 50,000 were based on clinical populations, largely in Europe [27, 28, 95]. While clinic-based data are important for the planning of clinic-based services, they underestimate the size of the broader population of gender diverse people. Nor is it clear from this approach how to determine the denominator for estimates of the population proportion.

In recent years, researchers have adopted population-based methods to estimate the number of trans people. For example, McFarland and colleagues [62] used two population-based methods to estimate the number of trans men living in San

Francisco [62]: the service multiplier method [55] and the wisdom of the crowds method [99]. The service multiplier method calculated the total population size as a count of trans men using a specified community-based organization service in a single year divided by the proportion of trans men in the survey who reported using the service in that same year. The wisdom of the crowds method asked survey participants "How many transgender men do you think there are living in San Francisco?" The median response was used as the population size estimate.

Other strategies include asking a representative sample of people from the general population about their gender identity and extrapolating results to the entire population. One example of this approach is the U.S. Behavioral Risk Factor Surveillance Study (BRFSS). The BRFSS collects data via interviews with more than 400,000 adults in all 50 states as well as the District of Columbia and three U. S. territories each year, making it the largest continuously conducted health survey system in the world [13]. In 2014, 19 states included the question, "Do you consider yourself to be transgender?" In 2016, the Williams Institute began to publish estimates of the transgender population based on these data, providing not only the number and proportion of the U.S. population who identify as transgender but also information on the age and racial distribution. The Williams Institutes estimated that 1.4 million adults (0.6% of the U.S. population) identify as transgender [39] as well as 150,000 U.S. youth, 0.7% of the population ages 13–17 years [46]. The population of adults who identified as transgender was more racially and ethnically diverse than the U.S. general population. Among adults who identified as transgender, 55% identified as White, 16% identified as African-American or Black, 21% identified as Latinx or Hispanic, and 8% identified as another race or ethnicity. Adults who are African-American or Black (0.8%), Latinx or Hispanic (0.8%), and of another race or ethnicity (0.6%) were more likely than White adults (0.5%) to identify as transgender [38].

A recent meta-analysis identified five population-based national surveys with 20 waves of data collection that reported on trans identities between 2006 and 2016 [63]. Questions used to collect data on trans identities varied by survey with questions ranging from "Do you identify as transgender?" to "Are you male, female, or transgender?" to "Which of the following best represents Do you think of yourself" with response options that include "transgender, transsexual, or gender variant." A meta-regression of these data suggests that the number and proportion of people who identify as gender diverse has been rising and will continue to rise over time. Winter et al. [95] used data from studies in five countries (U.S., U.K., Belgium, Netherlands, and New Zealand) where reported proportions of trans people ranged from 0.5 to 1.2%, and they applied the lower proportion to the global population to estimate 25 million transgender people worldwide [95]. However, global estimates are quite limited by lack of data from several regions, including Sub-Saharan Africa, Middle East/North Africa, and Eastern Europe/Central Asia. Sabin and colleagues [75] found that only 17 size estimates of trans women (not inclusive of trans men or non-binary individuals) had been conducted in all low and middle-income countries, with 6 of those studies having been conducted in 2014, the most recent year of the analysis [75].

The Center of Excellence for Transgender Health (COE) currently recommends using a two-step method that distinguishes sex assigned at birth from current gender [81]. While this is considered a best practice [85], it has limited ability to capture the growing number and complexities of emerging gender identities, particularly among youth. The widespread stigma against gender diverse people has been well documented and may prevent them from sharing their gender identities or gender histories with others, even on anonymous surveys and in confidential medical records [51, 86].

Future directions in trans research will require carefully fitting underlying research questions with sampling and ascertainment methods used to estimate the number of gender diverse people. For example, planning for clinical services would be an appropriate time to use electronic record data or other means to identify the proportion of the practice population that is trans or non-binary, if such data is routinely collected [52]. Questions that seek to describe the broader gender diverse population will need to use population-based, representative methods—which can be a challenge for small and stigmatized populations. As the exponential increase in studies with gender diverse populations indicate, these challenges have not, and should not, deter future and ongoing research to address the health of trans and non-binary people [72].

A Brief Review of Diagnostic Changes Over Time

The story of gender diversity and its relationship to social constructs is one that has undergone tremendous change over the course of the past 100 years. It is a story of controversies and rifts within medical and mental health communities and it is a story that has evolved from one of morality and criminality to one of medical access and self-advocacy. The terms 'transvestite' and 'transsexual' were first utilized by Magnus Hirschfeld, a leading sexologist and physician practicing in Berlin, Germany in 1910 [47] and in a journal article published in 1923, respectively [48]. Unfortunately, Hirschfeld's institute and records were destroyed when the Nazis came to power. The study of gender diversity fell into quiescence until the middle of the twentieth century with the work of Michael Dillon [30] and then Harry Benjamin, who went on to advocate for gender diverse individuals [92] to have access to gender-affirming medical care. Dr. Benjamin's work arose in the context of a history of treatment by the broader medical and mental health community that strove for many decades to define gender diversity as inherently pathological [14].

Within the mental health and medical communities, practitioners have looked to the DSM and ICD for a common language and set of descriptors to define a specific diagnosis. With consistent diagnostic criteria, the field is able to better define, and thus more accurately research the same set of concerns across contexts. Unfortunately, this also means that the inherent bias of those writing the criteria shapes how the diagnosis is described, and also may shape the stories that patients must tell in order to "qualify" for a diagnosis. Over the last several decades, trans and non-binary individuals have claimed platforms to share their experiences and have enriched the broader conversation about gender in our society. In concert with this change in the broader social context, the descriptions for gender diversity in the DSM and the ICD have been enriched over time.

There are ongoing robust debates about whether gender diversity should have an associated diagnosis. Proponents of a diagnosis point to the need for a diagnosis in order to access reimbursement of medical care and advance research initiatives, and some trans individuals describe a sense of relief that their experience is concretized into a diagnosis. Opponents of a diagnosis point to gender diversity as a normal aspect of human development that is not pathologic and assert that a diagnosis is stigmatizing and unnecessary for seeking care. This debate is beyond the scope of this chapter, but it is important to reflect that trans and non-binary individuals have not been members of the committees that finalize diagnostic criteria in the DSM and ICD until their most recent iterations.

Within the Diagnostic and Statistical Manual (DSM), gender identity was first addressed in the DSM-II (1968) and was classified in the chapter titled "Transvestism or Other Sexual Deviation" [3]. For DSM-III (1980), the term transsexualism was defined as a sense of discomfort and inappropriateness in one's anatomic sex that was persistent and continuous over a 2-year period [4]. This term was separate from transvestism, which was defined as a paraphilia, marked by "recurrent and persistent crossdressing by a heterosexual male…for the purpose of sexual excitement." (1980). It was not until the DSM-IIIR (1987) that childhood and adolescent gender identity was addressed [5]. In this edition, adults remained within the diagnosis of transsexualism, and children were given the diagnosis of atypical gender identity disorder (GID). Individuals meeting criteria for transvestism in DSM-III would met criteria for the diagnosis of "transvestic fetishism" in DSM-IIIR. The label of GID persisted until the DSM-5 (2013), at which point the diagnoses were changed to: Gender Dysphoria in Children, and Gender Dysphoria in Adolescents and Adults [6] (Tables 1.1 and 1.2).

There are stricter criteria for diagnosing prepubertal youth with Gender Dysphoria than for adolescents and adults. This is in part due to the process of gender development and in part due to the lack of specificity of previous diagnoses. In particular, prior to the DSM-5, the diagnostic criteria focused more on stereotypical, binary gender expression as opposed to gender identification. Much of the diagnostic criteria were focused on how children preferred to play and dress as opposed to how they described their gender identity. For example, in the DSM-IV,

Table 1 Gender identity in the DSM

	DSM-I—1952	DSM-II—1968	DSM-IIR—1973	DSM-III—1980	DSM-IIIR—1987	DSM-IV—1994	DSM-5—2013
Gender identity	N/A	Sexual deviation	Sexual deviation	Transsexuality (adults); atypical GID (children)	Transsexuality (adults); GID-NOS (children)	Gender identity disorder	Gender dysphoria

Table 2 DSM-IV versus DSM-5 diagnostic criteria [6, 7]

DSM-IV	DSM-5	DSM-5
Gender identity disorder A. A strong and persistent cross-gender identification (not merely a desire for any perceived cultural advantages of being the other sex). In children, the disturbance is manifested by four (or more) of the following: (1) Repeatedly stated desire to be, or insistence that he or she is, the other sex (2) In boys, preference for cross-dressing or simulating female attire; in girls, insistence on wearing only stereotypical masculine clothing (3) Strong and persistent preferences for cross-sex roles in make-believe play or persistent fantasies of being the other sex (4) Intense desire to participate in the stereotypical games and pastimes of the other sex (5) Strong preference for playmates of the other sex B. Persistent discomfort with his or her sex or sense of inappropriateness in the gender role of that sex C. The disturbance is not concurrent with a physical intersex condition D. The disturbance causes clinically significant distress or impairment in social, occupational, or other important areas of functioning	Gender dysphoria in children A. A marked incongruence between one's experienced/expressed gender and assigned gender, of at least 6 months duration, as manifested by at least six of the following (one of which must be Criterion A1): (1) A strong desire to be of the other gender or an insistence that one is the other gender (or some alternative gender different from one's assigned gender) (2) In boys (assigned gender), a strong preference for cross-dressing or simulating female attire; or in girls (assigned gender), a strong preference for wearing only typical masculine clothing and a strong resistance to the wearing of typical feminine clothing (3) A strong preference for cross-gender roles in make-believe play or fantasy play (4) A strong preference for the toys, games, or activities stereotypically used or engaged in by the other gender (5) A strong preference for playmates of the other gender (6) In boys (assigned gender), a strong rejection of typically masculine toys, games, and activities and a strong avoidance of rough-and-tumble play; or in girls (assigned gender), a strong rejection of typically feminine toys, games, and activities and a strong rejection of typically feminine toys, games, and activities (7) A strong dislike of one's sexual anatomy (8) A strong desire for the primary and/or secondary sex characteristics of the other gender B. The condition is associated with clinically significant distress or impairment in social, school, or other important areas of functioning	Gender dysphoria in adolescents and adults A. A marked incongruence between one's experienced/expressed gender and assigned gender, of at least 6 months duration, as manifested by at least two of the following: (1) A marked incongruence between one's experienced/ expressed gender and primary and/or secondary sex characteristics (2) A strong desire to be rid of one's primary and/or secondary sex characteristics, or a desire to prevent the development of the anticipated secondary sex characteristics (3) A strong desire for the primary and secondary sex characteristics of the other gender (4) A strong desire to be of the other gender (or some alternative gender different from one's assigned gender) (5) A strong desire to be treated as the other gender (6) A strong conviction that one has the typical feelings and reactions of the other gender B. The condition is associated with clinically significant distress or impairment in social, occupational, or other important areas of functioning

the applicable diagnosis was Gender Identity Disorder (GID) and because the diagnostic criteria were heavily weighted toward gender expression, one could be diagnosed with GID while still having an identity that aligned with birth sex. That is, a natal male who identifies as a boy who happens to prefer girls as friends, enjoys girls' toys and dressing in girls' clothes in play, and avoided more stereotypically masculine play, would still meet criteria for GID. As such, the diagnosis was highly nonspecific and captured both children who would later self-identify as trans and non-binary as well as children who would later identify as cisgender.

The new diagnostic criteria for Gender Dysphoria in the DSM-5 have shifted to focus more specifically on the alignment of gender identity and sex assigned at birth and take a stance that a trans identity in and of itself is not pathological, but the distress felt from Gender Dysphoria can negatively impact functioning. Additional changes include language that provides for more flexibility in recognizing non-binary identities and does not presume that a person whose identity does not align with their sex at birth has a gender identity that does align with a binary identity of female or male. The presence of Other Specified Gender Dysphoria and Unspecified Gender Dysphoria in the DSM-5 (and GID Not Otherwise Specified in the DSM-IV) provides additional opportunities to diagnostically capture the breadth of presentations by gender diverse individuals. These diagnoses allow for individuals. who do not meet full diagnostic criteria for Gender Dysphoria to still be able to access gender-affirming care [70].

There have been similar changes in diagnostic classification in the ICD as in the DSM. The current version of the ICD, ICD-10, came into use in 1994. In the ICD-10, "transsexualism" is described as a "disorder characterized by a strong and persistent cross-gender identification (such as stating a desire to be the other sex or frequently passing as the other sex) coupled with persistent discomfort with his or her sex" [53]. The proposed changes for the diagnoses in ICD-11 are twofold: the new diagnostic term will be Gender Incongruence, and it will be moved out of the section on mental and behavioral disorders and into the section on conditions related to sexual health.

As described previously, concretizing a set of experiences into diagnostic criteria that one is required to meet in order to access care may also ultimately shape the stories told by patients to their health care providers [16, 59]. As more gender diverse patients, activists, clinicians, educators, and researchers have been able to advocate and describe their own experiences as separate from the diagnostic criteria, professional service providers have been able to see the diversity of lived experiences of transgender populations and, slowly, the diagnostic criteria have begun to reflect this understanding.

An Evolution of Guidelines

As the field of transgender health has evolved, treatment guidelines [2] and standards of care [55] have developed to meet the needs of transgender people. These guidelines provide direction for professional conduct and decision-making and are intended to ensure that diagnosis, treatment, and research are optimized and standardized across settings. Every medical specialty has standards of care and the most widely accepted standards of care in the field of transgender health are the Standards of Care for the Health of Transsexual, Transgender, and Gender-Nonconforming People, Version 7, (SOC) published by the World Professional Association for Transgender Health [21]. The first version of the SOC was published in 1979 and filled one page. The seventh version, published online in 2011 is 112 pages [97]. Since 1979, the SOC have gone through six revisions and the organization has changed its name from The Harry Benjamin International Gender Dysphoria Association (HBIGDA) to the World Professional Association for Transgender Health (WPATH). The renaming of WPATH reflects its broad international constituency and a field that is increasingly focused upon health and well-being and away from diagnosis, dysfunction, and pathologization. Successive versions of the SOC reflect the evolution and development in treatment options, and the burgeoning interdisciplinary transgender movement which constitutes a vocal group of gender diverse people who have had input into the SOC as well as other standards and guidelines.

> The overall goal of the SOC is to provide clinical guidance for health professionals to assist transsexual, transgender, and gender-nonconforming people with safe and effective pathways to achieving lasting personal comfort with their gendered selves, in order to maximize their overall health, psychological well-being, and self-fulfillment. [21]

The SOC attempt to walk a fine line by providing both maximum flexibility for a diverse population and tangible and specific guidance for practice and policy. This is evident in the recommendation that when practitioners tailor the guidelines for individual treatment they are encouraged to acknowledge how they have deviated from the standard practice, to inform the patient that they are doing so, and to document this treatment both for legal and research purposes [21].

Within the WPATH SOC, there are several areas that have been most controversial. The first is the role of psychotherapy, mental health evaluation, and diagnosis [43]; related to that, is the potential of informed consent paradigms, the next is the need for a "real life experience" (RLE); and a third is the treatment of children and adolescents. The earliest versions of the SOC required individuals to have a period of psychotherapy prior to hormones and surgery. Version 7 of the SOC does not require people to have psychotherapy but do require a mental health evaluation and a diagnosis (which can be provided by either a medical or behavioral health professional). RLE, the practice of living in one's affirmed gender for a period of time before hormones or surgery, was a requirement for early versions of the SOC; and it continues to be a recommendation in many treatment protocols (such as those of many insurers and third-party payers in the U.S. which require RLE prior to surgery).

Because of the irreversible nature of the surgery, and to a lesser extent, hormones, individuals have been encouraged or required to live for a time in their affirmed gender prior to undergoing these procedures. Such protocols assume that social transition is more reversible than medical transition. This is often not the case because once a person comes out as transgender, the disruption to family, social life, and professional life may be irreversible. In addition, many people need some medical interventions in order to be able to effectively present in their affirmed gender. A period of hormones, chest masculinization surgery for transmasculine people, or feminizing facial surgery (FFS) for transfeminine people may be necessary in order for people to engage safely in RLE. In that case, it makes sense for medical interventions to precede RLE. There may also be individuals who do not need or want a social transition, but who do want medical interventions, and RLE would be contraindicated for them [33, 69, 91]. The SOC recommend a period of RLE as a criterion prior to genital surgery, though the SOC also say that they are meant to be interpreted as flexible recommendations.

> As in all previous versions of the SOC, the criteria put forth in this document for hormone therapy and surgical treatments for gender dysphoria are clinical guidelines: individual health professionals and programs may modify them. Clinical departures from the SOC may come about because of a patient's unique anatomic, social, or psychological situation; and experienced health professional's evolving method of handling a common situation; a research protocol; lack of resources in various parts of the world; or the need for specific harm-reduction strategies. These departures should be recognized as such, explained to the patient, and documented through informed consent for quality patient care and legal protection. This documentation is also valuable for the accumulation of new data which can be retrospectively examined to allow for health care – and the SOC – to evolve. [21]

Guidelines for the treatment of children and adolescents have changed quite dramatically over the course of the last three decades, as more research and clinical work has been done to better understand the trajectories and outcomes of gender diverse youth. Any guidelines for this population will be inherently more controversial given the ethics of medical decision-making for individuals without the legal capacity to consent, and the potential for disagreement between children and their parents. A notable set of guidelines for children and adolescents, created by the Royal College of Psychiatrists [19] focused on four main interventions—a full assessment, ongoing therapy, recognition and acceptance of the "gender identity problem," and decisions about the extent to which to support gender role transition. The authors described Gender Identity Disorders in childhood as rare and complex phenomena and recommended that any potentially irreversible interventions be delayed until after age 18. Since these guidelines were released, more and more children and adolescents are presenting for gender-affirming care, and because of changes in insurance coverage and a better understanding of the efficacy of medical interventions for youth with Gender Dysphoria, an increasing number of individuals under 18 are seeking medical and surgical interventions, and many children and adolescents are presenting initially for treatment having already socially transitioned.

The guidelines concerning access to care for children, adolescents, and adults have become less restrictive over the course of time so that fewer procedures require mental health evaluation, fewer recommendation letters are required, and more types of professionals are viewed as capable of providing such evaluations. Over the seven versions of the SOC, there has been increasing recognition that transgender individuals need holistic care—this may include not only provision of puberty blockers, hormones, and surgery, but also primary and preventative health care, reproductive care, vocal therapy, hair removal, support for partners and family, and advocacy in the world outside of medical settings. The SOC have also evolved in response to current conceptions of gender and gender identity, and the inclusion of non-binary identities is one of many core features of the current climate in transgender health.

Though the WPATH SOC are the most widely recognized standards internationally, there are, in fact, many clinical and treatment guidelines for the support of transgender people throughout the world. These guidelines are produced by professional organizations, national health services, human rights organizations, and community, public, and private health organizations. Some are so specific as to describe hormone regimens [23, 36, 44, 45], others are broad enough to apply to all medical specialties and centers serving this population [21, 83, 98]. Some are true treatment guidelines, and some provide general guidance for cultural competence. It is beyond the scope of this chapter to describe every guideline. It is enough to recognize that there have been guidelines of some sort developed for use by organizations operating within Asia, Canada, the Caribbean, Israel, Latin America, Australia and New Zealand, Europe, and the United States as described below.

One of the earliest guidelines to emerge from the transgender rights movement is the Health Law Standards of Care for Transsexualism [40]. These standards are composed of five principles and five standards focused upon depathologization of gender nonconformity, the right to self-determination, and freedom from barriers to care through informed consent as determined by the treating medical provider, and the elimination of the mental health provider as a gatekeeper. These themes have been addressed by all subsequent treatment protocols. By the early 2000s, identity-affirming care had become the primary orientation for specialists in the field of transgender health [21, 24, 33, 34, 54, 60, 78].

Some of the most widely used and influential guidelines have been developed by community-based healthcare centers that deliver care to thousands of transgender people every year. In the United States these centers include the Fenway Center in Boston, the Mazzoni Center in Philadelphia, the Tom Waddell Clinic in Los Angeles, Whitman-Walker Health in Washington, D.C. and the Callen Lorde Health Center in New York City, all of which have developed treatment guidelines and protocols for the provision of healthcare services to transgender people [18, 26, 61, 71]. One of the features of these clinical protocols is an emphasis on removing barriers to care by using an informed consent model for access to hormones [26]. The informed consent model approaches gender-affirming hormones like most other medical treatments and procedures, which require only a consultation with a medical provider to obtain informed consent for treatment. This model has emphatically eliminated any required period of psychotherapy, RLE, and in some cases, the need for a diagnosis of gender dysphoria. Depending upon the program, individuals may see a social worker or other mental health provider for a one- or two-session psychosocial evaluation, or a patient may meet only with a medical practitioner who discusses the risks and benefits of treatment options and ensures that the patient is fully informed and understands them. If the medical or behavioral health specialist who does the brief screening detects serious physical or mental health concerns or other reasons that an individual may not be ready for hormones, then the person may be referred to a specialist prior to treatment, with the goal being to support the person in becoming ready for the services they need. Most informed consent protocols have been developed in places that provide hormones, and they have documented the success of these programs as measured by patient satisfaction and absence of regret [26].

Increasingly, the development of guidelines is a discipline within itself and the evaluation of evidence that is used in constructing evidence-based guidelines is a specialized practice [8, 11, 29, 35, 84]. Evidence is evaluated using a formal rating system and treatment recommendations are given grades based upon the available evidence used to support them.

One of the most influential guidelines to employ an evidence-based review are the *Guidelines for the Primary and Gender-Affirming Care of Transgender and Gender Nonbinary People*, University of California—San Francisco [27, 28]. These guidelines offer a graded review in which each recommendation carries a description of the research which underlies that recommendation and a measure of the strength of that recommendation. They present a comprehensive model of care developed by the Center of Excellence for Transgender Health's Medical Advisory Board, "a diverse group of expert clinicians from a variety of academic and community based setting" [27, 28] and aim to include every aspect of transgender health and well-being that can be addressed in the context of health care. These guidelines, which attempt to build upon existing guidelines, such as the WPATH SOC v.7, are distinguished by their rigorous empirical basis, the diverse composition of the US consultants and authors, by covering healthcare needs broadly, by being less pathologizing, more inclusive, and removing barriers to care whenever possible.

Some treatment guidelines have been developed by professionals who work with community advisory boards, while other guidelines have been developed with community organizations as first authors. Examples of community-generated guidelines include the *Blueprint for the Provision of Comprehensive Care for Trans People and Trans Communities in Asia and the Pacific* [15], the *Blueprint for the Provision of Comprehensive Care for Trans Persons and Their Communities in the Caribbean and other Anglophone Countries* [67], *Por La Salud de las Personas Trans: Elementos para el desarrollo de la atención integral de personas trans y sus comunidades en Latinoamérica y el Caribe* [68], and *Implementing Comprehensive HIV and STI Programmes with Transgender People: Practical Guidance for Collaborative Interventions* (the "TRANSIT") [89].

In addition to general guidelines intended to support care across a range of treatment settings, some have been developed for very specific institutions. Guidelines developed to address the needs of transgender people housed in correctional facilities, detained by the US Department of Homeland Security, and serving in the military, reflect the institutional recognition that transgender people need affirmative care in every setting [10, 17, 20, 50, 76, 87, 88]. In 2011 and 2013, the US Department of Veterans Affairs, part of the US Veterans Health Administration in Washington, DC, approved a document which "established policy regarding the respectful delivery of health care to transgender and intersex Veterans who are enrolled in the Department of Veterans Affairs (VA) health care system or are otherwise eligible for VA care." This policy includes an introduction to basic terminology and guidance on how to be respectful of transgender patients, as well as what kinds of care are available and guidelines for how to provide that care [20]. Institutional guidelines, such as those of the Boston VA, often concern themselves with accommodations such as room assignments and gender-segregated facilities [90].

As the practice of transgender health and medicine has become more widespread, more specialty association have published guidelines for working with transgender and gender diverse populations. These specialty areas include: plastic surgery, endocrinology, urology, social work, psychology, psychiatry, nursing, voice and speech pathology/therapy, epidemiology, infectious disease, public health, pediatrics, and family practice. The websites for these professional organizations often display policy statements in support of the health and agency of transgender individuals.

Because of the interconnectedness of medical and social policy, and the specific needs of transgender individuals around the world, most standards of care and healthcare guidelines provide both clinical guidance and discussion of social policy. Writers of such guidelines recognize that it is not enough to offer gender-affirming health care. In response to the stigma and other challenges faced by transgender people, professionals who deliver care also advocate for their patients' very basic rights to access care, and for the recognition of identity in broader social policy, such as the ability to change gender markers on legal identity documents, to marry, adopt children, and receive protection from violence and from discrimination in employment, health care, and housing [42]. For example, the *Blueprint for the Provision of Comprehensive Care for Trans People and Trans Communities in Asia and the Pacific* states that

> The main purpose of the Blueprint is to improve access to competent primary and specialized care for trans people in Asia and the Pacific. A comprehensive evidence-based guide is an essential step in that process. This Blueprint will be a resource enabling health providers, program planners and managers, policymakers, community leaders, and other stakeholders to promote and address the health needs of trans people. At the same time, enhancing trans people's health and well-being requires a human rights approach that seeks to end discrimination and recognizes the dignity and equality of all. For that reason, the Blueprint builds the case for changing laws, policies, and practices to bring trans people back from the margins of society and ensure their full social inclusion in the life of the community at large. [15]

There are pros and cons to the existence of treatment guidelines. Guidelines are designed to ensure uniformly best care across settings, but once a protocol is standardized it may lose flexibility [96]. This is especially evident where insurance companies in the United States have instituted policies regarding third-party payment for gender-affirming hormones and surgery. The policy for Aetna Insurance is typical of those that require patients to meet certain criteria for their medical care to be reimbursed [1]. These criteria may be easily met by some patients and be completely inappropriate for others. For example, the insurance guidelines require a "real life experience" of 12 months prior to surgery, they also assume 12 months of hormones prior to surgery. In practice, many people will not want or need hormones before they request surgery, and the definition of "real life experience" may vary widely based on individual needs. As mentioned earlier, individuals who do not fit neatly into diagnostic categories may be forced to misrepresent their experience in order to access treatment.

Transgender medical options are used by a range of gender diverse individuals who fall outside of the better-known trans population of individuals who seek transition across the gender binary. The DSM-5 and SOC 7 both acknowledge the need for flexibility in support of non-binary individuals and others who challenge gender norms. One clear example of a population of individuals who need access to gender-affirming medical treatment are those who identify as Eunuchs—some of whom do not identify as male—and may need surgery and/or hormones in order to bring their bodies into alignment with their gender identities. Research shows that they are at great risk of self-surgery if denied treatment [69, 91]. The WPATH SOC version 8 (in the process) will include a section that addresses the need for recognition of this group and guidance for professionals who can provide for their safe access to gender-affirming care.

In summary, current and developing guidelines reflect trends in transgender health such as a turn away from pathology towards healthy identity, an increased focus on the needs of children and youth, provision of services for non-binary and other gender diverse individuals [12], a shift from strict treatment criteria toward flexible informed consent, and from a focus on hormones and surgery to a focus on whole-person health and well-being. Additionally, many comprehensive guidelines address the negative effects of social stigma and the positive effects of community and peer empowerment, and the increasing involvement of transgender consumers and transgender professionals as designers and consultants in the development of guidelines.

We have provided a brief social history of transgender people; reviewed the challenges and approaches to estimating the number of transgender people; provided an overview of the history of Gender Dysphoria as a diagnosis; and presented an overview of the evolution of the Standards of Care. As the field of transgender medicine continues to evolve, it will be important to remember how we got here and to understand how that historical path has influenced current standards as well as the way we move forward with gender-affirming care for transgender people.

References

1. Aetna Inc. Gender reassignment surgery. Clin Policy Bull. 2018. Retrieved from http://www.aetna.com/cpb/medical/data/600_699/0615.html. Accessed 15 Aug 2018.
2. American Academy of Family Physicians. Clinical practice guideline manual. 2017. Retrieved from https://www.aafp.org/patient-care/clinical-recommendations/cpg-manual.html#xiii. Accessed 15 Mar 2018.
3. American Psychiatric Association. Diagnostic and statistical manual of mental disorders. 2d ed. Washington, DC: American Psychiatric Association; 1968.
4. American Psychiatric Association. Diagnostic and statistical manual of mental disorders. 3d ed. Washington, D.C.: American Psychiatric Association; 1980.
5. American Psychiatric Association. Diagnostic and Statistical Manual of Mental Disorders, 3rd ed., Revised. Washington, DC American Psychiatric Association; 1987.
6. American Psychiatric Association. Diagnostic and statistical manual of mental disorders: DSM-IV. 4th ed. Washington, DC: American Psychiatric Association; 1994.
7. American Psychiatric Association. Diagnostic and statistical manual of mental disorders (DSM-5®). Washington, DC: American Psychiatric Association; 2013.
8. American Psychological Association. Criteria for evaluating treatment guidelines. In Guidelines for practitioners. 2000. Retrieved from http://www.apa.org/practice/guidelines/evaluating.aspx. Accessed 15 Mar 2018.
9. Arcelus J, Bouman WP, Van Den Noortgate W, Claes L, Witcomb G, Fernandez-Aranda F. Systematic review and meta-analysis of prevalence studies in transsexualism. Eur Psychiatry. 2015;30(6):807–15. https://doi.org/10.1016/j.eurpsy.2015.04.005.
10. Assistant Secretary of Defense. Guidance for treatment of gender dysphoria for active and reserve component service members. Department of Defense. 2016. Retrieved from https://www.defense.gov/Portals/1/features/2016/0616_policy/Guidance_for_Treatment_of_Gender_Dysphoria_Memo_FINAL_SIGNED.pdf. Accessed 15 Mar 2018.
11. Atkins D, Best D, Briss PA, Eccles M, Falck-Ytter Y, Flottorp S, …Grade Working Group. Grading quality of evidence and strength of recommendations. BMJ 2004; 328 (7454):1490. https://doi.org/10.1136/bmj.328.7454.1490.
12. Beek TF, Kreukels BP, Cohen-Kettenis PT, Steensma TD. Partial treatment requests and underlying motives of applicants for gender affirming interventions. J Sex Med. 2015;12 (11):2201–5. https://doi.org/10.1111/jsm.13033.
13. Behavioral Risk Factor Surveillance System. 2018. Retrieved from https://www.cdc.gov/brfss/questionnaires/index.htm. Accessed 15 Mar 2018.
14. Benjamin H. The transsexual phenomenon. Dusseldorf: Symposium Publishing (Original publication in 1966); 1966/1999.
15. Blueprint for the provision of comprehensive care for trans people and trans communities in Asia and the Pacific. Washington D.C.: Health Policy Project; 2015.
16. Bolin A. In search of eve: Transsexual rites of passage. South Hadley: Bergin & Garvey Publishers: Inc.; 1988.
17. Carter A. DoD instruction 1300.28: in-service transition for transgender service members (1300.28). Office of the Under Secretary of Defense for Personnel and Readiness; 2016. Retrieved from https://www.defense.gov/Portals/1/features/2016/0616_policy/DoD-Instruction-1300.28.pdf. Accessed 15 Mar 2018.
18. Cavanaugh T, Hopwood R, Lambert C. Informed consent in the medical care of transgender and gender-nonconforming patients. AMA J Ethics. 2016;18(11):1147–55. https://doi.org/10.1001/journalofethics.2016.18.11.sect1-1611.
19. Ceglie DD, Sturge C, Sutton A. gender identity disorders in children and adolescents guidance for management. Int J Transgenderism. 1998;2(2).

20. Charness ME. Management of transgender veteran patients. (11-046-LM). Department of Veterans Affairs, VA Boston Healthcare System; 2011. Retrieved from https://www.boston.va.gov/services/images/LGBT_PATIENT_CARE_MEMO_TRANSGENDER_CARE.pdf. Accessed 15 Mar 2018.
21. Coleman E, Bockting W, Botzer M, Cohen-Kettenis P, DeCuypere G, Feldman J, … Zucker K. Standards of care for the health of transsexual, transgender, and gender-nonconforming people, Version 7. Int J Transgenderism. 2012;13(4), 165–232. https://doi.org/10.1080/15532739.2011.700873.
22. Cooney K. *The woman who would be king*. Oneworld Publications; 2015.
23. Dahl M, Feldman J, Goldberg J, Jaberi A, Bockting W, Knudson G. Endocrine therapy for transgender adults in British Columbia: suggested guidelines. 2006. Retrieved from http://public.eblib.com/choice/publicfullrecord.aspx?p=3243278. Accessed 6 Aug 2018. Materials specified: Ebook Library http://public.eblib.com/choice/publicfullrecord.aspx?p=3243278.
24. De Cuypere G, Knudson G, Bockting W. Response of the World Professional Association for Transgender Health to the Proposed DSM 5 Criteria for Gender Incongruence. International Journal of Transgenderism. 2010;12(2):119–23. https://doi.org/10.1080/15532739.2010.509214.
25. de Erauso C. Lieutenant Nun: Memoir of a Basque Transvestite in the New World. Beacon Press; 2011.
26. Deutsch MB. Use of the informed consent model in the provision of cross-sex hormone therapy: a survey of the practices of selected clinics. Int J Transgenderism. 2012;13(3):140–6. https://doi.org/10.1080/15532739.2011.675233.
27. Deutsch MB. Guidelines for the primary and gender-affirming care of transgender and gender nonbinary people. 2nd ed. San Francisco, CA: University of California, San Francisco, Department of Family and Community Medicine Center of Excellence for Transgender Health; 2016.
28. Deutsch MB. Making it count: improving estimates of the size of transgender and gender nonconforming populations. LGBT Health. 2016;3(3):181–5. https://doi.org/10.1089/lgbt.2016.0013.
29. Deutsch MB, Radix A, Reisner S. What's in a guideline? Developing collaborative and sound research designs that substantiate best practice recommendations for transgender health care. AMA J Ethics. 2016;18(11):1098–106. https://doi.org/10.1001/journalofethics.2016.18.11.stas1-1611.
30. Dillon M. *Self: a study in ethics and endocrinology*. Amsterdam: Elsevier (Original published in 1946); 1946/2013.
31. Docter R. Becoming a woman: a biography of Christine Jorgensen: Routledge; 2013.
32. Docter RF. From man to woman: The transgender journey of Virginia prince. Docter Press; 2004.
33. Ehrbar RD, Gorton RN. Exploring provider treatment models in interpreting the standards of care. Int J Transgenderism. 2010;12(4):198–210. https://doi.org/10.1080/15532739.2010.544235.
34. Ettner R. Principles of transgender medicine and surgery. New York: Haworth Press; 2007.
35. Feldman JL. Medical management of transgender patients. In: Makadon HJ, Mayer KH, Potter J, Goldhammer H, editors. The Fenway guide to lesbian, gay, bisexual, and transgender health. 1st ed. Philadelphia, PA: American College of Physicians; 2007.
36. Feldman JLGJ. Transgender primary medical care: suggested guidelines for clinicians in British Columbia. 2006. Retrieved from http://public.eblib.com/choice/publicfullrecord.aspx?p=3243306. Accessed 15 Mar 2018.
37. Filice M. Two-Spirit. 26 Nov 2015. Retrieved from https://www.thecanadianencyclopedia.ca/en/article/two-spirit/. Accessed 6 Aug 2018.
38. Flores AR, Brown TN, Herman J. Race and ethnicity of adults who identify as transgender in the United States. Williams Institute, UCLA School of Law; 2016.

39. Flores AR, Herman JL, Gates GJ, Brown TNT. How many adults identify as transgender in the United States? 2016. Retrieved from http://williamsinstitute.law.ucla.edu/wp-content/uploads/How-Many-Adults-Identify-as-Transgender-in-the-United-States.pdf. Accessed 15 Mar 2018.
40. Frye PR. Health law standards of care for transsexualism. 1997. Retrieved from New York.
41. Glick JL, Theall K, Andrinopoulos K, Kendall C. For data's sake: dilemmas in the measurement of gender minorities. Cult Health Sex. 2018;1–16. https://doi.org/10.1080/13691058.2018.1437220.
42. Grant JM, Mottet LA, Tanis J, Harrision J, Herman JL, Keisling M. Injustice at every turn: a report of the National Transgender Discrimination Survey. 2011. Retrieved from http://www.thetaskforce.org/downloads/reports/reports/ntds_full.pdf. Accessed 15 Mar 2018.
43. Hale CJ. Ethical problems with the mental health evaluation standards of care for adult gender variant prospective patients. Perspect Biol Med. 2007;50(4):491–505. https://doi.org/10.1353/pbm.2007.0047.
44. Hembree WC, Cohen-Kettenis P, Delemarre-van de Waal HA, Gooren LJ, Meyer WJ 3rd, Spack NP, … Montori VM. Endocrine treatment of transsexual persons: an Endocrine Society clinical practice guideline. J Clin Endocrinol Metab. 2009;94(9):3132–54. https://doi.org/10.1210/jc.2009-0345.
45. Hembree WC, Cohen-Kettenis PT, Gooren L, Hannema SE, Meyer WJ, Murad MH, … T'Sjoen GG. Corrigendum for "Endocrine Treatment of Gender-Dysphoric/Gender-Incongruent Persons: An Endocrine Society Clinical Practice Guideline". The Journal of Clinical Endocrinology & Metabolism. 2018;103(2):699. https://doi.org/10.1210/jc.2017-02548.
46. Herman JL, Flores AR, Brown TN, Wilson BD, Conron KJ. Age of individuals who identify as transgender in the United States. Los Angeles, CA: The Williams Institute; 2017.
47. Hirschfeld M. *Transvestites: the erotic drive to cross dress*. 1910/1991.
48. Hirschfeld M. In Wolfgang Johann Schmidt, editor. Die intersexuelle Konstitution *Jahrbuch f,r sexuelle Zwischenstufen*, Neu ediert. Frankfurt am Main: Qumran; 1923. p. 3–27.
49. Hodgkinson L. Michael Nee Laura: the story of the world's first female to male transsexual. London: Columbus: Books Ltd.; 1989.
50. Homan T. Further guidance regarding the care of transgender detainees. Washington, D.C.: U. S. Immigration and Customs Enforcement. 2015. Retrieved from https://www.ice.gov/sites/default/files/documents/Document/2015/TransgenderCareMemorandum.pdf. Accessed 24 May 2018.
51. Hughto JMW, Reisner SL, Pachankis JE. Transgender stigma and health: a critical review of stigma determinants, mechanisms, and interventions. Soc Sci Med. 2015;147:222–31.
52. Ingraham N, Pratt V, Gorton N. Counting Trans* patients: a Community Health Center case study. TSQ: Transgender Stud Q. 2015;2(1):136–47. https://doi.org/10.1215/23289252-2848922.
53. International statistical classification of diseases and related health problems. 10th revision ed. Geneva: World Health Organization; 1992.
54. Israel GE, Tarver DE. Transgender care: recommended guidelines, practical information, and personal accounts. Philadelphia: Temple University Press; 1997.
55. Johnston LG, Prybylski D, Raymond HF, Mirzazadeh A, Manopaiboon C, McFarland W. Incorporating the service multiplier method in respondent-driven sampling surveys to estimate the size of hidden and hard-to-reach populations: case studies from around the world. Sex Trans Dis 2013;40(4).
56. Kates G. The transgendered world of the chevalier/chevaliere d'Eon. J Mod Hist. 1995;67(3):558–94.
57. Krafft-Ebing Rv. Psychopathia Sexualis, with special reference to contrary sexual instinct. Philadelphia and London: FA Davies and JR Berman, 1896. Ebook ed: Forgotten Books; 2012.
58. Labuski C, Keo-Meier C. The (Mis)measure of trans. TSQ: Transgender Stud Qu. 2015;2(1):13–33. https://doi.org/10.1215/23289252-2848868.

59. Lev AI. Transgender emergence. New York, NY: Haworth Clinical Practice Press; 2004a.
60. Lev AI. Transgender emergence: therapeutic guidelines for working with gender-variant people and their families. Binghamton, NY, US: Haworth Clinical Practice Press; 2004.
61. Mayer G, Radix A, Douglass K, Vavasis A, Mukerjee R, Weiss S, … Steever J. Protocols for the provision of cross-gender hormone therapy 2012 revision. 2012. Retrieved from http://tmeltzer.com/assets/callen-lorde-revised-protocols.pdf. Accessed 15 Mar 2018.
62. McFarland W, Wilson E, Fisher Raymond H. How many transgender men are there in San Francisco? J Urban Health. 2017. https://doi.org/10.1007/s11524-017-0150-5.
63. Meerwijk EL, Sevelius JM. Transgender population size in the United States: a meta-regression of population-based probability samples. Am J Public Health. 2017;107(2): e1–8. https://doi.org/10.2105/AJPH.2016.303578.
64. Meier SC, Labuski CM. The demographics of the transgender population. In: Baumle A, editor. The international handbook on the demography of sexuality. New York, NY: Springer Press; 2013. p. 289–327.
65. Mijatovic A. A brief biography of Elagabalus: the transgender ruler of Rome. 2013. Retrieved from http://outhistory.org/exhibits/show/tgi-bios/Elagabalus. Accessed 15 Aug 2018.
66. Nanda S. The Hijras of India: cultural and individual dimensions of an institutionalized third gender role. J Homosex. 1986;11(3–4):35–54.
67. Pan American Health Organization. Blueprint for the provision of comprehensive care for trans persons and their communities in the caribbean and other Anglophone countries. 2014a. Retrieved from http://www.who.int/hiv/pub/transgender/blueprint-trans-paho/en/. Accessed 15 Mar 2018.
68. Pan American Health Organization. Por La Salud de las Personas Trans: Elementos para el desarrollo de la atención integral de personas trans y sus comunidades en Latinoamérica y el Caribe. 2014b. Retrieved from http://www.who.int/hiv/pub/transgender/blueprint-trans-paho/en/. Accessed 15 Mar 2018.
69. Rachlin K. Medical transition without social transition: expanding options for the privately gendered body. Transgender Stud Q. 2018;5(2).
70. Rachlin K, Dhejne C, Brown GR. The future of GID NOS in the DSM 5: report of the GID NOS Working Group of a consensus process conducted by the World Professional Association for transgender health. Int J Transgenderism. 2010;12(2):86–93. https://doi.org/10.1080/15532739.2010.509209.
71. Reisner S, Bradford J, Hopwood R, Gonzalez A, Makadon H, Todisco D, Mayer K. Comprehensive transgender healthcare: the gender affirming clinical and public health model of Fenway Health. J Urban Health. 2015;92(3):584–92. https://doi.org/10.1007/s11524-015-9947-2.
72. Reisner SL, Deutsch MB, Bhasin S, Bockting W, Brown GR, Feldman J, Goodman M. Advancing methods for US transgender health research. Curr Opin Endocrinol Diabetes Obes. 2016;23(2):198–207. https://doi.org/10.1097/med.0000000000000229.
73. Richards C, Bouman WP, Seal L, Barker MJ, Nieder TO, T'Sjoen G. Non-binary or genderqueer genders. Int Rev Psychiatry. 2016;28(1):95–102. https://doi.org/10.3109/09540261.2015.1106446.
74. Roscoe W. Who are the two spirits? Q & A with Will Roscoe. 2010. Retrieved from http://www.willsworld.org/twospiritq-a.html. Accessed 15 Aug 2018.
75. Sabin K, Zhao J, Garcia Calleja JM, Sheng Y, Arias Garcia S, Reinisch A, Komatsu R. Availability and quality of size estimations of female sex workers, men who have sex with men, people who inject drugs and transgender women in low- and middle-income countries. PLoS ONE. 2016;11(5):e0155150. https://doi.org/10.1371/journal.pone.0155150.
76. Secretary of Defense. Directive-type Memorandum(DTM) 16-005, "Military Service of Transggender Service Members". (16-005). United States Department of Defense Office of the Secretary of Defense. 2016. Retrieved from https://www.hsdl.org/?view&did=794019. Accessed 15 March 2018.

77. Singer TB. The profusion of things: the "transgender matrix" and demographic imaginaries in US public health. TSQ: Transgender Stud Q. 2015;2(1):58–76. https://doi.org/10.1215/23289252-2848886.
78. Singh A, dickey lm. Affirmative counseling and psychological practice with transgender and gender nonconforming clients. Washington, DC, US: American Psychological Association; 2017.
79. Singh Y, Aher A, Shaikh S, Mehta S, Robertson J, Chakrapani V. Gender transition services for Hijras and other male-to-female transgender people in India: availability and barriers to access and use. Int J Transgenderism. 2014;15(1):1–15. https://doi.org/10.1080/15532739.2014.890559.
80. Smith B. Lou Sullivan: daring to be a man among men. Oakland: Transgress Press; 2016.
81. Tate CC, Ledbetter JN, Youssef CP. A two-question method for assessing gender categories in the social and medical sciences. J Sex Res. 2013;50(8):767–76. https://doi.org/10.1080/00224499.2012.690110.
82. Taylor LJ. Joan of Arc, the Church, and the Papacy, 1429-1920. The Catholic Historical Review. 2012;98(2):217–40.
83. Telfer MM, Pang K, Pace C, Tollit M. Australian standards of care and treatment guidelines for trans and gender diverse children and adolescents Version 1.1. 2018. Retrieved from http://www.sciencedirect.com/science/article/pii/S1054139X17306298 doi:https://doi.org/10.1016/j.jadohealth.2017.11.100. Accessed 15 Mar 2018.
84. Template for developing guidelines: interventions for mental disorders and psychosocial aspects of physical disorders. Albany, NY: American Psychological Association, Task Force on Psychological Intervention Guidelines; 1995.
85. The GenIUSS Group. Best practices for asking questions to identify transgender and other gender minority respondents on population-based surveys. Los Angeles, CA: The Williams Institute; 2014.
86. Thompson HM. Patient perspectives on gender identity data collection in electronic health records: an analysis of disclosure, privacy, and access to care. Transgend Health. 2016;1(1):205–15. https://doi.org/10.1089/trgh.2016.0007.
87. Transgender, transsexual, and gender nonconforming health care in correctional settings. 2009. Retrieved from https://www.ncchc.org/transgender-transsexual-and-gender-nonconforming-health-care. Accessed 15 Mar 2018.
88. Transgender, transsexual, and gender nonconforming health care in correctional settings. 2015. Retrieved from https://www.ncchc.org/transgender-transsexual-and-gender-nonconforming-health-care. Accessed 15 Mar 2018.
89. United Nations Development Programme. Implementing comprehensive HIV and STI programmes with transgender people: practical guidance for collaborative interventions. 2016. Retrieved from http://www.undp.org/content/undp/en/home/librarypage/hiv-aids/implementing-comprehensive-hiv-and-sti-programmes-with-transgend.html. Accessed 15 Mar 2018.
90. VA Boston Healthcare System. Lesbian, gay, bisexual and transgender veterans. 2018. Retrieved from https://www.boston.va.gov/services/Lesbian_Gay_Bisexual_and_Transgender_Veterans.asp. Accessed 15 Aug 2018.
91. Vale K, Johnson TW, Jansen MS, Lawson BK, Lieberman T, Willette KH, Wassersug RJ. The development of standards of care for individuals with a male-to-eunuch gender identity disorder. Int J Transgenderism. 2010;12(1):40–51. https://doi.org/10.1080/15532731003749095.
92. Walker P. Standards of care: the hormonal and surgical sex reassignment of gender dysphoric persons. Paper presented at the Sixth International Gender Dysphoria Symposium. 1979.
93. Wasson D. Elagabalus. 21 October 2013. Retrieved from https://www.ancient.eu/Elagabalus/. Accessed 15 Aug 2018.

94. Wiepjes CM, Nota NM, de Blok CJM, Klaver M, de Vries ALC, Wensing-Kruger SA, den Heijer M. The Amsterdam cohort of gender dysphoria study (1972–2015): trends in prevalence, treatment, and regrets. J Sex Med. 2018. https://doi.org/10.1016/j.jsxm.2018.01.016.
95. Winter S, Diamond M, Green J, Karasic D, Reed T, Whittle S, Wylie K. Transgender people: health at the margins of society. Lancet. 2016;388(10042):390–400. https://doi.org/10.1016/s0140-6736(16)00683-8.
96. Woolf SH, Grol R, Hutchinson A, Eccles M, Grimshaw J. Clinical guidelines: potential benefits, limitations, and harms of clinical guidelines. BMJ. 1999;318(7182):527–30.
97. World Professional Association for Transgender Health. Standards of care for the health of transsexual, transgender, and gender nonconforming people. Minneapolis, MN: World Professional Association for Transgender Health; 2011.
98. Wylie K, Barrett J, Besser M, Bouman WP, Bridgman M, Clayton A, Thornton J. Good practice guidelines for the assessment and treatment of adults with gender dysphoria. Sexual & Relationship Therapy. 2014;29(2):154–214. https://doi.org/10.1080/14681994.2014.883353.
99. Yi SK, Steyvers M, Lee MD, Dry MJ. The wisdom of the crowd in combinatorial problems. Cogn Sci. 2012;36(3):452–70. https://doi.org/10.1111/j.1551-6709.2011.01223.x.

Chapter 2
Review of Medical, Socioeconomic, and Systemic Barriers to Transgender Care

Joshua D. Safer and Kelly J. Chan

Transgender individuals face many barriers to accessing medical care. In this chapter, we review the major barriers to health care faced by transgender patients in three parts—issues within health care, socioeconomic considerations, and systemic barriers.

Background

In the United States, transgender people make up an estimated 0.5–0.6% of the population [1].

Collectively, transgender individuals face disproportionate challenges in accessing healthcare services and may experience medical mistreatment from providers through insensitivity, denied services, verbal abuse, and forced care. One study found that 50% of transgender people report having to teach their providers about transgender care, and 19% have been refused care due to their transgender identity [2]. In addition, transgender people face financial obstacles paying for hormone therapy and gender-confirming surgery that is not covered by insurance and may resort to taking hormones outside of a physician's care or even attempt self-surgery [3].

These persistent barriers to accessing appropriate and culturally competent care play a significant role in the health disparities experienced by transgender indi-

J. D. Safer (✉)
Center for Transgender Medicine and Surgery, Mount Sinai Health System and Icahn School of Medicine, New York, NY, USA
e-mail: jsafer0115@gmail.com

K. J. Chan
Boston Medical Center and Boston University School of Medicine, Boston, MA, USA

L. Poretsky and W. C. Hembree (eds.), *Transgender Medicine*, Contemporary Endocrinology, https://doi.org/10.1007/978-3-030-05683-4_2

viduals, such as increased rates of certain cancers, substance abuse, mental health concerns, infections, and chronic diseases. For example, transgender women (male to female) are recognized as a population that carries a disproportionately large burden of HIV infection, and 48 times more likely to be infected with HIV compared to adults of reproductive age [4]. Additionally, the Transgender Discrimination survey reports that 26% of respondents reported current or former alcohol or drug use to cope with mistreatment, and 41% report having attempted suicide compared to 1.6% of the general population.

Although some of these healthcare barriers are faced by other minority groups, many are unique and considerably magnified for transgender persons. Further, the socioeconomic considerations for transgender individuals—ranging from age, race, ethnicity, income to mental health—are complicated through the lens of intersecting identities, with transgender people of color facing greater obstacles in terms of harassment, homelessness, and unemployment rates [2].

On an institutional level, transgender individuals face health systems barriers such as inappropriate electronic records, forms, lab references, and clinic facilities. Issues in representative data collection also pose an issue, as well as the insurance policy coverage for gender confirmation care and surgeries, most of which vary between states with little uniformity. The purpose of this chapter is to review comprehensively the current literature characterizing major barriers to health care for transgender individuals, and to explore future directions in each topic to understand both the obstacles to care and potential recommendations to overcome them.

Barriers Within Health Care

Gaps in Medical Education

Historically, the treatment of transgender individuals has not been taught in conventional medical curricula and few physicians have the knowledge, comfort level, and cultural competency to provide appropriate care. Transgender patients report that lack of providers with expertise in transgender medicine is the most prominent barrier to accessing health care, such as safe hormonal therapy and general medical care [5]. Medical schools have used LGB and transgender-related educational sessions to gauge medical students' interest, finding that 87% considered these topics meaningful to their education [6].

However, physicians and medical students report having knowledge gaps in transgender health care due to insufficient education and exposure. Publications in the field have long documented the modest time investment in medical education for the health of LGB and transgender people. In 1991, Wallick et al. surveyed all U.S. medical schools to assess the number of curriculum hours devoted to the topic of homosexuality. They reported a national average of 3 h and 26 min across

4 years of undergraduate medical education per institution, most frequently presented in didactic lectures [7]. In 1998, Tesar et al. reported an average of 2.5 h for all 4 years of undergraduate medical education dedicated to the care of LGB and transgender patients, with 50% of all schools containing no content whatsoever in their curricula [8].

More recently, a 2011 study by Obedin-Maliver et al. found that among 176 allopathic and osteopathic medical schools in the United States and Canada, a median of 5 h was dedicated to teaching content related to LGB and transgender health but 33% of medical schools reported 0 h of LGBT-related content being taught during clinical years [9]. Topics relevant to lesbian, gay, and bisexual (LGB) patients were more commonly taught compared to those addressing care for transgender patients. Additionally, fewer than 35% provided content related to hormone therapy and transgender surgery [9, 10].

These gaps in medical education in addressing transgender health care have downstream effects on physician attitudes and ability in multiple realms. For example, 80% of practicing endocrinologists report having no training in transgender patient care. Of the 20% who did receive training, only 4% indicated that they received any during medical school [11]. A 2016 study found that in a cohort of mid-Atlantic endocrinologists, only 20% were "very" comfortable in discussing gender identity and self-rated their competency to treat transgender patients as "low" [12]. In addition, a needs assessment showed that Emergency Medicine residency training programs averaged 45 min of LGB and transgender-specific instruction, with a significant discrepancy between actual hours spent and desired hours by residents [13]. In a population that continues to be medically underserved, there is a clear need for medical schools to address these gaps across undergraduate and residency medical school curricula.

Future Directions—Addressing the Gaps

In recent years, public awareness regarding the health disparities faced by the transgender community has been increasing. The Institute of Medicine has pushed for further research on healthcare inequities faced by LGB and transgender patients by specifically addressing the shortage of LGBT medical education training. The Association of American Medical Colleges (AAMC) suggested specific curricular content for LGB and transgender patients consisting of supplements to didactic instruction, case-based learning, and virtual patients [14].

Over the past decade, several schools recognized the importance and need for improved education in transgender health care. Efforts were made to implement curriculum changes to meet and surpass the AAMC recommendations. The University of Louisville School of Medicine created 12–15 h of new content and enhanced three dozen hours of the existing curriculum, focusing on inclusive, affirmative language when taking a patient's sexual history and new content on the spectrum of human sexuality. First-year medical students at Case Western receive four hours of required instruction on LGBT patient care, learning about transgender terminology, the potential barriers to care, and personal biases they may have about transgender people [14].

Some supplements to the medical school curriculum have been shown to have positive outcomes on student attitudes. For example, Boston University School of Medicine (BUSM) first-year students in standard physiology learn about the biologic evidence for gender identity. In the second year, BUSM students are taught both classic treatment regimens and monitoring requirements for transgender hormone therapy as part of the standard, obligatory endocrinology curriculum. After the first 2 years, students reported a significant increase in willingness to care for transgender patients and a 67% decrease in discomfort with providing care to transgender patients [15].

Similarly, the University of Pennsylvania School of Medicine implemented a lecture on transgender health as part of the mandatory family medicine clerkship. After the lecture, students reported significantly higher levels of competency compared to students who had not taken the lecture in several realms: knowledge of health outcomes, skill in discussing, and performing appropriate medical evaluation of transgender patients [16].

Evidence for Experiential Learning

While increased LGB and transgender curricular content have demonstrated effectiveness relative to attitudes and provider comfort, there is a growing body of literature that suggests that in addition to evidence-based learning, experiential learning is integral to increasing medical student comfort and knowledge in working with transgender patients. In 2006, a study showed that medical knowledge of LGBT health and frequency of exposure to sexual history taking from LGBT patients were positively associated with the amount of clinical exposure to those populations, demonstrating that the number of hours in the curriculum may not be the only or best indicator of medical trainees' ability to provide care for LGBT patients [5]. Moreover, the AAMC 2014 guidelines advocate for investment across all levels of medical education within institutions in order to comprehensively address the healthcare needs and disparities faced by people who are or may be LGB, transgender, or gender nonconforming [14].

Several programs have found success with the inclusion of an experiential learning component, reporting that medical trainees with greater clinical exposure to transgender patients reported more comfort and greater knowledge than students with no clinical exposure [5, 17] (Morrison, Sanchez). BUSM supplemented the AAMC approach with evidence-based, transgender-specific medical education that was longitudinally integrated throughout the medical curriculum. Investigators found that student comfort in LGB patient care lags behind transgender patients, speculating that the disparity stems from lack of direct personal exposure compared to LGB patients.

BUSM demonstrated that clinical exposure to care for transgender patients would help close the gap in student comfort and knowledge in treating transgender

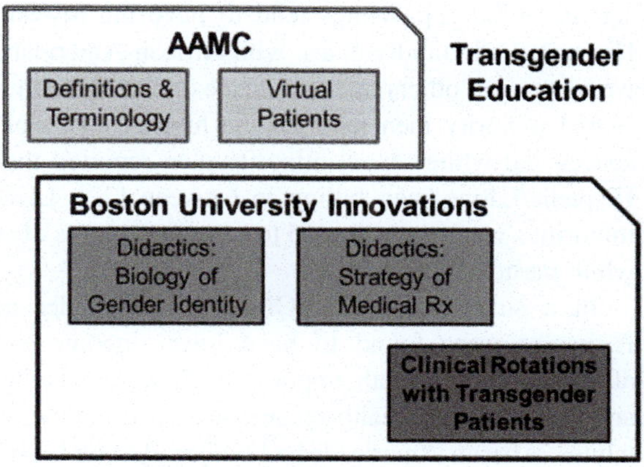

Fig. 2.1 Adapted from the Boston University model for teaching transgender medical care. Boston University's transgender education framework follows AAMC recommendations and further supplements them with own innovations [18]

patients and found that self-reported comfort/knowledge levels with transgender care rose significantly in fourth-year students after this clinical component (Fig. 2.1) [18].

Social Barriers and Considerations

Socioeconomic Considerations

The socioeconomic barriers facing transgender individuals are numerous and intersecting, ranging from age, race, ethnicity, income to mental health. The most comprehensive survey to date of transgender individuals surveyed 28,000 transgender respondents in all 50 states [2]. The findings revealed patterns of mistreatment and discrimination, permeating aspects of daily life such as employment, living, medical care, and the support of family and community. They found that a staggering number of transgender individuals live in extreme poverty, nearly one-third (29%) of respondents compared to 12% in the U.S. population. In terms of mental health, transgender respondents were nine times more likely to attempt suicide compared to the general population.

Differences in healthcare access by LGB and transgender individuals are further impacted by ethnicity and race. As described by Cronin and King, racial, ethnic, and social identities are distinct yet intersecting, serving as dimensions of social stratification that impact one's ability to achieve health [19]. The National Transgender Discrimination Survey in 2016 found that while of anti-transgender prejudice was prevalent throughout the entire sample, the interaction of discrimination and persistent structural racism was especially striking [2].

Overall, people of color fare worse than white participants across the board in measures such as unemployment rate, housing discrimination, harassment by teachers, employers, and homeless shelter staff, and ability to access healthcare services [20, 21]. Whites tend to have the lowest rates, followed by Asian and Hispanic/Latino individuals, with African-American transgender respondents faring worse than all others in every area examined. Additionally, a study found that black sexual minority men reported the highest levels of racial/ethnic stigma in LGBT spaces and white sexual minority men reported the lowest levels, with Asian and Hispanic/Latino men falling in between [22]. LGB and transgender racial/ethnic minorities were also reported to have lower rates of insurance coverage compared to white participants [23].

In a study on older LGB and transgender adults, African-Americans and Hispanics were found to have lower income, educational attainment, identity affirmation, and social support, which were associated with a decrease in physical and psychological health-related quality of life measures compared to non-Hispanic whites. African-Americans had higher lifetime LGBT-related discrimination, which was linked to a decrease in their physical and psychological quality measure [24].

Another study of black and Latina transgender women in major metropolitan areas found notable disparities in socioeconomic challenges faced by this population. Of 227 transgender women enrolled, most were economically and socially disadvantaged: 73% had an annual income of less than $15,000; 62% lacked health insurance; 61% were unemployed; and 46% reported being homeless in the past 12 months [25]. These findings indicate that the intersection of minority identities shape transgender individuals' experiences in health care, often in detrimental ways.

Transgender and Gender Nonconforming Youth

Transgender youth face unique barriers to accessing health care, in large part due to differing individual demographic characteristics and the values of their communities [26]. There is no consensus on the prevalence of gender nonconformity among children and adolescents, and studies face methodological difficulties ranging from recruitment to difficulties in standardized measurement of gender identity.

Overall, transgender and gender-nonconforming youth reported significantly poorer health, lower rates of preventive health checkups, and more nurse office visits than cisgender youth. They are also at high risk for mental health morbidities, often the result of hostile school and home environments that subsequently impact academic achievement, educational aspirations, and psychological well-being [27]. A study found that 73 transgender student subjects (92.4%) were diagnosed with one or more of the following conditions: depression, anxiety, post-traumatic stress disorder, eating disorders, autism spectrum disorder, and bipolar disorder. 74.7% reported suicidal ideation, 55.7% exhibited self-harm, and 30.4% had one or more suicide attempts. 58.2% subjects reported school victimization. Of the 27 patients prescribed gonadotropin-releasing hormone analogues, only 8 (29.6%) received insurance coverage [28].

Barriers to implementation of current clinical practice guidelines include the fact that pubertal blockers and cross-sex hormone treatments are off-label in gender dysphoric youth and are expensive, and coverage is often denied or excluded by insurance companies [27, 29]. While an increasing number of clinical programs have emerged in recent years, many are clustered around the Northeast and West coast. There are many Midwestern geographic regions in which such services do not exist, often requiring patients and families to travel long distances to seek care [30].

In addition, access to optimal care may be limited by a lack of training of pediatric providers and by prejudice and misunderstanding on the part of family, community, and medical and mental health professionals [31]. In a survey of both transgender youth and their caregivers, other barriers were identified, such as inconsistent use of chosen name/pronoun, uncoordinated care, and gatekeeping [32].

Despite increased awareness to the need for comprehensive medical and mental health care for transgender youth, adolescent medicine and pediatric endocrine providers report lack of confidence in their ability to provide care to this vulnerable population. A study of physician attitudes toward providing care to transgender youth showed 66.5% had provided care to transgender youth, and 62.4% felt comfortable with providing transgender medical therapy. While only 47.1% felt confident in doing so, most respondents were interested in learning more about transgender-related care [33]. Physicians have cited obstacles to providing care as lack of clinical training in transgender-specific care and lack of insurance coverage and reimbursement. Furthermore, physicians report a lack of mental health provider support in determining whether transgender youth is eligible for medical therapy [33, 34].

Future Directions

Several recommendations have been made to improve care for transgender youth, such as mandatory training on gender-affirming health care and cultural humility for providers/staff, development of protocols for the care, and roadmaps for families, more specifically, using and recording chosen names/pronouns and designating a navigator for transgender patients in clinic. Other important suggestions were to providing cross-sex hormones at an age that permits peer-congruent development and an increase in multidisciplinary gender clinics offering care [32].

Institutional and Systemic Barriers

Insurance Coverage and State Policies

An enormous barrier to care for transgender individuals lies in their insurance coverage and the policies for gender-confirming care and surgery, most of which vary between states. Even for those who are insured, barriers to care can persist as private insurers have historically excluded coverage for medical interventions related to gender transition, claiming that these procedures are "cosmetic" or "medically unnecessary" [35].

Insurers also have a history of denying claims for routine preventive services, such as prostate or cervical cancer screenings for transgender patients whose gender identification does not "match" their bodies. In 2015, the U.S. Transgender Survey found that of their roughly 28,000 respondents, more than half (55%) of those who sought coverage for transition-related surgery in the past year were denied, and 25% of those who sought coverage for hormones in the past year were denied [36].

Although the passage of a nondiscrimination clause in the Affordable Care Act (ACA) penalizes insurance companies for the absence of coverage for transition-related care, the limited availability of transgender-competent providers and the limited coverage for gender-affirming surgeries may force some transgender people to pay out-of-pocket for a provider outside their plan. This leads to exorbitant healthcare expenditures even for those that are insured [1].

Due to the many challenges surrounding affordability and access to health care for transgender individuals, transgender individuals encounter two primary barriers to care: inadequate insurance coverage and lack of financial resources. For example, both transgender men and women are more likely to be uninsured than their cisgender counterparts, and more likely to have unmet medical care needs due to cost, and no routine checkup in the prior year [37]. In a survey of transgender women in New York City, specific barriers were identified as the cost of medical care, access to specialists, and a paucity of transgender-friendly and transgender-knowledgeable providers [5].

On a national level, the federal government does not have specific laws protecting transgender people from discrimination in employment, housing, health care, and adoption. Consequently, transgender individuals face greater barriers to health care in some areas of the country. In 2008, the National Transgender Discrimination Survey found that only 11 states (Hawaii, Illinois, Indiana, Maine, Montana, New Jersey, New Mexico, Oregon, Rhode Island, Vermont, and Washington) and the District of Columbia had policies providing protections against gender identity-based discrimination in public accommodations, including healthcare settings [38]. As of 2018, 22 states feature legislation that prohibits discrimination based on gender identity in either employment, housing, and/or public accommodations [39, 40].

However, such legislation remains absent in Southern U.S. states [38]. Southern states have historically been slow to implement policies that ban transgender exclusions in both private insurance and Medicaid coverage. Prior to the enactment of the nondiscrimination provision of the ACA, no Southern state had insurance policy protections against transgender exclusions [41]. This is compared to the states with such policies existing in place: four states in the East (Massachusetts, New York, Connecticut, and Rhode Island) and Washington, D.C. in the Northeast, four states in the West (Washington, California, Oregon, and Colorado), and one state in the Midwest (Illinois) [42].

Further, a multilevel analysis investigating lifetime healthcare refusal using national data from 5831 U.S. transgender adults showed a greater proportion of states in the Southern and Western United States with transgender residents at increased odds of experiencing care refusal, relative to other regions of the United States. After adjusting for state-level factors, the percentage of the state population voting Republican was positively associated with care refusal among the transgender respondents [43].

Beyond transgender protective policies, several Southern states (i.e., Arkansas, Mississippi, North Carolina) also currently have policies that explicitly prevent the passage or enforcement of local nondiscrimination laws [38]. For example, in 2016, Mississippi and Tennessee passed laws that allow healthcare providers to refuse to serve LGB and transgender people and same-sex couples based on religious or moral objection [44]. The First Amendment Protection Act—first conceived in 2015 and reintroduced into Congress in March 2018—would prohibit the federal government from intervening against any business or person that discriminates against LGBTQ people on the basis of religious beliefs [40, 45].

Future Directions

Many transgender Americans continue to remain uninsured or are underinsured because of refusal to cover medically necessary, gender-affirming healthcare services such as hormone replacement therapy, mental health counseling services, and reconstructive surgeries. Coverage refusal results in higher costs and poor health outcomes among transgender people who cannot access gender-affirming care [46]. In the rapidly changing landscape of healthcare systems, the care of transgender individuals faces challenges such as imprecise quality measures, sex-specific criteria, and pushback from payers [47, 48].

While there is a general lack of data investigating the economic effects of health insurance coverage to transgender enrollees, a study by Padula et al. analyzed the cost-effectiveness of insurance coverage for medically necessary transgender-related services over 5- and 10-year periods. They concluded that the additional expenses are ultimately cost-effective in reducing the risk of negative endpoints without health benefits—HIV, depression, suicidality, and drug abuse [47]. More studies must be conducted on a larger scale to incorporate transgender individuals into measures that use sex-specific criteria, and careful consideration of existing guidelines and recommendations. Unless these health policies are updated, systems designed to disregard transgender individuals will exacerbate existing healthcare disparities and become a larger collective burden [43].

Health Systems Barriers and Data Collection Issues

Many of the barriers faced by transgender and gender nonconforming adults are rooted in inadequate and dated public policy [37]. Within healthcare systems, barriers take the form of inappropriate or non-inclusive electronic records, forms, lab references, and clinic facilities. The lack of inclusiveness in these realms impacts both access to care and data collection of transgender patients, in part due to inadequate information systems that fail to capture identity data [49].

This lack of cohesive data on the transgender community in part stems from difficulties in data collection and methodology. Issues such as the lack of large observational studies and intervention trials, limited data on risks and benefits of gender affirmation care or surgical intervention, and inconsistent use of definitions across studies hinder evidence-based care for transgender people [50]. Further, health disparities in this group may be under-recognized due to difficulties categorizing those who do not identify with these labels. For example, men who have sex with men (MSM) who identify as heterosexual or people questioning their gender identity may be reluctant to disclose certain behaviors to providers. In turn, providers may fail to inquire about health concerns for which sexual or gender minorities are at higher risk [23].

Future Plans

The growing adoption of electronic health records provides a vital opportunity to optimize care for LGB and transgender individuals via routine collection of patient sexual orientation, gender identity, preferred name, and pronoun in structured form. In 2015, University of California, Davis, Health System (UCDHS) became the first U.S. academic health center to incorporate patient sexual orientation and gender identity data into its electronic health records to reduce LGB and transgender health disparities. Their strategies were targeted at improving institutional culture, such as senior leadership involvement, key informant interviews, educational outreach during grand rounds, resident workshops, and inviting healthcare providers to self-identify [51].

Additionally, nurse informaticists play an increasingly vital role in the process of developing new electronic health records that are sensitive to the needs and identities of the LGB and transgender communities, while bridging gaps in provider knowledge and discomfort through inter-professional collaboration. More inclusive electronic health records will allow providers to monitor risk behavior, assess progress toward the reduction of disparities, and provide health care centered around the needs of the patient and family [49].

In terms of data collection, Reisner et al. recommend that systematic high-quality observational and intervention-testing studies may be carried out using several approaches, including general population-based, health systems-based, clinic-based, venue-based, and hybrid designs. More specific criteria aimed at identification, recruitment, and long-term follow-up of transgender people of different ages, racial, ethnic, and socioeconomic backgrounds and with diverse gender identities will benefit the data pool [29, 50].

In addition to improving care provided, increasing the presence of gender-inclusive language may help patients feel more comfortable, as well as collection of structured sexual orientation and gender identity information will facilitate important public health data collection efforts that can be used to further identify and reduce healthcare disparities in this underserved population [52]. Ultimately, a harmonization of research and clinical efforts in this field is needed to provide a comprehensive view of the transgender community.

Conclusion

While health disparities in the LGB and transgender population persist, it becomes increasingly important to identify and target these major barriers, as well as discuss recommendations for future steps to be taken.

References

1. Conron KJ, Mimiaga MJ, Landers SJ. A population-based study of sexual orientation identity and gender differences in adult health. Am J Public Health. 2010;100(10):1953–60. https://doi.org/10.2105/ajph.2009.174169.
2. Grant JM, Mottet LA, Tanis J, Harrison J, Herman JL, Keisling M. Injustice at every turn: a report of the national gender discrimination survey. http://www.thetaskforce.org/static_html/downloads/reports/reports/ntds_full.pdf. Accessed 12 Apr 2018.
3. Rotondi NK, Bauer GR, Scanlon K, Kaay M, Travers R, Travers A. Nonprescribed hormone use and self-performed surgeries: "do-it-yourself" transitions in transgender communities in Ontario, Canada. Am J Public Health. 2013;103(10):1830–6. https://doi.org/10.2105/ajph.2013.301348.
4. Poteat T, Reisner SL, Radix A. HIV epidemics among transgender women. Curr Opin HIV AIDS. 2014;9(2):168–73. https://doi.org/10.1097/coh.0000000000000030.
5. Sanchez N. Medical students' ability to care for lesbian, gay, bisexual, and transgendered patients. https://www.stfm.org/fmhub/fm2006/january/nelson21.pdf. Accessed 2 Mar 2018.
6. Sequeira GM, Chakraborti C, Panunti BA. Integrating lesbian, gay, bisexual, and transgender (LGBT) content into undergraduate medical school curricula: a qualitative study. Ochsner J. 2012;12(4):379–82. https://doi.org/10.1043/1524-5012-12.4.379.
7. Wallick MM, Cambre KM, Townsend MH. How the topic of homosexuality is taught at U.S. medical schools. Acad Med. 1992;67(9):601–3.
8. Tesar CM, Rovi SL. Survey of curriculum on homosexuality/bisexuality in departments of family medicine. Fam Med. 1998;30(4):283–7.
9. Obedin-Maliver J, Goldsmith ES, Stewart L, et al. Lesbian, gay, bisexual, and transgender-related content in undergraduate medical education. JAMA. 2011;306(9):971–7. https://doi.org/10.1001/jama.2011.1255.
10. Criniti S, Opurum I, Sandra Urdaneta HS, Montgomery O, Woodland M. Perspectives on sexuality instruction among medical residents. Contraception. 2013;88(3):441. https://doi.org/10.1016/j.contraception.2013.05.047.
11. Davidge-Pitts C, Nippoldt TB, Danoff A, Radziejewski L, Natt N. Transgender health in endocrinology: current status of endocrinology fellowship programs and practicing clinicians. J Clin Endocrinol Metab. 2017;102(4):1286–90. https://doi.org/10.1210/jc.2016-3007.

12. Irwig MS. Transgender care by endocrinologists in the United States. Endocr Pract. 2016;22 (7):832–6. https://doi.org/10.4158/ep151185.or.
13. Moll J, Krieger P, Moreno-Walton L, et al. The prevalence of lesbian, gay, bisexual, and transgender health education and training in emergency medicine residency programs: what do we know? Acad Emerg Med. 2014;21(5):608–11. https://doi.org/10.1111/acem.12368.
14. Implementing curricular and institutional climate changes to improve health care for individuals who are LGBT, gender nonconforming, or born with DSD. https://members.aamc.org/eweb/upload/LGBTDSD%20Publication.pdf. Accessed 3 Mar 2018.
15. Gardner IH, Safer JD. Progress on the road to better medical care for transgender patients. Curr Opin Endocrinol Diabetes Obes. 2013;20(6):553–8. https://doi.org/10.1097/01.med.0000436188.95351.4d.
16. Dowshen N, Nyguyen G, Gilbert K, Feiler A, Margot K. Improving transgender health education for future doctors/stroumsa responds. ProQuest. https://search.proquest.com/openview/e4754a2ea987d1a343b761b87da7cea8/1?pq-origsite=gscholar&cbl=41804. Accessed 3 Mar 2018.
17. Morrison SD, Dy GW, Chong HJ, et al. Transgender-related education in plastic surgery and urology residency programs. J Grad Med Educ. 2017;9(2):178–83. https://doi.org/10.4300/jgme-d-16-00417.1.
18. Park JA, Safer JD. Clinical exposure to transgender medicine improves students' preparedness above levels seen with didactic teaching alone: a key addition to the Boston University model for teaching transgender healthcare. Transgender Health. 2018;3(1):10–6. https://doi.org/10.1089/trgh.2017.0047.
19. Cronin A, King A. Power, inequality and identification: exploring diversity and intersectionality amongst older LGB adults. 2010. http://journals.sagepub.com/doi/10.1177/0038038510375738. Accessed 21 Jun 2018.
20. Bry LJ, Mustanski B, Garofalo R, Burns MN. Resilience to discrimination and rejection among young sexual minority males and transgender females: a qualitative study on coping with minority stress. J Homosex. 2018;65(11):1435–56. https://doi.org/10.1080/00918369.2017.1375367.
21. Levitt HM, Ippolito MR. Being transgender: navigating minority stressors and developing authentic self-presentation. Psychol Women Q. 2014;38(1):46–64. https://doi.org/10.1177/0361684313501644.
22. McConnell EA, Janulis P, Phillips G, Truong R, Birkett M. Multiple minority stress and LGBT community resilience among sexual minority men. Psychol Sex Orientat Gend Divers. 2018;5(1):1–12. https://doi.org/10.1037/sgd0000265.
23. Macapagal K, Bhatia R, Greene GJ. Differences in healthcare access, use, and experiences within a community sample of racially diverse lesbian, gay, bisexual, transgender, and questioning emerging adults. LGBT Health. 2016;3(6):434–42. https://doi.org/10.1089/lgbt.2015.0124.
24. Kim H-J, Jen S, Fredriksen-Goldsen KI. Race/ethnicity and health-related quality of life among LGBT older adults. Gerontologist. 2017;57(Suppl 1):S30–9. https://doi.org/10.1093/geront/gnw172.
25. Denson DJ, Padgett PM, Pitts N, et al. Health care use and HIV-related behaviors of Black and Latina transgender women in 3 US metropolitan areas: results from the transgender HIV behavioral survey. J Acquir Immune Defic Syndr. 2017;75(Suppl 3):S268–75. https://doi.org/10.1097/qai.0000000000001402.
26. Kosciw JG, Greytak EA, Diaz EM. Who, what, where, when, and why: demographic and ecological factors contributing to hostile school climate for lesbian, gay, bisexual, and transgender youth. J Youth Adolesc. 2009;38(7):976–88. https://doi.org/10.1007/s10964-009-9412-1.
27. PhD AHG, PhD ARD. Transgender youth. J Homosex. 2006;51(1):111–28. https://doi.org/10.1300/j082v51n01_06.

28. Rider GN, McMorris BJ, Gower AL, Coleman E, Eisenberg ME. Health and care utilization of transgender and gender nonconforming youth: a population-based study. Pediatrics. 2018;141(3):e20171683. https://doi.org/10.1542/peds.2017-1683.
29. Institute of Medicine (US) Committee on Lesbian, Gay, Bisexual, and Transgender Health Issues and Research Gaps and Opportunities. The health of lesbian, gay, bisexual, and transgender people: building a foundation for better understanding. Washington (DC): National Academies Press (US); 2011. http://www.ncbi.nlm.nih.gov/books/NBK64806/. Accessed 24 Aug 2018.
30. Pediatrics AA. Child and adolescent gender center: a multidisciplinary collaboration to improve the lives of gender nonconforming children and teens. Pediatr Rev. 2012;33(6): 273–5. https://doi.org/10.1542/pir.33-6-273.
31. Rosenthal SM. Approach to the patient: transgender youth: endocrine considerations. J Clin Endocrinol Metab. 2014;99(12):4379–89. https://doi.org/10.1210/jc.2014-1919.
32. Gridley SJ, Crouch JM, Evans Y, et al. Youth and caregiver perspectives on barriers to gender-affirming health care for transgender youth. J Adolesc Health. 2016;59(3):254–61. https://doi.org/10.1016/j.jadohealth.2016.03.017.
33. Vance SR, Halpern-Felsher BL, Rosenthal SM. Health care providers' comfort with and barriers to care of transgender youth. J Adolesc Health. 2015;56(2):251–3. https://doi.org/10.1016/j.jadohealth.2014.11.002.
34. Winoker JS, Kent MA, Grotas AB. MP44-19 the current landscape of transgender patient care in urology: an evaluation of attitudes, knowledge, and practice patterns among urologists. J Urol. 2018;199(4, Supplement):e595–6. https://doi.org/10.1016/j.juro.2018.02.1438.
35. People FT, Gehi PS, Arkles G. Unraveling injustice: race and class impact of medicaid exclusions of transition-related health care.
36. National Transgender Discrimination Survey. National center for transgender equality. https://transequality.org/issues/national-transgender-discrimination-survey. Accessed 24 Aug 2018.
37. Gonzales G, Henning-Smith C. Barriers to care among transgender and gender nonconforming adults. Milbank Q. 2017;95(4):726–48. https://doi.org/10.1111/1468-0009.12297.
38. Currah P. Transgender law and policy institute: scope of explicitly transgender-inclusive anti-discrimination laws. Jul 2008. http://www.thetaskforce.org/static_html/downloads/reports/fact_sheets/TI_antidisc_laws_7_08.pdf. Accessed 13 Jul 2018.
39. Stroumsa D. The state of transgender health care: policy, law, and medical frameworks. Am J Public Health. 2014;104(3):e31–8. https://doi.org/10.2105/ajph.2013.301789.
40. Campaign HR. First Amendment Defense Act. Human Rights Campaign. http://www.hrc.org/resources/first-amendment-defense-act/. Accessed 24 Aug 2018.
41. Transgender Law and Policy Institute. U.S. jurisdictions with laws prohibiting discrimination on the basis of gender identity or expression. State by state guide to laws that prohibit discrimination against transgender people. http://www.nclrights.org/wp-content/uploads/2013/07/StateLawsThatProhibitDiscriminationAgainstTransPeople.pdf. Accessed 24 Aug 2018.
42. Mapping LGBT equality in America. Movement Advancement Project | Equality Maps. http://www.lgbtmap.org/equality-maps. Accessed 24 Aug 2018.
43. White Hughto JM, Murchison GR, Clark K, Pachankis JE, Reisner SL. Geographic and individual differences in healthcare access for U.S. transgender adults: a multilevel analysis. LGBT Health. 2016;3(6):424–33. https://doi.org/10.1089/lgbt.2016.0044.
44. Wang T, Geffen S, Cahill S. The current wave of anti-LGBT legislation: historical context and implications for LGBT health. The Fenway Institute; 2016. http://fenwayhealth.org/wp-content/uploads/The-Fenway-Institute-Religious-Exemption-Brief-June-2016.pdf. Accessed 13 Jul 2018.
45. Cahill SR. Legal and policy issues for LGBT patients with cancer or at elevated risk of cancer. Semin Oncol Nurs. 2018;34(1):90–8. https://doi.org/10.1016/j.soncn.2017.12.006.
46. Coleman E, Bockting W, Botzer M, et al. Standards of care for the health of transsexual, transgender, and gender-nonconforming people, version 7. Int J Transgenderism. 2012;13(4):165–232. https://doi.org/10.1080/15532739.2011.700873.

47. Padula WV, Heru S, Campbell JD. Societal implications of health insurance coverage for medically necessary services in the U.S. transgender population: a cost-effectiveness analysis. J Gen Intern Med. 2016;31(4):394–401. https://doi.org/10.1007/s11606-015-3529-6.
48. Khan L. Transgender health at the crossroads: legal norms, insurance markets, and the threat of healthcare reform. Yale J Health Policy Law Ethics. 2013;11(2). https://digitalcommons.law.yale.edu/yjhple/vol11/iss2/4.
49. Bosse JD, Leblanc RG, Jackman K, Bjarnadottir RI. Benefits of implementing and improving collection of sexual orientation and gender identity data in electronic health records. Comput Inform Nurs CIN. 2018;36(6):267–74. https://doi.org/10.1097/cin.0000000000000417.
50. Reisner SL, Deutsch MB, Bhasin S, et al. Advancing methods for U.S. transgender health research. Curr Opin Endocrinol Diabetes Obes. 2016;23(2):198–207. https://doi.org/10.1097/med.0000000000000229.
51. Callahan EJ, Sitkin N, Ton H, Eidson-Ton WS, Weckstein J, Latimore D. Introducing sexual orientation and gender identity into the electronic health record: one academic health center's experience. Acad Med J Assoc Am Med Coll. 2015;90(2):154–60. https://doi.org/10.1097/acm.0000000000000467.
52. Donald C, Ehrenfeld JM. The opportunity for medical systems to reduce health disparities among lesbian, gay, bisexual, transgender and intersex patients. J Med Syst. 2015;39(11):178. https://doi.org/10.1007/s10916-015-0355-7.

Chapter 3
Biology of Gender Identity and Gender Incongruence

Oksana Hamidi and Todd B. Nippoldt

Concepts of Gender Identity Development

Gender is one of the most fundamental societal principles, and it is central to how people view themselves, interact with others, and experience their social world. The terms *gender identity* (a person's inner sense and perception of self as male, female, or other) and *gender role* (the role, behavior, attributes, and personality traits attributed to one's gender as determined by the prevailing cultural norms and constructs) were first introduced in the medical literature in the 1950s when gender identity development was studied in individuals with differences of sex development (DSD) and gender dysphoria.

How we learn about our gender is unclear. Nonetheless, gender learning is a gradual process that starts early and ensues through various stages over many years [1]. Awareness of gender differences emerges in infancy [2]. Most children develop the ability to label faces as male or female between 18 and 24 months of age. By 2–4 years of age, children understand gender differences, use gendered pronouns such as "him" and "her," and label themselves as a boy or girl [1]. This cognitive stage of gender development is thought to be at the core of future gender-related roles. By 4–5 years of age, most children achieve gender stability, understand the lasting nature of gender, and express their gender identity by playing with toys and games that correlate with their anatomic sex [3].

At initial stages, gender identity may be viewed as fluid and subject to change. However, by age 6–7 years, gender identity becomes stable and unlikely to change

O. Hamidi
Department of Endocrinology and Metabolism, UT Southwestern Medical Center, Dallas, TX, USA

T. B. Nippoldt (✉)
Department of Endocrinology, Diabetes and Nutrition, Mayo Clinic, Rochester, MN, USA
e-mail: nippoldt.todd@mayo.edu

L. Poretsky and W. C. Hembree (eds.), *Transgender Medicine*, Contemporary Endocrinology, https://doi.org/10.1007/978-3-030-05683-4_3

even if environmental or physical changes occur. At this stage, children assume gender stereotypes and begin sex segregation by developing preference for same-sex playmates, and gender identity becomes more constant [2, 4, 5]. Although gender-conforming behaviors become more flexible in the school-age years, peer groups generally continue to be same sex [6]. Gender identity is more malleable before puberty than later in adolescence or in adulthood [7]. Further gender role identification in boys and girls intensifies throughout adolescence and is thought to be mediated by pubertal hormones. Increased pressure to conform to culturally endorsed gender roles, fitting in, and peer group acceptance is important in school-aged children [8]. For most adolescents, gender identity seems to be fairly fixed from early childhood and is largely congruent with the physical gender characteristics, assigned natal sex, and culturally expected gender role behaviors [9].

Development of Gender Variant Identity

Exploring sexuality and experimenting with gender roles, such as interest in cross-gender toys and games and cross-dressing, are a normal part of child development [10, 11]. However, little is known about gender development among persons with a gender variant identity. Children with gender incongruence appear to lag in gender learning and have the same, but slower, sequence of cognitive gender development compared to children without gender variant behaviors or interests [12]. From clinical experience, most children with gender variant identity have the ability to label their natal sex but are not able to identify with it. They may verbalize their preference for the other gender as soon as they learn to talk. Moreover, as young as age 2 years, they may indicate that they want to be the other gender, dislike the gender associated with their natal sex, and express anatomic dysphoria ("I do not want to have a penis" or "I do not want to have breasts") [13].

Based on available evidence from prospective follow-up studies, gender nonconformity in childhood does not inevitably persist in adolescence and adulthood (desistence), and only approximately 15% (range 2–27%) of children continue to experience gender incongruence by adolescence [14]. The relatively high rate of desistence in this group can be explained by relatively broad DSM-IV-TR criteria for the diagnosis of gender identity disorder and consequent inclusion of mildly gender nonconforming children in these studies. Children with a strong incongruent gender identity and/or gender dysphoria are more likely to persist into adolescence [15]. Adolescence, particularly between 10 and 13 years of age, is a critical period among children with early onset gender variant identity. Gender incongruence in this age group may persist or desist based on three possible contributing factors: (1) physical puberty; (2) changing environment and being more explicitly treated as one's natal sex (e.g., first year of high school); and (3) the discovery of sexuality [14]. Irrespective of the underlying mechanism of gender variant identity, adolescence may either consolidate an already existing gender incongruence or serve as an initial time point in the development of gender nonconformity [16].

Psychosocial Factors Related to Gender Identity

Early literature from nearly 50 years ago proposed that the development of gender nonconformity was primarily, if not exclusively, an outcome of certain parental characteristics such as a maternal wish for a daughter, paternal absence, parental reinforcement patterns, or a symbiotic relationship between mother and son [17, 18]. Some of these hypotheses were tested, but either did not receive empirical support or lacked interpretable outcomes.

More recent psychosocial theories incorporate complex cumulative parent- and child-related factors contributing to the development of gender incongruence [19, 20]. During a critical period in the child's life, the presence and degree of psychopathology in the parents and anxiety in the child were shown to play a role in gender identity outcome [21–23]. Evidence of the role of specific child and parental factors on the development of gender incongruence is limited. It has been suggested that the physical appearance of being a more feminine and beautiful boy, or a more masculine-looking girl, fear of male aggression, and lack of limit setting by mothers, particularly with respect to cross-gender behaviors, are factors that influence gender identity outcome [20, 24].

Differences in Sexual Development and the Role of Androgen Exposure in Gender Identity Development

DSD are congenital conditions involving the reproductive system, in which the development of chromosomal, gonadal, or anatomic sex is atypical [25]. In DSD, external genitalia may not correspond with the gonads and/or sex chromosomes. Gender identity may or may not be congruent with the chromosomes, the gonads, or the external genitalia. Gender identity and sexual orientation variants in individuals with DSD were first reported in 1945 [26]. A decade later, the term *gender identity* was proposed to make a clear distinction between the terms *sex* and *gender* [27].

46,XX Individuals with Congenital Adrenal Hyperplasia (CAH)

Although most transgender patients do not have DSD, studies carried out in individuals with atypical prenatal hormone levels, such as individuals with some DSD, have looked at the effects of prenatal and postnatal sex hormones on gender identity development. Specifically, prenatal androgen exposure and gender identity outcomes have been extensively studied in 46,XX individuals with classical CAH, caused by a mutation in the *CYP21A2* gene, leading to complete or near-complete deficiency of 21-hydroxylase and, in turn, prenatal exposure of the brain to elevated levels of androgens and also resulting in varying degrees of external genital masculinization [28]. 46,XX individuals with CAH raised as females show more masculine interests and behaviors than control girls and women without CAH [29]. However, despite the association of lower rates of feminine gender expression, the effect of the prenatal androgen exposure on gender identity seems to be less robust [30]. Although the studies demonstrate that patients with CAH have higher than expected prevalence of gender incongruence or gender dysphoria, the vast majority of women with CAH identify as females [30–33]. In an interview study of 43 patients, ages 3–18 years, gender identity scores indicated that 11.6% of patients with CAH had scores outside the range of control girls. There was no correlation between gender identity and degree of prenatal androgen exposure (i.e., degree of genital virilization) or age at the time of genital surgery [30]. Another study demonstrated that despite elevated androgen levels and genital virilization among 46,XX patients with CAH, 5.2% (13 out of 250) reported gender incongruence [32]. Gender identity outcome did not correlate with the degree of genital masculinization and did not seem to occur more frequently in patients raised as males compared to those raised as females. In contrast, the severity of salt-wasting form of classical 21-hydroxylase deficiency has been demonstrated to correlate with gender identity outcome with 3 of 42 patients (7.1%) identifying as male; whereas no gender incongruence was seen in individuals with less severe CAH variants (the study included 42 46,XX patients with the salt-wasting variant, 21 with the simple virilizing variant, 82 women with the non-classic variant, and 24 related non-CAH sisters and female cousins as controls) [34]. These and other studies demonstrate that most 46,XX patients with virilizing CAH appear to have a female gender identity and that gender identity development in these individuals seems to be remarkably adaptive. However, the finding that 5.2–11.6% of such patients have gender incongruence, much more common than expected based on the reported prevalence of female-to-male transgenderism, implies that prenatal/postnatal androgen exposure plays some role in the development of gender identity [30, 32, 34].

Androgen Insensitivity Syndromes

Complete androgen insensitivity syndrome (CAIS) results from a mutation in the androgen receptor (*AR*) gene leading to an inactive receptor. Individuals with CAIS have a 46,XY karyotype and produce normal or high male levels of androgens, but typically have an unambiguous female phenotype. 46,XY individuals with CAIS are generally assigned female sex at birth, develop a female gender identity, and because of their feminine physical appearance, are perceived and treated as females throughout their lives [35]. The absence of androgen effects on the brains of these XY women with CAIS, as well as female-based socialization, may contribute to the development of the usually encountered female gender identity. Nonetheless, despite the multitude of factors reinforcing female gender identity, XY individuals with CAIS are reported to score lower on a female gender identity scale compared to controls [36]. Moreover, a case report of a 46,XY individual with CAIS (due to an *AR* gene mutation resulting in a premature stop codon), who developed severe gender dysphoria and underwent female-to-male gender transition, challenges the concept that androgens are essential in male gender identity development [37].

In contrast to individuals with CAIS, gender transitions are considerably more prevalent among XY persons born with partial androgen insensitivity syndrome (PAIS) [35]. Gender dysphoria seems to affect nearly 25% of individuals with PAIS and develops at similar rates whether they are raised as boys or girls [38]. Moreover, related distress seems to be equally severe, regardless of the magnitude of the discrepancy between their anatomic development and gender identity.

Defects in Androgen Biosynthesis and Structural DSD

The effects of prenatal and postnatal exposure to androgens on development of gender identity have also been evaluated in other DSD. For instance, 5α-reductase-2 deficiency (5α-RD-2) is an autosomal recessive condition in which 46,XY individuals with bilateral testes and normal testosterone synthesis have defective conversion of testosterone to dihydrotestosterone and consequently impaired virilization of external genitalia during embryogenesis. Similarly, 17 β-hydroxysteroid dehydrogenase-3 deficiency (17β-HSD-3) secondary to a deletion or mutation of the underlying gene affects masculinization of the male external genitalia via impaired testosterone biosynthesis, which in turn leads to formation of female appearing or ambiguous genitalia. In both conditions, affected 46,XY children are usually raised as girls. While in 5α-RD-2, the brain is prenatally exposed to normal male testosterone levels, in 17β-HSD-3 prenatal brain exposure to testosterone is deficient. In these conditions, masculinization of the body and genitalia does occur, to varying degrees, at the time of puberty. Individuals with 5α-RD-2 raised as females who undergo gonadectomy prior to puberty generally maintain a female gender identity [39]. Notably, the prevalence of gender incongruence among those who are raised as girls (male gender identity) is considerably higher in the individuals with 5α-RD-2 and 17β-HSD-3, particularly if the condition is not diagnosed before the development of male secondary sex characteristics [40]. Gender role changes from female to male are reported in 56–63% of 46,XY patients with 5α-RD-2 (generally after puberty) and in 39–64% of 46,XY individuals with 17β-HSD-3 [40]. Among patients with 5α-RD-2 and 17β-HSD-3, those who underwent gender role change from female to male had intact testes, bolstering the potential role of androgen exposure in gender identity outcomes [41, 42]. Similar to those with PAIS, individuals with 5α-RD-2 and 17β-HSD-3 demonstrate somewhat masculine appearance, behaviors, and interests, and as a result may develop a nonconforming gender role. Moreover, such individuals may be perceived more masculine by their family members and peers, especially around the time of masculinization at puberty, further impacting the development of gender identity variant. Cultural and societal context therefore should not be overlooked.

Gender identity outcome has also been studied in patients with structural (non-hormonal) causes of DSD (e.g., cloacal exstrophy, penile ablation, and penile agenesis) [33, 43]. In individuals with 46,XY cloacal exstrophy who underwent neonatal sex reassignment (surgically, socially, and legally) to female, 8 of the 14 subsequently reported a male gender identity. Two patients who did not have surgery and were raised as males reported a male gender identity [43]. In a study of 51 individuals with cloacal exstrophy who were assigned female, most (65%) identified as female, whereas 14% were living as female but were suspected to have gender dysphoria, and nearly 22% identified and lived as male [33]. Moreover, among 16 46,XY individuals with penile agenesis assigned female at birth and 7 males with penile ablation reassigned female in infancy or early childhood, the majority were living as female [33]. This inability to predict the eventual gender identity underlies the continued controversy regarding management of infants with DSD [44].

In summary, prenatal androgen exposure of the brain appears to have an influence on the development of gender identity and male-typical behaviors. Although gender identity outcome in hormonal and structural DSD is not solely dependent on sex hormone exposure, gender incongruence is significantly higher than in general population, supporting at least modest role of androgens in the gender identity outcome. The interplay between androgen exposure and gender identity is, however, complex and not linear—individuals with prenatal exposure to high levels of testosterone but raised as girls generally maintain female gender identity [32], yet male gender identity may develop in the absence of prenatal testosterone exposure [37].

Genetics and Gender Identity

Hereditability of transgenderism has been suggested by observing concordance of gender incongruence in monozygotic twin pairs and in father–son and brother–sister pairs [45, 46]. Based on survey responses from parents, clinically significant gender incongruence was demonstrated in 2.3% of twins, with 62% of the gender variance attributed to hereditability (96 monozygotic pairs and 61 dizygotic pairs, ages 7–14 years) [47]. A role of genetics in gender identity development was further supported by demonstrating a 39% concordance for gender variant in 23 monozygotic female and male twin pairs, with no concordance in 21 same-sex dizygotic female and male twin pairs or in 7 opposite-sex twin pairs [48]. Fascinatingly, there were three sets of twins among the probands who were raised separately but were concordant for gender incongruence. In a study of 112 pairs of twins evaluating gender incongruence, there was a 33.3% concordance among monozygotic male twins and a 22.8% concordance among monozygotic female twins [49].

Several studies have reported a co-occurrence of gender nonconformity in families. For instance, in a sample of 995 transgender individuals, there were 12 pairs of non-twin siblings [50]. This prevalence of gender nonconformity in siblings (1/211 siblings) is much higher than expected from the local prevalence data on transgender identity, suggesting that siblings of transgender individuals may have a higher chance of developing gender incongruence than the general population. Interestingly, the study reported a 4.5-fold higher probability of gender nonconformity in siblings of transwomen compared to siblings of transmen, and a 3.9-fold higher probability for brothers rather than sisters of transgender probands.

Emerging research has shown that biological differences between men and women are mediated by genetic factors, which in turn directly affect behavioral and brain sex differences [51]. However, data on specific genes associated with transgenderism are inconsistent and lack strong statistical significance. For instance, a longer dinucleotide CA repeat in intron 5 of the estrogen receptor-beta (*ERβ*) gene was found in 29 transgender women (male-to-female), when compared to 229 cisgender male controls ($P = 0.03$), but no associations were present with polymorphism in the *AR* (CAG repeat length) and the aromatase (*CYP19*) (TTTA repeat length) genes [52]. However, another study showed no association between transgenderism and the *ERβ* gene or the *CYP19* gene, although transgender women had a significantly longer trinucleotide CAG repeat in exon 1 of the *AR*, compared with controls (112 transgender women and 258 cisgender male controls) [53]. Gender identity outcome did not correlate with polymorphisms in five candidate genes (*AR*, *CYP19*, *ERα*, *ERβ*, and the progesterone receptor) in a study evaluating 74 transgender women and 168 transgender men with 106 cisgender male and 169 cisgender female controls [54]. In another study, a positive association was detected between a single-nucleotide polymorphism in the *CYP17* gene and transgender men but not in transgender women [55]. In summary, results of these studies demonstrate a contribution of genetic factors in the development of gender identity. How these are influenced by hormonal, environmental, and psychosocial factors remains unclear and warrant further investigation.

Neurobiological Basis for Gender Nonconforming Identity

Neuroanatomical differences in transgender individuals have been reported in numerous studies. "Sexually dimorphic" brain structures are well established in the medical literature. Specifically, cell groups in the anterior hypothalamus—interstitial nucleus of the anterior hypothalamus 3 (INAH 3) and the central part of the bed nucleus of the stria terminalis (BSTc)—have different morphological characteristics in males and females [56, 57]. The first anatomical studies of brains at autopsy reported differences in the BSTc of male-to-female transgender individuals when compared to heterosexual and homosexual cisgender male brains [57]. Subsequent studies demonstrated that the volume and neuron number of INAH 3 and BSTc in transgender women was indeed similar to those in the cisgender women, and significantly smaller than those of cisgender men [58]. The study was criticized for assessing transgender individuals treated with cross-sex hormone therapy, which in turn questioned whether the volume differences in the BSTc were attributed to the hormone use. However, the study also described important controls, such as a cisgender male with a feminizing adrenal tumor producing high concentrations of estrogen, yet maintaining the male BSTc pattern, as did two testosterone-deficient males due to orchiectomy for prostate cancer. Furthermore, a female with virilizing adrenal tumor producing high concentrations of androstenedione and testosterone nonetheless had the female BSTc pattern, as did an 84-year-old transgender woman who had never received feminizing or anti-androgen hormone therapy [59]. The association between the anatomy of BSTc and transgenderism bolstered the concept that gender identity evolves as a consequence of the interaction of the developing brain and sex hormones.

Another hypothalamic nucleus located in the preoptic area, the intermediate nucleus (InM), was identified to relate to gender identity [60]. Postmortem brain tissue in transgender women (on feminizing hormone therapy) was found to have intermediate total neuron and volume values compared to those of cisgender men and women. Intriguingly, the study included five men who underwent castration for prostate cancer and showed that total neuron numbers were similar to cisgender males, implying that the change in adult circulating testosterone levels does not seem to explain the intermediate values in the transwoman group. The inclusion of critical controls with sex steroid variations and untreated transgender individuals provides additional evidence that the observed brain structure differences in the transgender individuals are intrinsic and not simply a consequence of hormone exposure. Yet, it should be noted that the sexually dimorphic differentiation of the BSTc and InM in humans is not present until puberty [61, 62]. Therefore, the relationship between BSTc volume and gender identity is unclear, as most transgender adolescents experience significant gender incongruence prior to the onset of puberty.

With regard to neuroanatomical differences, structural and functional imaging studies examining anatomic variance of the corpus callosum revealed no differences between anatomic sex and gender identity [63]. However, the majority of participants in this study received cross-sex hormone therapy. Sexually dimorphic white matter structures (e.g., parts of the superior longitudinal fasciculus) in the transgender participants prior to initiating cross-sex hormones were closer to controls with the same gender identity rather than the same natal sex [64].

Similarly, gray matter volumes by magnetic resonance imaging noted that the dimensions of right putamen in transgender women prior to cross-sex hormone therapy were larger than in cisgender males and within the average range for cisgender females [65]. A subsequent study, however, reported that the putamen volume in transgender female individuals was smaller than in both cisgender male and female controls [66]. A functional imaging study examined the hypothalamic activation pattern of smelling two aromatic steroids, one present in the sweat, saliva, and semen of cisgender men, and the other in the urine of pregnant women. Heterosexual cisgender men and heterosexual cisgender women showed a different pattern of activation after smelling these compounds. The pattern of hypothalamic activation present in male-to-female transgender subjects (with sexual orientation to females) did not differ from that seen in heterosexual cisgender women [67]. Additional studies showed similarities in brain activation patterns due to visual erotic stimuli [68] and in quantitative EEG analysis [69] in transgender women and cisgender female volunteers. Moreover, regional cerebral blood flow in the left anterior cingulate cortex and right insula [70] and brain network activation patterns during a standardized mental rotation task [71] differed in untreated transgender individuals compared to controls of their natal sex. A potential limitation in these gray and white matter studies is related to brain functional plasticity, as the changes in both white and gray matter can be induced by training and/or experience in healthy human adults [72, 73].

Conclusions

Historically, gender identity and gender role were conceptualized as a dichotomous construct, rather than a wide and fluid spectrum of gender identity labels. More recently, the dimensionality of gender incongruence has received increasing attention in the medical literature and public media. The nonconforming individuals do not necessarily experience a binary transgender identity and do not always need medical intervention. Despite increasing interest in gender nonconforming children and adults, the understanding of gender identity development is limited.

Research has demonstrated that gender identity is not simply a psychological entity. Hormones and genes cause differences in morphology and physiology that in turn may lead to different interactions with the environment. Although prenatal and postnatal hormone exposure plays an important role in gender identity development, these effects are not straightforward. Data from neuropsychological and imaging studies support that biological factors are fundamentally associated with specific gender identities, but are insufficient to form a concrete theory of the development of gender identity variance. Moreover, the current evidence lacks a causal relationship between brain development and gender identity development. Psychological and environmental factors have also been shown to have important associations in gender nonconforming individuals. Gender identity development most likely occurs from a complex interplay between biological, environmental, cultural, and psychological factors.

References

1. Kohlberg L. A cognitive-developmental analysis of children's sex-role concepts and attitudes, in the development of sex differences. In: Maccoby EE, editor. Stanford University Press; 1966.
2. Martin CR, Ruble D. Children's search for gender cues. CDPS. 2004;13:67.

3. Zosuls KM, et al. The acquisition of gender labels in infancy: implications for gender-typed play. Dev Psychol. 2009;45(3):688–701.
4. Lobel TE, et al. Gender schema and social judgments: a developmental study of children from Hong Kong. Sex Roles. 2000;43(1/2):19–42.
5. Egan SK, Perry DG. Gender identity: a multidimensional analysis with implications for psychosocial adjustment. Dev Psychol. 2001;37(4):451–63.
6. Carver PR, Yunger JL, Perry DG. Gender identity and adjustment in middle childhood. Sex Roles. 2003;49(3/4):95–109.
7. Byne W, et al. Report of the American Psychiatric Association task force on treatment of gender identity disorder. Arch Sex Behav. 2012;41(4):759–96.
8. Hill JP, Lynch ME. The intensification of gender-related role expectations during early adolescence, in girls at puberty. 1983. p. 201–28.
9. Diamond LM, Butterworth M. Questioning gender and sexual identity: dynamic links over time. Sex Roles. 2008;59(5–6):365–76.
10. Bullough VL. Children and adolescents as sexual beings: a historical overview. Child Adolesc Psychiatr Clin N Am. 2004;13(3):447–59.
11. Mallon GP, DeCrescenzo T. Transgender children and youth: a child welfare practice perspective. Child Welfare. 2006;85(2):215–41.
12. Zucker KJ, et al. Gender constancy judgments in children with gender identity disorder: evidence for a developmental lag. Arch Sex Behav. 1999;28(6):475–502.
13. Cohen-Kettenis PT. Gender identity disorders. In: Gillberg C, Steinhausen HC, Harrington R, editors. A clinician's handbook of child and adolescent psychiatry. Cambridge: Cambridge University Press; 2006. p. 695–725.
14. Steensma TD, et al. Desisting and persisting gender dysphoria after childhood: a qualitative follow-up study. Clin Child Psychol Psychiatry. 2011;16(4):499–516.
15. Wallien MS, Cohen-Kettenis PT. Psychosexual outcome of gender-dysphoric children. J Am Acad Child Adolesc Psychiatry. 2008;47(12):1413–23.
16. Steensma TD, et al. Gender identity development in adolescence. Horm Behav. 2013;64 (2):288–97.
17. Green R. Sexual identity conflict in children and adults. New York: Basic Books; 1974.
18. Stoller RJ. Sex and gender. New York: Science House; 1968.
19. Coates S. Ontogenesis of boyhood gender identity disorder. J Am Acad Psychoanal. 1990;18 (3):414–38.
20. Zucker KJ, Bradley S. Gender identity disorder and psychosexual problems in children and adolescents. New York: Guilford; 1995.
21. Marantz S, et al. Mothers of boys with gender identity disorder: a comparison of matched controls. J Am Acad Child Adolesc Psychiatry. 1991;30(2):310–5.
22. Zucker KJ, Bradley SJ, Lowry Sullivan CB. Traits of separation anxiety in boys with gender identity disorder. J Am Acad Child Adolesc Psychiatry. 1996;35(6):791–8.
23. Cohen-Kettenis PT, et al. Demographic characteristics, social competence, and behavior problems in children with gender identity disorder: a cross-national, cross-clinic comparative analysis. J Abnorm Child Psychol. 2003;31(1):41–53.
24. Zucker KJ, et al. Physical attractiveness of boys with gender identity disorder. Arch Sex Behav. 1993;22(1):23–36.
25. Lee PA, et al. Consensus statement on management of intersex disorders. International Consensus Conference on Intersex. Pediatrics. 2006;118(2):e488–500.
26. Ellis A. The sexual psychology of human hermaphrodites. Psychosom Med. 1945.
27. Money J. The concept of gender identity disorder in childhood and adolescence after 39 years. J Sex Marital Ther. 1994;20(3):163–77.
28. Merke DP, Bornstein SR. Congenital adrenal hyperplasia. The Lancet. 2005;365 (9477):2125–36.

29. Cohen-Bendahan CCC, van de Beek C, Berenbaum SA. Prenatal sex hormone effects on child and adult sex-typed behavior: methods and findings. Neurosci Biobehav Rev. 2005;29(2):353–84.
30. Berenbaum SA, Bailey JM. Effects on gender identity of prenatal androgens and genital appearance: evidence from girls with congenital adrenal hyperplasia. J Clin Endocrinol Metab. 2003;88(3):1102–6.
31. de Vries AL, Doreleijers TA, Cohen-Kettenis PT. Disorders of sex development and gender identity outcome in adolescence and adulthood: understanding gender identity development and its clinical implications. Pediatr Endocrinol Rev. 2007;4(4):343–51.
32. Dessens AB, Slijper FM, Drop SL. Gender dysphoria and gender change in chromosomal females with congenital adrenal hyperplasia. Arch Sex Behav. 2005;34(4):389–97.
33. Meyer-Bahlburg HFL. Gender identity outcome in female-raised 46,XY persons with penile agenesis, cloacal exstrophy of the bladder, or penile ablation. Arch Sex Behav. 2005;34(4):423–38.
34. Meyer-Bahlburg HF, et al. Gender development in women with congenital adrenal hyperplasia as a function of disorder severity. Arch Sex Behav. 2006;35(6):667–84.
35. Mazur T. Gender dysphoria and gender change in androgen insensitivity or micropenis. Arch Sex Behav. 2005;34(4):411–21.
36. Richter-Appelt H, Discher C, Gedrose B. Gender identity and recalled gender related childhood play-behaviour in adult individuals with different forms of intersexuality. Anthropol Anz. 2005;63(3):241–56.
37. T'Sjoen G, et al. Male gender identity in complete androgen insensitivity syndrome. Arch Sex Behav. 2011;40(3):635–8.
38. Warne GL. Long-term outcome of disorders of sex development. Sex Dev. 2008;2(4–5):268–77.
39. Hines M. Gonadal hormones and sexual differentiation of human brain and behavior. In: Pfaff DW, editor. Hormones, brain and behavior. San Diego: Academic Press; 2009, p. 1869–1910.
40. Cohen-Kettenis PT. Gender change in 46,XY persons with 5alpha-reductase-2 deficiency and 17beta-hydroxysteroid dehydrogenase-3 deficiency. Arch Sex Behav. 2005;34(4):399–410.
41. Rösler A, Silverstein S, Abeliovich D. A (R80Q) mutation in 17 beta-hydroxysteroid dehydrogenase type 3 gene among Arabs of Israel is associated with pseudohermaphroditism in males and normal asymptomatic females. J Clin Endocrinol Metab. 1996;81(5):1827–31.
42. Imperato-McGinley J, et al. Androgens and the evolution of male-gender identity among male pseudohermaphrodites with 5α-reductase deficiency. N Engl J Med. 1979;300(22):1233–7.
43. Reiner WG, Gearhart JP. Discordant sexual identity in some genetic males with cloacal exstrophy assigned to female sex at birth. N Engl J Med. 2004;350(4):333–41.
44. Mouriquand PDE, et al. Surgery in disorders of sex development (DSD) with a gender issue: if (why), when, and how? J Pediatr Urol. 2016;12(3):139–49.
45. Hyde C, Kenna JC. A male M Z twin pair, concordant for transsexualism, discordant for schizophrenia. Acta Psychiatr Scand. 1977;56(4):265–73.
46. Green R. Family cooccurrence of "gender dysphoria": ten sibling or parent-child pairs. Arch Sex Behav. 2000;29(5):499–507.
47. Coolidge FL, Thede LL, Young SE. The heritability of gender identity disorder in a child and adolescent twin sample. Behav Genet. 2002;32(4):251–7.
48. Heylens G, et al. Gender identity disorder in twins: a review of the case report literature. J Sex Med. 2012;9(3):751–7.
49. Diamond M. Transsexuality among twins: identity concordance, transition, rearing, and orientation. Int J Transgenderism. 2013;14(1):24–38.
50. Gomez-Gil E, et al. Familiality of gender identity disorder in non-twin siblings. Arch Sex Behav. 2010;39(2):546–52.
51. Ngun TC, et al. The genetics of sex differences in brain and behavior. Front Neuroendocrinol. 2011;32(2):227–46.

52. Henningsson S, et al. Sex steroid-related genes and male-to-female transsexualism. Psychoneuroendocrinology. 2005;30(7):657–64.
53. Hare L, et al. Androgen receptor repeat length polymorphism associated with male-to-female transsexualism. Biol Psychiat. 2009;65(1):93–6.
54. Ujike H, et al. Association study of gender identity disorder and sex hormone-related genes. Prog Neuropsychopharmacol Biol Psychiatry. 2009;33(7):1241–4.
55. Bentz E-K, et al. A polymorphism of the CYP17 gene related to sex steroid metabolism is associated with female-to-male but not male-to-female transsexualism. Fertil Steril. 2008;90 (1):56–9.
56. LeVay S. A difference in hypothalamic structure between heterosexual and homosexual men. Science. 1991;253(5023):1034–7.
57. Zhou JN, et al. A sex difference in the human brain and its relation to transsexuality. Nature. 1995;378(6552):68–70.
58. Swaab DF. Sexual differentiation of the human brain in relation to gender identity and sexual orientation. Funct Neurol. 2009;24(1):17.
59. Kruijver FP, et al. Male-to-female transsexuals have female neuron numbers in a limbic nucleus. J Clinical Endocrinol Metab. 2000;85(5):2034–41.
60. Garcia-Falgueras A, et al. Galanin neurons in the intermediate nucleus (InM) of the human hypothalamus in relation to sex, age, and gender identity. J Comp Neurol. 2011;519 (15):3061–84.
61. Chung WC, De Vries GJ, Swaab DF. Sexual differentiation of the bed nucleus of the stria terminalis in humans may extend into adulthood. J Neurosci. 2002;22(3):1027–33.
62. Chung WC, Swaab DF, De Vries GJ. Apoptosis during sexual differentiation of the bed nucleus of the stria terminalis in the rat brain. J Neurobiol. 2000;43(3):234–43.
63. Emory LE, et al. Anatomic variation of the corpus callosum in persons with gender dysphoria. Arch Sex Behav. 1991;20(4):409–17.
64. Rametti G, et al. White matter microstructure in female to male transsexuals before cross-sex hormonal treatment. A diffusion tensor imaging study. J Psychiatr Res. 2011;45(2):199–204.
65. Luders E, et al. Regional gray matter variation in male-to-female transsexualism. Neuroimage. 2009;46(4):904–7.
66. Savic I, Arver S. Sex dimorphism of the brain in male-to-female transsexuals. Cereb Cortex. 2011;21(11):2525–33.
67. Berglund H, et al. Male-to-female transsexuals show sex-atypical hypothalamus activation when smelling odorous steroids. Cereb Cortex. 2007;18(8):1900–8.
68. Gizewski ER, et al. Original research—intersex and gender identity disorders: specific cerebral activation due to visual erotic stimuli in male-to-female transsexuals compared with male and female controls: an fMRI study. J Sex Med. 6(2): 440–48.
69. Flor-Henry P. EEG analysis of male to female transsexuals: discriminant function and source analysis. Clin EEG Neurosci. 2010;41(4):219–22.
70. Nawata H, et al. Regional cerebral blood flow changes in female to male gender identity disorder. Psychiatry Clin Neurosci. 2010;64(2):157–61.
71. Schöning S, et al. Neuroimaging differences in spatial cognition between men and male-to-female transsexuals before and during hormone therapy. J Sex Med. 2010;7 (5):1858–67.
72. Scholz J, et al. Training induces changes in white-matter architecture. Nat Neurosci. 2009;12 (11):1370.
73. Draganski B, et al. Neuroplasticity: changes in grey matter induced by training. Nature. 2004;427(6972):311.

Chapter 4
Primary Care of Transgender Adults

Asa Radix

Introduction

Transgender and gender nonbinary people have become more visible and accepted in society, however, their transition-related and primary care medical needs are frequently unmet [1]. Several professional associations, such as the American Academy of Pediatrics (AAP), The American College of Obstetricians and Gynecologists (ACOG), The American College of Physicians (ACP) and the American Academy of Family Medicine (AAFP) have issued policy statements proposing that medical providers should be competent to care for transgender individuals [2–5]. However, primary care medical providers often lack knowledge about how to provide appropriate and culturally competent health care, both transition-related care as well as preventive care services to transgender clients [6, 7]. This lack of medical provider knowledge, in addition to other barriers to care, such as discrimination in healthcare settings, denial of services, verbal harassment, and physical assault, results in many transgender and gender non-binary individuals avoiding or delaying preventive care services [8–10]. Studies have indicated, for example, that transgender men are less likely to have been screened for breast and cervical cancer [11, 12] and transgender men and women may be less likely to be screened and therefore aware of their HIV status [13, 14].

The intent of this chapter is to enable medical providers to modify gender- and anatomy-based preventive care recommendations to patients of transgender experience, in particular, those who have undertaken gender-affirming medical and surgical interventions. Medical providers first need to be aware of and understand the basics of the medical and surgical aspects of gender-affirming care, including health outcomes related to hormone therapy (see Chap. 19). They should also be aware of the unique health disparities affecting transgender people, such as higher

A. Radix (✉)
Department of Medicine, Callen-Lorde Community Health Center, New York, NY, USA
e-mail: a.radix@nyumc.org

L. Poretsky and W. C. Hembree (eds.), *Transgender Medicine*, Contemporary Endocrinology, https://doi.org/10.1007/978-3-030-05683-4_4

rates of mood disorders, tobacco and substance use, and higher rates of HIV and sexually transmitted infections [1, 15–18] that will impact patient education needs and preventive care screenings.

Clinical Guidelines and Primary Care

Professional bodies that publish hormone guidelines for transgender health include The World Professional Association of Transgender Health (WPATH) [19], The Endocrine Society [20] and the UCSF Center of Excellence for Transgender Health [21]. Several international guidelines provide hormone protocols that are specific to national or regional contexts and reflect available formularies and medical infrastructure (Table 4.1).

Although these guidelines provide information necessary for the initiation and maintenance of hormone regimens, such as information about adverse effects and monitoring considerations, guidance on preventive care is frequently lacking. The reason is that there are few high-quality prospective studies that examine long-term health outcomes in transgender populations. A recent review indicated that although the number of published articles about transgender health has significantly increased over the past 50 years, there are significant gaps in published articles pertaining to general health, especially published research conducted in older age groups, where issues of cancer screenings and other preventive care interventions are paramount [22]. There are several clinical preventive care interventions that are recommended for adults in the United States and published by the United States Preventive Services Task Force (USPSTF), a body that develops recommendations based on a review of high-quality scientific evidence [23]. The recommended preventive care interventions include screening for colon, breast, and cervical cancer, hypertension and cholesterol disorders, tobacco use, and provision of influenza vaccinations. Uptake of these interventions among US adults is routinely monitored through the Behavioral Risk Factor Surveillance System (BRFSS), an ongoing, state-based survey of adults residing in the United States [24]. A recent review of research on preventive care utilization in transgender populations demonstrated that only 41 publications in the United States had addressed these preventive care interventions. The majority of published studies focused on HIV-related topics with very few addressing tobacco, pelvic health, hypertension or cholesterol-related issues. In this review, no studies had examined colorectal health, mammography or influenza vaccination [25]. Research in transgender populations has mostly been limited to small observational, usually retrospective, studies and case reports [26, 27]. There are no randomized prospective controlled trials, for example, that examine the efficacy of breast cancer screening using mammography for transgender women receiving hormones. This recommendation, therefore, is not

Table 4.1 Hormone protocols and guidelines

Year of publication	Guideline	Agency
2011	Standards of Care (SOC) for the health of transsexual, transgender, and gender nonconforming people (https://www.wpath.org/publications/soc)	World Professional Association for Transgender Health (WPATH)
2013	Good practice guidelines for the assessment and treatment of adults with gender dysphoria, 2013 (http://www.teni.ie/attachments/14767e01-a8de-4b90-9a19-8c2c50edf4e1.PDF)	Royal College of Psychiatrists, London, UK
2014	Blueprint for the provision of comprehensive care for trans persons and their communities in the Caribbean and other anglophone countries (http://www.who.int/hiv/pub/transgender/blueprint-trans-paho/en/)	Pan American Health Organization
2015	Blueprint for the provision of comprehensive care for trans people and trans communities in Asia and the Pacific (http://www.asiapacific.undp.org/content/dam/rbap/docs/Research%20&%20Publications/hivaids/rbap-hhd-2015-asia-pacific-trans-health-blueprint.pdf)	Health Policy Project, Asia Pacific Transgender Network, United Nations Development Programme
2016	Guidelines for the primary and gender-affirming care of transgender and gender nonbinary people (http://transhealth.ucsf.edu/protocols)	UCSF Center of Excellence for Transgender Health
2017	Endocrine Treatment of gender-dysphoric/gender-incongruent persons: an endocrine society. Clinical practice guideline 2017 (https://academic-oup-com.ezproxy.cul.columbia.edu/icem/article/102/11/3869/4157558)	The Endocrine Society

based on the evidence but on expert opinion and consensus, which is the case for many of the recommendations regarding transgender health when high-quality evidence does not exist [20, 26].

Research investigating health outcomes in transgender people who have accessed gender-affirming care is complicated by considerable variation in treatment plans including the types and doses of hormones used, duration of use as well as variations in surgical procedures performed by different surgeons. This chapter, therefore, will discuss current recommendations for primary preventive care that are predominantly based on expert opinion after evaluation of available research, both in transgender and general populations.

Provider/Staff–Patient Interactions

In order for medical providers to deliver optimal preventive care services to transgender adults, they first need to ensure that the clinical environment is welcoming. This begins by not making assumptions about a patient's gender identity or sexual orientation. Medical providers and other health facility staff should avoid referring to patients as "Sir" "Ma'am" or other gendered language, whether in person or over the phone [28–32]. There are several strategies that clinicians can employ, such as ensuring that registration forms allow patients to document their gender identity as well as sex assigned at birth, called a "two-step question" [28, 33]. The two-step question has been validated, both in LGBT as well as non-LGBT populations and has been found to be acceptable, allowing for correct identification of transgender people, including in electronic health records [33, 34]. Patients should be asked to provide their pronoun and chosen name, in addition to their legal name and gender marker used for insurance purposes. Other strategies include displaying signage about nondiscrimination policies. Indications of a trans-inclusive environment include having gender-neutral or all-gender restrooms and patient health promotion materials that are intentionally inclusive of transgender people [32]. This is particularly important for patient education materials that focus on preventive care services [28, 32].

Initial Encounter

Available research has indicated that transgender people frequently avoid or delay preventive medical services due to past episodes of discrimination or anticipated stigma [8]. During the initial visit, the primary care provider should gently probe for information on past medical encounters and experience with the healthcare system. Establishing trust and rapport is a goal of this visit. The initial encounter should focus on all aspects of general health care in addition to transition-related care. The medical provider should undertake a comprehensive health assessment including past medical history, surgical history, review of systems with particular attention to conditions that may be exacerbated by hormonal therapy, e.g., risk factors for cardiovascular and venous thromboembolic disease. The medical provider should discuss the need for a complete physical exam. However, due to past negative experiences and patient discomfort, this may need to be deferred to a later visit. The medical provider should also investigate past preventive care screenings, such as cervical and colorectal cancer screenings as well as immunization history. For patients in the USA, preventive care screenings and laboratory testing should be conducted in accordance with the USPSTF and recommendations from professional societies, such as The Endocrine Society [20, 23]. Since some of the USPSTF guidelines are gender-based, additional guidance is required for transgender people who may have undergone gender-affirming hormonal or surgical interventions.

Cardiovascular Risk

In 2013, The American College of Cardiology/American Heart Association (ACC/AHA) developed a new cardiovascular (CVD) risk assessment tool, recommending that all adult patients be assessed for CVD risk [35]. The tool includes traditional cardiovascular risk factors such as age, sex, total cholesterol, and high-density lipoprotein (HDL) cholesterol levels, history of diabetes mellitus, systolic blood pressure, and smoking status.

Several studies have indicated that transgender status and hormonal therapy may impact traditional CVD risk factors. Transgender people have elevated rates of tobacco use when compared to the general population, one of the strongest predictors of adverse CVD outcomes [36, 37]. A systematic review and meta-analysis of the effect of hormonal regimen on lipids found that testosterone was associated with increases in serum triglycerides and low-density lipoprotein cholesterol (LDL) as well as a drop in HDL cholesterol [38]. For transgender women on feminizing regimens, there is a risk of an increase in serum triglycerides [38]. Transgender women on hormonal therapy may be at higher risk for diabetes with studies showing a decrease in insulin sensitivity and an increase in weight gain [39–41]. To date, there has not been evidence of increased incidence of adult-onset type 2 diabetes mellitus. One small study conducted at a gender clinic in Ghent, Belgium revealed that 9 of 1081 transgender persons had been previously diagnosed with type 1 diabetes mellitus and another person had been diagnosed with latent autoimmune diabetes of adulthood. However, this may be a spurious finding and a causal relationship, if any, is not understood [42].

Despite the higher prevalence of CVD risk factors, the consensus is that higher rates of CVD have not consistently been shown among transgender people [43]. A cohort of patients, followed at a gender clinic in Amsterdam, provided morbidity and mortality data on over 1300 clients [37]. Although no increase in all-cause mortality was noted for transgender men, transgender women had an elevated mortality risk [standardized mortality ratio (SMR) 1.51 (95% confidence interval (CI):1.47–1.55)]. The increase in deaths was attributed to suicide, drug-related causes, acquired immunodeficiency syndrome (AIDS) and ischemic heart disease, the latter showing an increased standardized mortality rate of 1.64 (95% CI; 1.43–1.87) [37]. A sub-analysis revealed that the increase in cardiac deaths only occurred in those using ethinylestradiol, which has mostly been discontinued as a source of estrogen in hormonal protocols.

There has not been any consensus about which gender to use when applying gender-based risk calculators. Since hormonal therapy does not appear to significantly impact CVD risk in transgender populations, using sex assignment at birth in risk calculators may be the correct course. In transgender women at elevated risk for CVD, using transdermal estradiol may be the safest option due to reduced risk of thromboembolism [41, 43].

In summary, the evidence does not point to the elevated risk of CVD among transgender people using current hormonal regimens, i.e., oral, injectable, or transdermal estradiol [43]. Medical providers should continue to assess CVD risk, encourage active lifestyles, and intervene in modifiable risk factors such as tobacco use, dyslipidemias, and hypertension.

Cancer Screening

The USPSTF has screening guidelines in place for cancer of the cervix and breast (cisgender women), and lung and colorectal cancer screening for all individuals at risk [23]. There are no federal guidelines that address cancer screening in transgender populations.

Cervical Cancer Screening

Transgender men and gender non-binary individuals assigned female at birth should undergo cervical cancer screening using the same recommendations as for cisgender women [44]. In the United States, the recommendations are to screen for cervical cancer in women age 21–65 years with cytology (Pap smear) every 3 years. For women age 30–65 years the screening interval can be extended to every 5 years if the Pap smear is done in combination with human papillomavirus (HPV) testing [45]. Transgender men often avoid cervical cancer screening due to stigma and discrimination experienced in medical settings, discomfort with medical examinations as well as believe they are not at risk for HPV-related disease, including cervical cancer [8, 11, 32, 46]. This has been shown not to be the case with a recent study revealing that 16% of transgender men had evidence of high-risk HPV infection [47]. In addition, after changing the gender marker on insurance and identification cards, some transgender men may have challenges getting insurance coverage for procedures that have female indications, such as Pap smears and mammograms. Transgender men who use testosterone are more likely to have inadequate or unsatisfactory specimens, likely due to atrophy producing effects of testosterone on cervical tissue [48].

Primary care providers can employ several strategies to improve the uptake of cervical cancer screening among transmasculine patients, including asking the patient's choice of terminology for body parts, use of non-gendered language during the exam (e.g., internal organs instead of uterus/ovaries), and allowing a partner or friend to be present during the exam [32]. Some medical providers have advocated the use of intravaginal estrogen creams 5 days before the Pap smear [32].

This is done to lessen the discomfort due to testosterone-induced atrophic vaginitis, and to possibly reduce unsatisfactory cytology results. This outcome has not been formally studied [32]. For transgender men who decline Pap smears, a recent study has shown that patient-collected swabs to test for high-risk HPV may be a viable option for primary cervical cancer screening [47]. In the event that insurance companies decline coverage for Pap smears on the basis that the patient is male, primary care providers should advocate by submitting an appeal on their behalf. In the United States, patients who obtain public insurance under the Affordable Care Act (ACA) or The Centers for Medicaid and Medicare (CMS) cannot be denied insurance coverage for most transition-related care or for procedures that do not align with a person's gender identity [49].

Breast Cancer

There are several guidelines in existence that address breast cancer screening in cisgender women and that provide different recommendations concerning the frequency of screening and the age at which to start [50, 51]. The USPSTF recommends that breast cancer screening, using mammography, starts at age 50 years for cisgender women at average risk. Two observational studies have investigated breast cancer risk among transgender women, and neither demonstrated an increase in breast cancer risk [37, 52]. A recent review of the literature found 26 case reports of breast cancer among transgender women between 1968 and 2017 [53]. Current recommendations are that transgender women receiving feminizing hormonal therapy should undergo breast cancer screening in accordance with guidelines for cisgender women [20] and after at least 5–10 years of hormone use [21]. Medical providers should be aware that mammography may present challenges, especially for those who have not yet changed their gender marker to female on the insurance company and/or their identification documents. In addition, use of injectable soft tissue fillers, a common practice among transgender women [54], that can lead to difficulty interpreting mammographic results. In these situations, the recommendation is to image with MRI [55].

Transgender men who have not had a chest masculinization procedure (mastectomy) should follow the breast cancer screening guidelines for cisgender women [21]. A retrospective study investigated breast cancer outcomes among 795 transgender men attending a transgender clinic in Amsterdam. Breast cancer incidence was lower than for cisgender women [56]. There are case reports of transgender men who have developed breast cancer despite having surgery, which is likely due to residual breast tissue remaining after mastectomy procedures [53]. Mammography may be technically difficult after surgery and transgender men may be unwilling to undergo a screening that does not align with their gender identity. Current recommendations include having discussions with patients about the risks and benefits of mammography and conducting routine chest wall examinations [21].

Colorectal Cancer

Colorectal cancer screening guidelines are not gender-based and therefore no differences in screening recommendations are expected for transgender populations. The USPSTF recommends screening for colorectal cancer starting at age 50 years and continuing until age 75 years [57]. A recent study has shown that transgender women are less likely to be up-to-date with colorectal cancer screening compared with cisgender individuals [58]. This may be due to fears about healthcare discrimination or apprehension about undergoing screening by colonoscopy. In these situations, medical providers can offer alternative recommended methods for colon cancer screening such as the guaiac-based fecal occult blood test (gFOBT), fecal immunochemical tests (FITs), or multitargeted stool DNA testing (FIT-DNA) that can be performed at home [57].

Prostate Cancer

Prostate cancer is common among cisgender men. Transgender women who have undergone vaginoplasty still retain the prostate and therefore are potentially at risk for cancer. Prostate cancer incidence, however, appears to be low in transgender women who have undergone orchiectomy or who have received feminizing therapy with estrogens and androgen blockers [59]. A study conducted among 2306 transgender women attending an Amsterdam gender clinic between 1975 and 2006 (51,173 person-years) revealed only one case of prostate cancer, that occurred in a 63-year old who had started hormones at age 53; the cancer was probably preexisting [59]. The incidence of prostate cancer was determined to be extremely low 0.04% in this population and may be due to androgen deprivation as a result of hormone regimens and/or orchiectomy. Medical providers can continue to follow the screening recommendations for cisgender men. However, they should know that the prostate-specific antigen (PSA) test is unreliable when androgen blockers have been used; for example, five-alpha-reductase inhibitors (e.g., finasteride/dutasteride) lower PSA levels [60, 61]. Spironolactone is a selective androgen receptor modulator (SARM) and can increase or decrease PSA [62, 63]. One author recommends doubling the measured PSA value for interpretation when on five-alpha-reductase inhibitors [64]. The pros and cons of prostate cancer screening should be discussed with all patients who have a prostate. For patients who have had a vaginoplasty, the prostate can be examined intravaginally, palpating the anterior wall.

Bone Health

Multiple recommendations exist for osteoporosis screening in cisgender populations, including the USPSTF, ACOG, The Endocrine Society, and The American Association of Clinical Endocrinologists. These organizations provide variable guidance on who to screen, when to screen, and frequency of screening [65–68]. Osteoporosis screening recommendations are age and sex based, and therefore present additional questions when applied to transgender people who have used hormone therapy. Known risk factors for osteoporosis include older age, Caucasian or Asian race, alcohol >10 drinks/week, low body mass index, smoking, corticosteroid use, hypogonadism, rheumatoid arthritis, hyperparathyroidism, immobility, vitamin D deficiency, and HIV infection. In fact, the current recommendation for people living with HIV is to screen for osteoporosis starting at age 50 [69].

Studies investigating bone mineral density changes in transgender women receiving feminizing hormones have shown inconsistent results possibly as a consequence of non-standardized hormone regimens and duration of follow-up [70–72]. One study that evaluated transgender women demonstrated that low bone mineral density was evident even before the initiation of hormones, and attributed these findings to low levels of physical activity and hypovitaminosis D [73]. Medical providers should be aware that the period of time that has the highest risk for low BMD is after gonadectomy, especially if hormone therapy is decreased or stopped. Transgender men receiving testosterone appear to maintain pretreatment BMD [20, 74]. Loss of BMD may occur if hormones are stopped after oophorectomy.

Current osteoporosis screening guidelines from the Endocrine Society recommend that clinicians obtain BMD measurements on transgender patients when risk factors for osteoporosis exist, specifically in those who stop sex hormone therapy after gonadectomy [20]. The primary care guidelines from UCSF suggest that transgender people (regardless of birth-assigned sex) should begin bone density screening at age 65, with earlier screening for those with established risk factors, including gonadectomy and 5 years or more without hormones [74].

There are no studies to determine whether clinicians should use the assigned birth sex or affirmed gender for assessment of osteoporosis. When using the FRAX® tool (http://www.shef.ac.uk/FRAX/), the consensus is that assigned birth sex should be used as bone mass has usually peaked for transgender people who initiate hormones in early adulthood [20, 74].

Medical providers should advise patients to optimize bone health. This includes tobacco cessation, calcium intake in line with current guidelines, correction of low vitamin D levels, maintaining an active lifestyle, weight-bearing activity, and consuming alcohol in moderation.

Sexual and Reproductive Health

Primary care includes assessment of risk for sexually transmitted infections, including HIV, as well as providing advice about fertility, pregnancy planning, and contraception.

Both the USPSTF and the Centers for Disease Control and Prevention recommend screening adults for HIV [23, 75]. However, recent reports show that many transgender individuals have never been screened [14]. HIV is especially a concern for transgender women, who have an estimated HIV prevalence over 20% in the USA [18]. This figure is even higher in African-American communities [13]. The rates of HIV infection have not been as well described in transgender men, however those who have sex with cisgender men appear to have an elevated risk [76]. Other research has indicated that once diagnosed, transgender women are less likely to adhere to antiretroviral medicines, resulting in elevated HIV viral loads compared with cisgender men [77]. Adherence issues may be due to many psychosocial factors such as homelessness, poverty, mental health issues, and substance use. Another factor that may also contribute to lower adherence is a fear of drug–drug interactions between hormones and antiretroviral therapy [78]. Patients at increased risk for HIV, including those who have condomless anal sex, a serodiscordant sexual partner, or use of injection drugs, should be offered HIV pre-exposure prophylaxis (PrEP) with a fixed dose combination of emtricitabine/tenofovir disoproxil fumarate. PrEP has been recommended by the CDC since 2012 to reduce the incidence of HIV among people at risk for HIV [79].

In addition to HIV screening, medical providers should assess patients for exposure to sexually transmitted infections and screen accordingly based on current anatomy and sexual behaviors [80]. Medical providers should not make assumptions about the gender(s) of their patients' sexual partners or their sexual practices. Using gender-neutral language to describe the anatomy and asking patients for their preferred language will facilitate openness and disclosure. Medical providers can modify sexual health interviewing to be trans inclusive (Table 4.2).

Several studies have indicated that transgender women have higher rates of STIs such as syphilis, gonorrhea, chlamydia, hepatitis C compared with non-transgender people [81–85]. There have been few studies that have evaluated STIs among transgender men. However, studies that have been completed demonstrated a wide variety of infections, including anal, vaginal, and oropharyngeal gonorrhea, chlamydia, and syphilis [86, 87]. Transgender individuals at elevated risk for STIs should undergo screening every 3–6 months in accordance with CDC guidelines. Transgender women who have had vaginoplasty surgery can acquire neovaginal STIs such as gonorrhea or HPV [88–90] and should be asked about symptoms such as discharge, pain, or bleeding. As part of routine primary care providers should inspect the neovagina using a small speculum or anoscope on an annual basis [21].

Discussions about fertility preservation should occur with all transgender people contemplating hormones or surgery that can impact fertility. The effects of

Table 4.2 Taking a sexual health history with transgender individuals

Pronouns	What pronouns do you use?
Parts	To understand your risk for STDs I need to know if you have had any genital or bottom surgeries. Have you had any surgeries?
Partners	What are the genders of your partners? In the past 2 months, how many partners have you had sex with? Is it possible that any of your sex partners in the past 12 months had sex with someone else while they were still in a sexual relationship with you?
Prevention of pregnancy	What are you doing to prevent pregnancy?
Protection from STDs	What do you do to protect yourself from STDs?
Practices	To understand your risks for STDs, I need to understand the kind of sex you have had recently." "Have you had vaginal/frontal sex?" If yes, "Do you use condoms: never, sometimes, or always?" "Have you had anal sex, meaning 'penis in rectum/anus'"
Past history of STDs	"Have you ever had an STD?" "Have any of your partners had an STD?"
PrEP	Do you take, or have you ever taken PrEP to prevent HIV?

Modified from: The Five P's: Partners, Prevention of Pregnancy, Protection from STDs, Practices, and Past History of STDs https://www.cdc.gov/std/treatment/sexualhistory.pdf

testosterone include cessation of menses as well as reduced fertility. Estrogens and androgen blockers reduce semen production. Discussions should include gamete cryopreservation, embryo freezing, and other options for parenting. Medical providers should also discuss pregnancy potential and contraception with transgender men, since pregnancies have occurred while receiving testosterone [91]. Acceptable options include depot medroxyprogesterone and long-acting reversible contraceptives (LARCS), such as intrauterine contraceptives and hormonal implants.

Immunizations

The Advisory Committee on Immunization Practices (ACIP) provides updated recommended immunization schedules for adults [92]. These can also be applied to transgender individuals. Providers should be aware that some vaccines are contraindicated in pregnancy. Transgender men requiring live vaccines such as measles, mumps, rubella, varicella, and zoster vaccines should be assessed for pregnancy risk before receiving these immunizations. Transgender men who are pregnant should receive tetanus, diphtheria, and acellular pertussis vaccine (Tdap) during pregnancy and influenza vaccination following guidelines for cisgender women. Medical providers should offer vaccinations against HPV through age 45 and immunization against hepatitis A and B, if not received in childhood.

Summary

Transgender individuals often delay or avoid medical services due to fear of discrimination in healthcare settings. Medical providers can improve engagement in care by becoming knowledgeable about the healthcare needs of transgender individuals, creating culturally competent healthcare environment and through thoughtful application and modification of primary care recommendations (Table 4.3).

Table 4.3 Comparison of preventive care guidelines for transgender individuals

Screening	Gender	UCSF	ES
Osteoporosis	Transgender men	Start BMD screening at age 65 or 50–64 with established risk factors or $\geq$5 years without hormone replacement after gonadectomy	Start BMD screening if established risk factors exist or After gonadectomy if the patient stops or is noncompliant with hormone replacement
	Transgender women	Start BMD screening at age 65 or 50–64 years with established risk factors or $\geq$5 years without hormone replacement after gonadectomy	Consider BMD testing at baseline and $\geq$60 years or those who are not compliant with hormone therapy
Cervical cancer	Transgender men	Follow recommendations for non-transgender women	Follow recommendations for non-transgender women
Prostate cancer	Transgender women	Follow guidelines for non-transgender men PSA: Reduce the upper limit of normal 1.0 ng/ml	Follow individualized screening according to personal risk for prostatic disease and prostate cancer
Breast cancer	Transgender men (after bilateral mastectomy)	Discuss the possible risk of residual breast tissue and technical limitations of mammography	Conduct sub- and periareolar annual breast examinations
	Transgender women	Screening mammography every 2 years starting at age 50 and at least 5–10 years of feminizing hormones	Follow breast-screening guidelines recommended for those designated female at birth

References

1. Institute of Medicine (US) Committee on Lesbian, gay, bisexual, and transgender health issues and research gaps and opportunities. 2011.
2. American Academy of Pediatrics, Committee on Adolescence. Office-based care for lesbian, gay, bisexual, transgender, and questioning youth. Pediatrics. 2013;132(1):198–203.
3. The American College of Obstetricians and Gynecologists. Committee Opinion no. 512: health care for transgender individuals. Obstet. Gynecol. 2011;118(6):1454–8.
4. Daniel H, Butkus R. Lesbian, gay, bisexual, and transgender health disparities: executive summary of a policy position paper from the American College of Physicians. Ann Intern Med. 2015;163(2):135–7.
5. Society for Adolescent Health and Medicine. Recommendations for promoting the health and well-being of lesbian, gay, bisexual, and transgender adolescents: a position paper of the Society for Adolescent Health and Medicine. J Adolesc Health: official publication of the Society for Adolescent Medicine. 2013;52(4):506–10.
6. Shires DA, Stroumsa D, Jaffee KD, Woodford MR. Primary care providers' willingness to continue gender-affirming hormone therapy for transgender patients. Fam Pract. 2017.
7. Unger CA. Care of the transgender patient: a survey of gynecologists' current knowledge and practice. J Womens Health (Larchmt). 2015;24(2):114–8.
8. Grant JM, Mottet LA, Tanis J. National transgender discrimination survey report on health and health care. Washington, DC: National Center for Transgender Equality and the National Gay and Lesbian Task Force; 2010. Contract No.: Report.
9. Jaffee KD, Shires DA, Stroumsa D. Discrimination and delayed health care among transgender women and men: implications for improving medical education and health care delivery. Medical Care. 2016.
10. Glick JL, Theall KP, Andrinopoulos KM, Kendall C. The role of discrimination in care postponement among trans-feminine individuals in the U.S. National Transgender Discrimination Survey. LGBT Health. 2018;5(3):171–9.
11. Peitzmeier SM, Khullar K, Reisner SL, Potter J. Pap test use is lower among female-to-male patients than non-transgender women. Am J Prev Med. 2014;47(6):808–12.
12. Bazzi AR, Whorms DS, King DS, Potter J. Adherence to mammography screening guidelines among transgender persons and sexual minority women. Am J Public Health. 2015;105 (11):2356–8.
13. Herbst JH, Jacobs ED, Finlayson TJ, McKleroy VS, Neumann MS, Crepaz N, et al. Estimating HIV prevalence and risk behaviors of transgender persons in the United States: a systematic review. AIDS Behav. 2008;12(1):1–17.
14. Pitasi MA, Oraka E, Clark H, Town M, DiNenno EA. HIV testing among transgender women and men—27 states and Guam, 2014–2015. MMWR Morb Mortal Wkly Rep. 2017;66 (33):883–7.
15. Bockting WO, Miner MH, Swinburne Romine RE, Hamilton A, Coleman E. Stigma, mental health, and resilience in an online sample of the US transgender population. Am J Public Health. 2013;103(5):943–51.
16. Buchting FO, Emory KT, Scout Kim Y, Fagan P, Vera LE, et al. Transgender use of cigarettes, cigars, and e-cigarettes in a national study. Am J Prev Med. 2017;53(1):e1–7.
17. Reisner SL, Greytak EA, Parsons JT, Ybarra ML. Gender minority social stress in adolescence: disparities in adolescent bullying and substance use by gender identity. J Sex Res. 2015;52(3):243–56.
18. Baral SD, Poteat T, Stromdahl S, Wirtz AL, Guadamuz TE, Beyrer C. Worldwide burden of HIV in transgender women: a systematic review and meta-analysis. Lancet Infect Dis. 2012.
19. Coleman E, Bockting W, Botzer M, Cohen-Kettenis P, DeCuypere G, Feldman J, et al. Standards of care for the health of transsexual, transgender, and gender-nonconforming people, Version 7. Int J Transgenderism. 2011;13:165.

20. Hembree WC, Cohen-Kettenis PT, Gooren L, Hannema SE, Meyer WJ, Murad MH, et al. Endocrine treatment of gender-dysphoric/gender-incongruent persons: an endocrine society* clinical practice guideline. J Clin Endocrinol Metab. 2017;102(11):3869–903.
21. Deutsch MB. Guidelines for the primary and gender-affirming care of transgender and gender nonbinary people. San Francisco, CA: Center of Excellence for Transgender Health, Department of Family and Community Medicine, University of California San Francisco; 2016. Available from: www.transhealth.ucsf.edu/guidelines. Accessed 3/1/2018.
22. Wanta JW, Unger CA. Review of the transgender literature: where do we go from here? Transgend Health. 2017;2(1):119–28.
23. U.S. Preventive Services Task Force. Rockville, MD: U.S. Dept. of Health & Human Services, Agency for Healthcare Research and Quality. Available from: https://www.uspreventiveservicestaskforce.org/Page/Name/home. Accessed 3/1/2018.
24. Centers for Disease Control and Prevention. Behavioral risk factor surveillance system. Available from: https://www.cdc.gov/brfss/about/index.htm. Accessed 3/1/2018.
25. Edmiston EK, Donald CA, Sattler AR, Peebles JK, Ehrenfeld JM, Eckstrand KL. Opportunities and gaps in primary care preventative health services for transgender patients: a systemic review. Transgend Health. 2016;1(1):216–30.
26. Madeline B, Deutsch AR, Sari Reisner. What's in a guideline? Developing collaborative and sound research designs that substantiate best practice recommendations for transgender health care. AMA J Ethics. 2016;18(11):1098–106.
27. MacCarthy S, Reisner SL, Nunn A, Perez-Brumer A, Operario D. The time is now: attention increases to transgender health in the United States but scientific knowledge gaps remain. LGBT Health. 2015;2(4):287–91.
28. Croghan CF, Moone RP, Olson AM. Working with LGBT Baby boomers and older adults: factors that signal a welcoming service environment. J Gerontol Soc Work. 2015;58 (6):637–51.
29. Bockting W, Coleman E, Deutsch MB, Guillamon A, Meyer I, Meyer W 3rd, et al. Adult development and quality of life of transgender and gender nonconforming people. Curr Opin Endocrinol Diabetes Obes. 2016;23(2):188–97.
30. Reisner SL, Bradford J, Hopwood R, Gonzalez A, Makadon H, Todisco D, et al. Comprehensive transgender healthcare: the gender affirming clinical and public health model of Fenway Health. J Urban Health Bull NY Acad Med. 2015;92(3):584–92.
31. Reisner SL, Radix A, Deutsch MB. Integrated and gender-affirming transgender clinical care and research. J Acquir Immune Defic Syndr. 2016;72(Suppl 3):S235–42.
32. Potter J, Peitzmeier SM, Bernstein I, Reisner SL, Alizaga NM, Agénor M, et al. Cervical cancer screening for patients on the female-to-male spectrum: a narrative review and guide for clinicians. J Gen Intern Med. 2015;30(12):1857–64.
33. Cahill S, Singal R, Grasso C, King D, Mayer K, Baker K, et al. Do ask, do tell: high levels of acceptability by patients of routine collection of sexual orientation and gender identity data in four diverse American Community Health Centers. PLoS ONE. 2014;9(9):e107104.
34. Deutsch MB, Green J, Keatley J, Mayer G, Hastings J, Hall AM. Electronic medical records and the transgender patient: recommendations from the World Professional Association for Transgender Health EMR Working Group. J Am Med Inf Assoc JAMIA. 2013;20(4):700–3.
35. Goff DC Jr, Lloyd-Jones DM, Bennett G, Coady S, D'Agostino RB Sr, Gibbons R, et al. 2013 ACC/AHA guideline on the assessment of cardiovascular risk: a report of the American College of Cardiology/American Heart Association Task Force on Practice Guidelines. J Am Coll Cardiol. 2014;63(25 Pt B):2935–59.
36. Institute of Medicine Committee on Lesbian GB, Transgender Health I, Research G, Opportunities. The National Academies Collection: Reports funded by National Institutes of Health. The health of lesbian, gay, bisexual, and transgender people: building a foundation for better understanding. Washington, DC; 2011.
37. Asscheman H, Giltay EJ, Megens JA, de Ronde WP, van Trotsenburg MA, Gooren LJ. A long-term follow-up study of mortality in transsexuals receiving treatment with cross-sex hormones. Eur J Endocrinol/Eur Fed Endocr Soc. 2011;164(4):635–42.

38. Maraka S, Singh Ospina N, Rodriguez-Gutierrez R, Davidge-Pitts CJ, Nippoldt TB, Prokop LJ, et al. Sex Steroids and cardiovascular outcomes in transgender individuals: a systematic review and meta-analysis. J Clin Endocrinol Metab. 2017;102(11):3914–23.
39. Elbers JMH, Giltay EJ, Teerlink T, Scheffer PG, Asscheman H, Seidell JC, et al. Effects of sex steroids on components of the insulin resistance syndrome in transsexual subjects. Clin Endocrinol. 2003;58:562.
40. Polderman KH, Gooren LJ, Asscheman H, Bakker A, Heine RJ. Induction of insulin resistance by androgens and estrogens. J Clin Endocrinol Metab. 1994;79(1):265–71.
41. Gooren LJ, Wierckx K, Giltay EJ. Cardiovascular disease in transsexual persons treated with cross-sex hormones: reversal of the traditional sex difference in cardiovascular disease pattern. Eur J Endocrinol/Eur Fed Endocr Soc. 2014;170(6):809–19.
42. Defreyne J, De Bacquer D, Shadid S, Lapauw B, T'Sjoen G. Is type 1 diabetes mellitus more prevalent than expected in transgender persons? A local observation. Sex Med. 2017;5(3): e215–8.
43. Streed CG Jr, Harfouch O, Marvel F, Blumenthal RS, Martin SS, Mukherjee M. Cardiovascular disease among transgender adults receiving hormone therapy: a narrative review. Ann Intern Med. 2017;167(4):256–67.
44. Committee on Health Care for Underserved W. Committee Opinion no. 512: health care for transgender individuals. Obstet Gynecol. 2011;118(6):1454–8.
45. Moyer VA. on behalf of the USPSTF. Screening for cervical cancer: U.S. Preventive Services Task Force recommendation statement. Ann Intern Med. 2012;156(12):880–91.
46. Reisner SL, Gamarel KE, Dunham E, Hopwood R, Hwahng S. Female-to-male transmasculine adult health: a mixed-methods community-based needs assessment. J Am Psychiatr Nurses Assoc. 2013;19(5):293–303.
47. Reisner SL, Deutsch MB, Peitzmeier SM, White Hughto JM, Cavanaugh TP, Pardee DJ, et al. Test performance and acceptability of self- versus provider-collected swabs for high-risk HPV DNA testing in female-to-male trans masculine patients. PLoS ONE. 2018;13(3): e0190172.
48. Peitzmeier SM, Reisner SL, Harigopal P, Potter J. Female-to-male patients have high prevalence of unsatisfactory Paps compared to non-transgender females: implications for cervical cancer screening. J Gen Intern Med. 2014;29(5):778–84.
49. Baker KE. The future of transgender coverage. N Engl J Med. 2017;376(19):1801–4.
50. The American College of Obstetricians and Gynecologists. Practice Bulletin Number 179: Breast cancer risk assessment and screening in average-risk women. Obstet Gynecol. 2017;130(1):e1–16.
51. US Preventive Services Task Force GD, Curry SJ, Owens DK, Bibbins-Domingo K, Caughey AB, Davidson KW, Doubeni CA, Ebell M, Epling JW Jr, Kemper AR, Krist AH, Kubik M, Landefeld CS, Mangione CM, Silverstein M, Simon MA, Siu AL, Tseng CW. Screening for breast cancer: U.S. Preventive Services Task Force recommendation statement. Ann Intern Med. 2009;151(10):716–26, w-236.
52. Brown GR, Jones KT. Incidence of breast cancer in a cohort of 5,135 transgender veterans. Breast Cancer Res Treat. 2015;149(1):191–8.
53. Deutsch MB, Radix A, Wesp L. Breast cancer screening, management, and a review of case study literature in transgender populations. Semin Reprod Med. 2017;35(5):434–41.
54. Wilson E, Rapues J, Jin H, Raymond HF. The use and correlates of illicit silicone or "fillers" in a population-based sample of transwomen, San Francisco, 2013. J Sex Med. 2014;11 (7):1717–24.
55. Scaranelo AM, de Fatima Ribeiro Maia M. Sonographic and mammographic findings of breast liquid silicone injection. J. Clin. Ultrasound JCU. 2006;34(6):273–7.
56. Gooren LJ, van Trotsenburg MAA, Giltay EJ, van Diest PJ. Breast cancer development in transsexual subjects receiving cross-sex hormone treatment. J Sex Med. 2013;10 (12):3129–34.
57. US Preventive Services Task Force. Screening for colorectal cancer: US Preventive Services Task Force recommendation statement. JAMA. 2016;315(23):2564–75.

58. Tabaac AR, Sutter ME, Wall CSJ, Baker KE. Gender identity disparities in cancer screening behaviors. Am J Prev Med. 2018;54(3):385–93.
59. Gooren L, Morgentaler A. Prostate cancer incidence in orchidectomised male-to-female transsexual persons treated with oestrogens. Andrologia. 2013.
60. Matzkin H, Barak M, Braf Z. Effect of finasteride on free and total serum prostate-specific antigen in men with benign prostatic hyperplasia. Br J Urol. 1996;78(3):405–8.
61. Etzioni RD, Howlader N, Shaw PA, Ankerst DP, Penson DF, Goodman PJ, et al. Long-term effects of finasteride on prostate specific antigen levels: results from the prostate cancer prevention trial. J Urol. 2005;174(3):877–81.
62. Sundar S, Dickinson PD. Spironolactone, a possible selective androgen receptor modulator, should be used with caution in patients with metastatic carcinoma of the prostate. BMJ Case Reports. 2012;2012.
63. Andriole GL, Bostwick D, Brawley OW, Gomella L, Marberger M, Montorsi F, et al. The effect of dutasteride on the usefulness of prostate specific antigen for the diagnosis of high grade and clinically relevant prostate cancer in men with a previous negative biopsy: results from the REDUCE study. J Urol. 2011;185(1):126–31.
64. Andriole GL, Guess HA, Epstein JI, Wise H, Kadmon D, Crawford ED, et al. Treatment with finasteride preserves usefulness of prostate-specific antigen in the detection of prostate cancer: results of a randomized, double-blind, placebo-controlled clinical trial. PLESS Study Group. Proscar Long-term Efficacy and Safety Study. Urology. 1998;52(2):195–201; discussion-2.
65. Camacho PM, Petak SM, Binkley N, Clarke BL, Harris ST, Hurley DL, et al. American Association of Clinical Endocrinologists and American College of Endocrinology Clinical Practice Guidelines for the diagnosis and treatment of postmenopausal osteoporosis—2016. Endocr Pract: Official journal of the American College of Endocrinology and the American Association of Clinical Endocrinologists. 2016;22(Suppl 4):1–42.
66. Watts NB, Adler RA, Bilezikian JP, Drake MT, Eastell R, Orwoll ES, et al. Osteoporosis in men: an Endocrine Society clinical practice guideline. J Clin Endocrinol Metab. 2012;97 (6):1802–22.
67. The American College of Obstetricians and Gynecologists. ACOG Practice Bulletin N. 129. Osteoporosis. Obstetrics and Gynecology. 2012;120(3):718–34.
68. U.S. Preventive Services Task Force. Screening for osteoporosis: U.S. Preventive Services Task Force recommendation statement. Ann Intern Med. 2011;154(5):356–64.
69. Aberg JA, Gallant JE, Ghanem KG, Emmanuel P, Zingman BS, Horberg MA. Primary care guidelines for the management of persons infected with HIV: 2013 update by the HIV Medicine Association of the Infectious Diseases Society of America. Clin Infect Dis. 2014;58 (1):1–10.
70. Wierckx K, Mueller S, Weyers S, Van Caenegem E, Roef G, Heylens G, et al. Long-term evaluation of cross-sex hormone treatment in transsexual persons. J Sex Med. 2012;9 (10):2641–51.
71. Lapauw B, Taes Y, Simoens S, Van Caenegem E, Weyers S, Goemaere S, et al. Body composition, volumetric and areal bone parameters in male-to-female transsexual persons. Bone. 2008;43(6):1016–21.
72. van Kesteren PJ, Asscheman H, Megens JA, Gooren LJ. Mortality and morbidity in transsexual subjects treated with cross-sex hormones. Clin Endocrinol. 1997;47(3):337–42.
73. Van Caenegem E, Taes Y, Wierckx K, Vandewalle S, Toye K, Kaufman JM, et al. Low bone mass is prevalent in male-to-female transsexual persons before the start of cross-sex hormonal therapy and gonadectomy. Bone. 54(1):92–7.
74. Radix A, Deutsch MB. Bone health and osteoporosis. In: Deutsch MB, editor. Guidelines for the primary and gender-affirming care of transgender and gender nonbinary people. 2nd ed. San Francisco: Center of Excellence for Transgender Health, Department of Family and Community Medicine, University of California; 2016.
75. Branson BM, Handsfield HH, Lampe MA, Janssen RS, Taylor AW, Lyss SB, et al. Revised recommendations for HIV testing of adults, adolescents, and pregnant women in health-care

settings. MMWR Recommendations and reports: morbidity and mortality weekly report. Recommendations and Reports/Centers for Disease Control. 2006;55(RR-14):1–17; quiz CE1-4.
76. Habarta N, Wang G, Mulatu MS, Larish N. HIV testing by Transgender Status at Centers for disease control and prevention-funded sites in the United States, Puerto Rico, and US Virgin Islands, 2009–2011. Am J Public Health. 2015;105(9):1917–25.
77. Mizuno Y, Frazier EL, Huang P, Skarbinski J. Characteristics of transgender women living with HIV receiving medical care in the United States. LGBT Health. 2015;2(3):228–34.
78. Braun HM, Candelario J, Hanlon CL, Segura ER, Clark JL, Currier JS, et al. Transgender women living with HIV frequently take antiretroviral therapy and/or feminizing hormone therapy differently than prescribed due to drug-drug interaction concerns. LGBT Health. 2017;4(5):371–5.
79. Centers for Disease Control and Prevention: US Public Health Service. Preexposure prophylaxis for the prevention of HIV infection in the United States—2017 Update: a clinical practice guideline.
80. Workowski KA, Bolan GA. Sexually transmitted diseases treatment guidelines, 2015. MMWR recommendations and reports: morbidity and mortality weekly report. Recommendations and reports/Centers for Disease Control. 2015;64(RR-03):1–137.
81. Nuttbrock L, Bockting W, Rosenblum A, Hwahng S, Mason M, Macri M, et al. Gender abuse, depressive symptoms, and HIV and other sexually transmitted infections among male-to-female transgender persons: a three-year prospective study. Am J Public Health. 2013;103(2):300–7.
82. Gupte S, Daly C, Agarwal V, Gaikwad SB, George B. Introduction of rapid tests for large-scale syphilis screening among female, male, and transgender sex workers in Mumbai. India. Sex Transm Dis. 2011;38(6):499–502.
83. Shrivastava SR, Bobhate PS. Prevalence of HIV and syphilis in patients attending sexually transmitted infections (STI) clinic in an urban slum. J Res Health Sci. 2012;12(1):7–14.
84. Brown B, Monsour E, Klausner JD, Galea JT. Sociodemographic and behavioral correlates of anogenital warts and human papillomavirus-related knowledge among men who have sex with men and transwomen in Lima, Peru. Sex Transm Dis. 2015;42(4):198–201.
85. Bastos FI, Bastos LS, Coutinho C, Toledo L, Mota JC, Velasco-de-Castro CA, et al. HIV, HCV, HBV, and syphilis among transgender women from Brazil: assessing different methods to adjust infection rates of a hard-to-reach, sparse population. Medicine. 2018;97(1S Suppl 1): S16–s24.
86. Reisner SL, White JM, Mayer KH, Mimiaga MJ. Sexual risk behaviors and psychosocial health concerns of female-to-male transgender men screening for STDs at an urban community health center. AIDS Care. 2014;26(7):857–64.
87. Stephens SC, Bernstein KT, Philip SS. Male to female and female to male transgender persons have different sexual risk behaviors yet similar rates of STDs and HIV. AIDS Behav. 2011;15(3):683–6.
88. Bodsworth NJ, Price R, Davies SC. Gonococcal infection of the neovagina in a male-to-female transsexual. Sex Transm Dis. 1994;21(4):211–2.
89. van der Sluis WB, Bouman MB, Gijs L, van Bodegraven AA. Gonorrhoea of the sigmoid neovagina in a male-to-female transgender. Int J STD AIDS. 2015;26(8):595–8.
90. Matsuki S, Kusatake K, Hein KZ, Anraku K, Morita E. Condylomata acuminata in the neovagina after male-to-female reassignment treated with CO_2 laser and imiquimod. Int J STD AIDS. 2015;26(7):509–11.
91. Light AD, Obedin-Maliver J, Sevelius JM, Kerns JL. Transgender men who experienced pregnancy after female-to-male gender transitioning. Obstet Gynecol. 2014;124(6):1120–7.
92. Kim DK, Riley LE, Hunter P, on behalf of the Advisory Committee on Immunization. Recommended immunization schedule for adults aged 19 years or older, United States, 2018*. Ann Intern Med. 2018;168(3):210–20.

Chapter 5
Primary Care of Transgender Children and Adolescents

Brittany J. Allen

Introduction

While there was a time when many primary care providers (PCPs) may have said that they would not care for a transgender patient in their career, the ability to provide affirming, appropriate care to TNG youth in a primary care setting is now widely recognized as the standard of care. The increasing visibility of transgender, nonbinary, and gender nonconforming (TNG) youth, who historically have been both oppressed (in medical settings and out) and vastly under-recognized, has made it clear that PCPs may expect to care for TNG youth or their families in their career. As has been outlined by multiple professional organizations, every primary care physician should have the tools to provide appropriate care and an affirming medical home for TNG people [1–4].

As is well outlined in other chapters, medical affirmation of gender in TNG youth has been a rapidly emerging area of medicine in the last two decades. Specialty care has been available to youth in the Netherlands since the late 1980s [5] and specific guidelines related to gender care in TNG youth were published in Great Britain in 1998 [6]. Prior to 2009, however, gender care services for youth in the United States were generally limited to few specialty clinics or individual providers in select larger cities, including Boston [7], Los Angeles, and Chicago. This can be attributed in large part to the lack of clinical guidance that was available prior to the publication of the Endocrine Society guidelines in 2009 [8]. Following the publication of these guidelines, which were then referenced in the World Professional Association for Transgender Health Standards of Care in 2012 [9], many providers—particularly in specialty roles—have been empowered to utilize

B. J. Allen (✉)
Department of Pediatrics, University of Wisconsin School of Medicine and Public Health, Madison, WI, USA
e-mail: bjallen@pediatrics.wisc.edu

L. Poretsky and W. C. Hembree (eds.), *Transgender Medicine*, Contemporary Endocrinology, https://doi.org/10.1007/978-3-030-05683-4_5

this guidance to provide medical gender care for TNG youth. This is reflected in a veritable explosion of gender clinics in the United States that provide care for TNG youth [10, 11].

While this trend in provision of gender-affirming medical care for TNG youth in the United States has lived largely in specialty centers, primary care is likely to play an increasingly foundational role in this area in the future. PCPs have not only the obligation to provide competent primary care—in supporting overall well-being throughout development with affirming health supervision and screenings—but also have the opportunity to gain skills in medical gender affirmation and subsequently increase access to care that can be life-changing and lifesaving for TNG youth.

This chapter will discuss some of the challenges TNG youth face in accessing affirming primary care settings as well as steps to take to create affirming healthcare environments. I will also discuss gender identity in a developmental context, a PCP's role in advocating for family and school support, and the role of the primary care physician in facilitating health maintenance and access to appropriate gender-affirming medical care for TNG youth.

Challenges in Primary Care

In establishing relationships with TNG patients, providers should recognize that these young people may have had negative interactions with the healthcare system in the past. TNG people have historically experienced oppression and incompetence in medical settings, and often live in spaces and communities that do not recognize that their identities exist. People that are cisgender, with gender identity aligning with the sex that they were assigned at birth, are often assumed to be the norm in comparison to TNG people. *Cisnormativity*, the term used to describe this false assumption, is pervasive throughout mainstream culture, despite evolving understanding that TNG identities are healthy and normal [12].

TNG people consistently report experiences of harassment, discrimination, and lack of knowledge in healthcare settings. In 2016, nearly one quarter (24%) of TNG adults who had sought healthcare in the last year reported having to teach their provider about TNG healthcare [13]; TNG youth report even higher rates of needing to educate their providers (55.1%) [14]. More than 1 in 20 TNG adults (6%) reported verbal harassment by medical professionals in the last year and more than one-third of TNG adults had experienced more than one negative experience in a medical office in the last year [13]. TNG adults also report high lifetime rates of care refusal (27%) and verbal and physical harassment in medical settings (21 and 8%, respectively) [15]. TNG people, particularly those that are lower income, also report low levels of access to gender-related care, including medications, surgeries, and mental health [13]. Though experiences of TNG youth are not as robustly described, they report similar care experiences. In addition to care refusal, TNG youth report high rates of providers using insulting language or denying their TNG identities by telling them that they are not transgender [14].

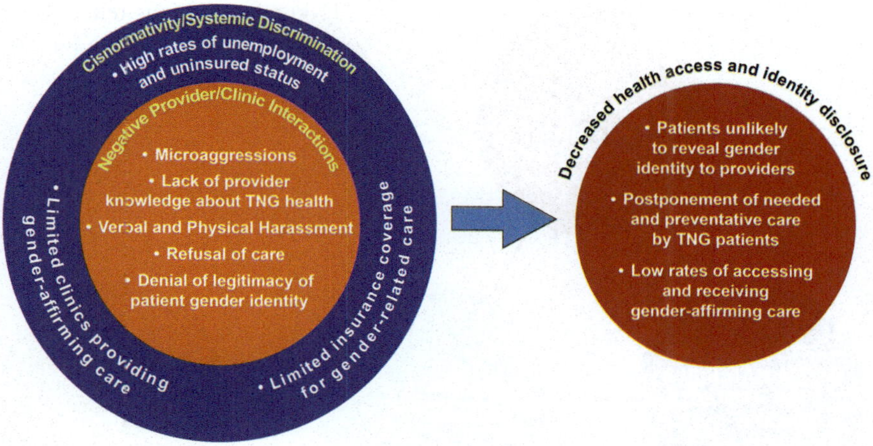

Fig. 5.1 Social and historical context that may inform TNG patients' relationships with healthcare

It is perhaps this cumulative effect of cisnormativity and systematic discrimination that often leads TNG people to conceal their gender identities from their providers (Fig. 5.1). Both TNG youth and adults report low rates of coming out to PCPs, with 21–38% of adults reporting that none of the providers that cared for them were aware of their gender identity [13, 16]. Similarly, among TNG youth in Wisconsin, only 28% had a PCP with whom they felt comfortable discussing their gender identity, and only half (50%) had discussed their gender identity with their PCP [14].

This history of discrimination, microaggressions, inadequate knowledge, and sometimes trauma in healthcare settings cannot be erased, and is important to acknowledge when caring for a TNG patient. In order to break this cycle of negative health care experiences, it is critical that providers actively engage in creating affirming clinical environments, with particular attention to addressing cisnormativity and unconscious bias for all staff that encounter a patient during their visit.

Affirming Environments/Facilitating Coming Out

Creating Affirming Spaces

There is general consensus around the importance of affirming spaces for all LGBTQ+ patients, including TNG youth. Organizations that have specifically addressed the importance of this in healthcare organizations include The Joint Commission [17], the American Academy of Pediatrics [1], the American Association of Family Physicians [2], and the American College of Physicians [3]. General recommendations for an approach to creating such spaces will be summarized here and in Fig. 5.2, but is also well outlined in detail by these organizations and others (see Appendix).

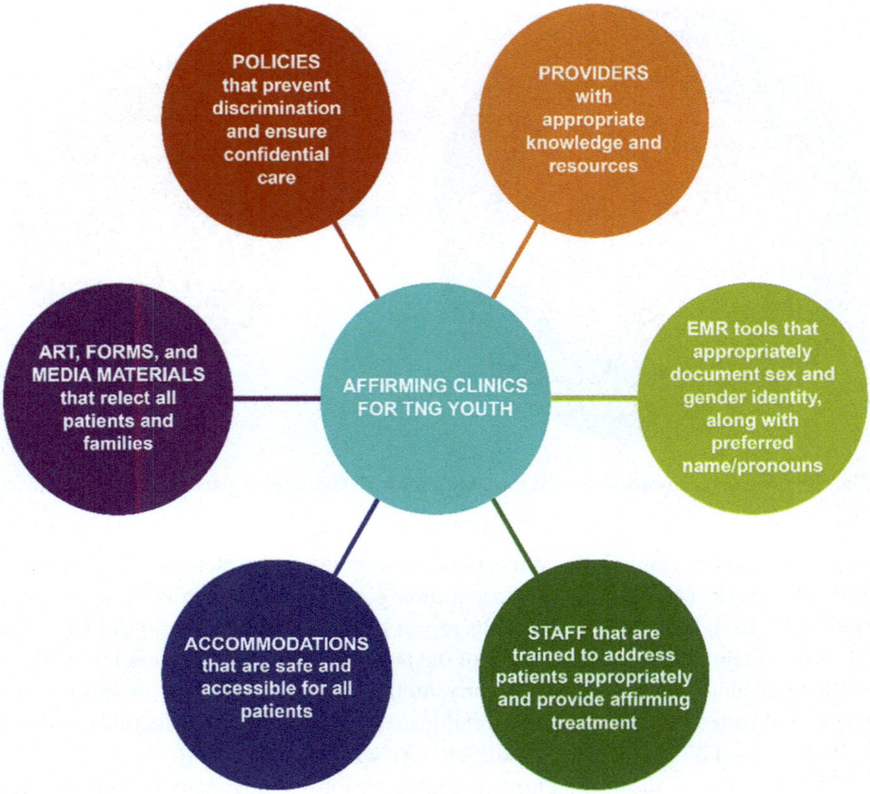
POLICIES
that prevent discrimination and ensure confidential care
PROVIDERS
with appropriate knowledge and resources
ART, FORMS, and MEDIA MATERIALS
that relect all patients and families
AFFIRMING CLINICS FOR TNG YOUTH
EMR tools that appropriately document sex and gender identity, along with preferred name/pronouns
ACCOMMODATIONS
that are safe and accessible for all patients
STAFF that are trained to address patients appropriately and provide affirming treatment

Fig. 5.2 Key components of an affirming clinic for TNG youth

In general, such environmental changes are based on creating accessible and affirming physical space and images and emphasizing the importance of positive, unbiased interactions between patients and *everyone a patient encounters in a clinical experience*.

In assessing physical space, it is important to consider what it may be like for a TNG patient or family member to navigate that healthcare setting. What images occupy the space, and who is represented in those educational, promotional, and artistic works? Is the diversity of the community and patient experience represented? How are families portrayed? When a patient or guardian completes forms in your clinic, are their identities validated and included? Are there safe and affirming places for them to use the bathroom or change clothes if needed? A "walk-through" of a clinic that mirrors the path of patients and families to assess areas where people might experience cisnormativity can be helpful and informative in identifying areas for change. Table 5.1 outlines areas that can be targeted to be more open and affirming.

Table 5.1 Creating affirming clinical spaces

Area for intervention	Action
Policy	Post the organization's nondiscrimination policy prominently. If an institution's nondiscrimination policy does not include gender identity or sexual orientation, advocacy for a policy that outlines protections for LGBTQ+ patients can be an important early step
Reflecting identity	Including representation of TNG people in educational or promotional images and artwork or waiting room materials Using forms to appropriately capture information about sex and gender identity by including separate questions for each of these categories and by providing options beyond "M" and "F," including write-in options. Forms can also be a great place to capture name and pronouns in use Post visual cues that care has been taken to create an affirming space for TNG people in waiting and exam rooms, such as rainbow or safe space stickers
Patient interactions	Avoid unnecessary gendered interactions, such as being addressed as "miss," "ma'am," or "sir," where misgendering can occur and lead to stress. In pediatrics, using language such as "child," "kid," or "young person" rather than "little boy/girl" or "young man/woman" may be helpful Create a system that allows patients to be identified by their preferred name or name in use. Asking all patients, "What would you like to be called?" during check-in or rooming can help with this. See "Electronic Medical Record" section below for more information Develop workflows that include sensitive, gender-neutral language during rooming or clinical interactions, such as when asking about particular medications (contraceptives, testosterone, estradiol), last menstrual period, or need for particular types of contraception. There is no workflow that can prevent all assumptions or confusion, so helping staff practice apologizing for confusion or use of inappropriate name, pronouns, or gender descriptions is a critical skill Use the words that patients use to describe themselves, particularly in relation to identity Remember that confidentiality around gender identity may be important to patients and that not all patients are "out" in all settings. Develop workflows to facilitate the use of appropriate name and pronoun in all communications that respect that patient's privacy, and talk with the patient about realistic approaches to honor both their identity and their confidentiality, when appropriate
Accommodations	Ensure access to bathrooms for people of all genders. If possible, single stall bathrooms can be helpful for many patients, including TNG patients, families with small children, or people with disabilities or those that require more space for other reasons. All-gender restrooms should be labeled with appropriate signage. If all-gender or single gender facilities are not an option, post a sign that clarifies that patients can use the bathroom that they feel is appropriate based on their gender identity

Adapted from [17]

It is important to note that experiences of discrimination in healthcare do not only occur for TNG patients or family members. Lack of representation is also a common experience for people of color or with disability as well as other members of the LGBTQ+ community. A clinic assessment and subsequent change plan to create affirming space for all can benefit all patients and staff.

Documentation and Use of the Electronic Medical Record (EMR)

Developing a standardized approach to documentation of name and pronouns in use as well as gender identity within the electronic medical record is a critical factor in creating affirming clinical spaces for TNG patients. In 2015, the Center for Medicare and Medicaid Services with the Office of the National Coordinator for Health Information Technology required that electronic medical records develop the capacity to collect information about gender identity and sexual orientation under Stage 3 Meaningful Use requirements [18]. Guidelines clearly outline a two-step approach for asking about and documenting sex assigned at birth as well as the patient's gender identity [19]. Different versions of the EMR may have different areas where a clinician or staff can document name and pronouns in use in a way that can be referenced to ensure that appropriate name and pronouns are used throughout the patient's time in a healthcare setting.

Inside the Clinician–Patient Interaction

Promoting and environment of trust and safety within the clinical interaction is perhaps the most critical aspect of providing affirming care for TNG youth. As with any adolescent, the importance of strength-based, confidential care is paramount. Use of name and pronouns in use both affirm acknowledgement and acceptance of the youth's identity and also can serve as role-modeling for parents that are struggling to adapt to or accept their child's gender identity. Language that affirms that TNG youth have gender identities that are healthy and normal can also help redirect concern on the part of the patient or family that questioning of gender identity is a problem to be "fixed."

Some youth may struggle to come out to their families, school, friends, or communities. A PCP can help facilitate conversation with family (see Promoting Family Support below) or communicate with the school around best practices to help facilitate a positive experience when the young person chooses to share this aspect of their identity. As with many aspects of identity, a young person may choose to keep their gender identity confidential for myriad reasons, including concerns about safety. Maintaining appropriate confidentiality is critical—and may even be lifesaving—for TNG youth.

Gender Identity Development for the PCP

Caring for youth of all genders requires a foundational understanding of gender in a developmental context. Gendering by others occurs well before birth, with the most current fad being prenatal "gender-reveal parties" that are pink or blue in theme. Assigned assumed differences in gender by others are well demonstrated in the first year of life. Parents have been noted to describe newborn infants of the same weight and gestational age, but different sexes assigned at birth, with different attributes, describing assigned females as softer, less attentive, and smaller than their male counterparts [20]. Parents similarly underestimate the crawling skills of female 11-month-old infants in comparison with male infants of the same age, though all infants studied perform equally well on measure of this skill [20]. Society projects particular expectations about gender and gender identity from the earliest moments of life.

Literature related to recognition of difference of sex, gender, and gender identity, though limited by basis on binary understandings of gender, show that children recognize differences in male and female voices and faces before age 1 and begin to use gender labels just before age 2, at which time children may begin to articulate their gender identity [20]. Children of all gender identities may start to verbally identify and sometimes display more stereotypical gender expression around age 3–4 [20], an age wherein children are rapidly recognizing and utilizing many of the categories and descriptions to define boundaries in their world. In the preschool years, children often start to display a preference for playmates of the same gender that persists in the school-aged years [20]. As they move through school-aged years, children develop a more flexible understanding of gender, gender expression, and gender roles.

Gender Development for TNG Youth: Persistence of TNG Identity

There is much interest in predictors of "persistence" of TNG gender identity based on characteristics or behaviors at younger ages. Studies describing development of TNG youth are limited, and there is much debate about whether and how to identify children that may persist as transgender into adulthood. Prepubertal gender non-conforming youth have shown rates of "persistence" in transgender gender identity of 25–37% [21, 22], though these studies have been limited by definitions of gender nonconformity and small sample sizes. Young children that are gender nonconforming are more likely to persist in their gender identity if they meet criteria for gender dysphoria, if they have increased measures of gender incongruity or dysphoria (in multiple areas or to a greater degree), or if they use particular language (stating, for example, "I am a girl" as opposed to "I wish I were a girl") [21, 22]. Additionally, children with gender incongruity assigned a female sex at birth are more likely to persist in gender identity than those assigned a male sex at birth [22]. While it is important not to conflate gender identity and sexual orientation, patterns of gender expression have been noted: children assigned a male sex at birth that show gender incongruity but do not have a transgender identity after puberty have higher rates of same-sex attraction than the general population [21, 22].

Clinicians should use these "predictors" cautiously given the numerous influences that can affect whether and how a child understands and articulates their gender identity. Studies of gender identity and expression are complicated by binary understandings of sex/gender stereotypic behavior. It is important to emphasize that there is no "right" way to be a man or woman, boy or girl, and that children should be supported in exploring interests, clothing, hair, and peer groups whether or not this is related more to exploration of gender expression or gender identity. PCPs should assess children and their gender journeys in a developmental context and anticipate that various possible paths ahead for their gender based on what is known. Regardless of whether a child "persists" in a TNG identity, family support in exploring their identities is central to the wellness of all children.

Gender Development for TNG Youth: Puberty

Puberty can be a difficult and defining time for TNG adolescents. As their body starts to develop in ways that may be incongruous with their gender identity and they experience ongoing minority stress, TNG adolescents experience increased rates of depression, suicidal ideation, and self-harm, including suicide attempts [23, 24]. Relatedly, they may demonstrate increased risk behaviors, including sexual activity and substance use [25].

In contrast to studies of younger children, clinical experience and research demonstrate that youth that identify as TNG at the onset of puberty have a high likelihood of persistence in their identity [26, 27]. A study of 70 TNG youth receiving medical gender-affirming medical care in a specialty gender program in the Netherlands showed that none had regret and all had persistence in their identity into adulthood [27].

Gender Development: A Lifelong Journey

Given the complex interplay of gender identity and expression as well as the impact of family, cultural, social, and societal dynamics, there is no age by which a person's "true" gender identity should be expected to emerge. While some children may express and articulate their gender identity clearly at a young age, youth or adults that come out or identify their gender identity later should not be considered less legitimate in their identity.

Family Support

Regardless of the developmental stage at which a TNG person first discusses their identity, appropriate support—from family and medical and mental health providers—is critical to long-term outcomes related to mental health, physical experience in their body, and quality of life. Perhaps the most critical role that every PCP can play in the life of a TNG young person is facilitating conversations that emphasize that TNG identities are normal and healthy, while helping families to support their children as fully as possible. Family support of LGBT people generally and transgender people specifically clearly correlates with improved health outcomes as well as higher levels of self-esteem and lower levels of substance use and depression [28].

Emphasizing the positive impact that a family can have in their child's development can give families a way to feel empowered in supporting their youth. The provider's role in this process may range from offering to be present as a resource and support when a young person first discusses their identity with their parents, to recommending community resources to help parents looking to connect with others that have parented TNG youth (see Appendix), to meeting with families over time to help parents explore and articulate their feelings about their child's gender identity. If parents are struggling with their child's gender identity, a PCP can help them identify what they *are* able to do to support their child at a given point in time—such as utilizing a name in use at home, or attending a support group for parents of TNG youth—and to grow these areas of support over time.

Many parents may grieve the loss of what they expected for their child. While exploring these feelings can be a critical process for parents or guardians, it is often helpful for parents to have opportunities to do so without their children present, and a PCP can suggest mental health providers or support groups that lend themselves to this process.

Social Transition

For both transgender youth and adults, a decision about when to socially transition—or live authentically as one's gender identity, which may include presenting this gender identity to others both in gender expression (including choices around clothes and hair) and name and pronouns in use—often includes weighing many factors. Though a fully reversible step, there has been some debate over time about at what age TNG youth should be encouraged to socially transition, and there is no template for whether and when this should occur for a given youth or family.

Current guidelines recommend that decisions about social transition be made with the assistance of a mental health provider experienced with TNG youth [9, 26, 29]. Such mental health support can be helpful for both the child and family, but it should be noted that such expertise may be relatively inaccessible in some places based on the limited number of mental health providers with experience both with young children and with the range of healthy gender identities. Whether or not mental resources are available, the experience of the child should be centered, and social transition should be strongly considered in children that demonstrate a high level of distress related to their experiences being identified as the gender associated with their sex assigned at birth.

Some feel that earlier social transition is both an opportunity to affirm and support a child's gender identity as well as a fully reversible process that can allow the child to experience living in their affirmed gender prior to any medical intervention [30]. TNG children that transition at younger ages show higher rates of "persistence" of transgender identity following puberty [22]. This likely reflects more distinct or severe gender dysphoria in children that socially transition at earlier ages, a factor that has also been associated with higher rates of persistence in TNG identity [21].

As with all interventions related to TNG youth, it is critical to consider the potential negative impacts of *not* facilitating social transition in addition to the impact of moving forward with this process. Limited evidence available shows that TNG children that socially transition prior to puberty have depression measures similar to their cisgender siblings and peers and only minimal increased measures of anxiety, a significant reduction in the mental health inequities broadly demonstrated in TNG youth [31, 32].

The PCP can play a central role in helping the family consider many factors related to social transition, including the child's level of distress and safety in the environments that they move through on a day-to-day basis. Lack of affirming environments should be addressed, when possible, and should not stand alone as a reason for a child not to socially transition. It is important to acknowledge, however, that TNG children in some communities could face real and serious threats to safety. When this degree of safety concern is encountered, a child, family and provider may consider whether there are avenues to improve safety prior to social transition or whether there are limited, safer settings in which the child can be themselves.

When a TNG child is socially transitioning, a PCP can assist the family in connecting them to organizations with a focus on advocacy for safe schools for TNG youth (see Appendix) and may provide a "carry letter" that the child can have available to document that it is appropriate and important for the child to be acknowledged as their affirmed gender and allowed to access spaces, such as bathrooms, that are in line with their gender identity. Similarly, a provider can play a critical role in helping families assess whether new environments, such as summer camps, are affirming of all gender identities, and can provide documentation and resources to ensure that youth are safe and affirmed in all environments.

Health Maintenance for Transgender and Gender Nonconforming Children and Adolescents

As for all youth, providing care for TNG youth involves understanding their whole person in a developmental context. This includes ongoing assessment of their growth, social contexts, relationships, risk behaviors, and health habits. While particular questions or challenges may arise for TNG youth and their families as they grow, a patient-centered, strength-based approach is the cornerstone of excellent care for TNG youth as it is for all children.

School Experiences

School may be a place where TNG youth can thrive when affirmed in their identity, but many TNG youth experience unsafe school environments. TNG youth report rates of victimization based on either sexual orientation or gender expression even higher than their lesbian, gay, and bisexual cisgender peers [33]. A large majority of TNG youth (85.7%) have heard remarks that were specifically transphobic at school and more than 40% (40.8%) heard transphobic comments frequently or often [34]. Students are also often asked to suppress their authentic gender expression and identity in school settings: more than half (50.9%) of transgender students report that they have not been able to use their preferred name or pronoun in the school setting and one in five (22.2%) have been stopped from wearing clothing that is considered inappropriate based on their sex assigned at birth [34].

The PCP should screen for victimization in TNG youth as for all young people and should be aware that cisnormativity may be systemically integrated in a way that leads to day-to-day microaggressions and stress. Bullying and victimization may be addressed through routine avenues, but additional advocacy or resources may be needed to change school culture to truly support the safety of TNG youth. As noted above, "carry letters" can provide helpful documentation from the PCP to support a TNG youth in being acknowledged as their affirmed gender and allowed to access spaces in line with their gender identity. To support long-term culture change, providers can identify allies within school districts and connect them with best practice resources to work toward a culture of inclusivity through curricular and staff development (see Appendix, School Resources). Providers may also leverage their positions as a community members and healthcare providers to advocate for affirming, enumerated policies inclusive of TNG students in their local school district.

Sports Participation

Participation in athletics may be a defining experience for youth, as it can connect young people to activity, community, and opportunities for leadership. TNG youth may encounter unique barriers to athletic participation in sex- or gender-segregated sports. Such barriers to participation may discourage TNG youth from engaging in athletics. This not only excludes them from a sometimes central part of their community but also may decrease physical activity, an important part of both physical and mental health.

Recognizing TNG athletes and incorporating them into athletics that are traditionally sex- or gender-segregated is an area that is currently evolving on community, interscholastic, collegiate, and professional levels. The International Olympic Committee (IOC) issued guidelines in 2015 that dictate that transwoman must have testosterone levels below a particular cutoff for a set period of time in order to compete and that transman may compete in the "male category without restriction" [35]; gender-affirming surgery had previously been a requirement for participation [36]. Other organizations, such as the National Collegiate Athletic Association (NCAA), have followed suit with similar guidelines [37], though regulations for different sports and levels of play may vary widely.

While a TNG athlete may be at the mercy of the rules of their athletic organizations (see Appendix, Sport), working for safe participation in athletics for all children is central to the role of a pediatric PCP. Providers may advocate for inclusion by providing supporting documentation. Doing this for prepubertal children may be less controversial, as all genders have low levels of sex steroids at this age. For pubertal youth, a practitioner may also consider advocacy for participation that is, at minimum, in line with guiding principles of the IOC or NCAA, or where requirements (such as a requirement for gender-affirming surgery) seem out of proportion to general goals of fairness and maximizing youth participation.

Mental Health

Experiences of gender dysphoria and minority stress put TNG youth at very high risk of mental health concerns, including depression and self-harm, eating disorders, substance use, and multiple psychiatric diagnoses [16, 23–25, 38]. TNG adults report high levels of psychological distress, with rates nearly 8 times higher than the general population in the United States [13]. Gender dysphoria or questioning of gender identity should be considered as a potential contributor to depression, anxiety, or behavioral concerns in any child. PCPs should follow recommendations for depression screening with a standardized tool in youth 12 and older [39] with low threshold for additional mental health evaluation in younger children or youth with symptoms of other mental health concerns. As for all adolescents, a provider should screen for mental health concerns and risk behaviors, including substance use, in a confidential setting and follow local legislation related to adolescent confidentiality.

Increased rates of depression and self-harm in TNG youth are clearly demonstrated and are a significant cause of morbidity and mortality amongst TNG people. TNG youth have high rates of depressive symptoms, with 40–50% reporting these symptoms compared to 10–20% of their cisgender peers [23]. Increased rates of suicidality, including strikingly high rates of suicide attempts, have been demonstrated for TNG people worldwide [40]. TNG youth report rates of suicide attempt and self-harm as high as 30 and 42%, respectively [24]; rates in these areas are 3–4 times higher than those seen in cisgender peers [23]. There are also racial disparities seen in suicidality in TNG adult populations. TNG adults that identify as American Indian, multiracial, Black, or Latino/a/x show the highest rates of history of suicide attempt, which is a pattern that is different than that seen in the general U.S. population [16].

PCPs should also be aware that TNG youth have higher rates of eating disorders compared to the general population [38], with rates as high as 2–16% [23]. In some cases, restriction may be spurred by pubertal changes—such as breast development, menstrual periods, or changes in fat distribution—that may be stopped or decreased with low weight or caloric intake. In a large survey of college students, transgender students were more likely to report a diagnosis of an eating disorder or disordered eating or weight control behaviors than their cisgender peers [38]. Regular review of growth curves along with screening tools, such as the SCOFF questionnaire, can help identify patients with eating disorders [41].

Considerations in Management of Mental Health Concerns

General management approaches to depression, self-harm, suicidality, or eating disorders do not differ from the approach that a provider would take with a cisgender young person in the use of multimodal therapies, such as medications and psychotherapy as well as escalating care as needed to protect safety. In addition, however, practitioners should be aware that failure to address gender dysphoria or triggers of stress associated with the day-to-day lived experience of TNG people may limit the efficacy of the overall treatment plan. As discussed previously, this process may involve social transition or facilitating family support and acceptance; for a young person at or beyond the onset of puberty, this should also involve consideration of medical interventions for gender affirmation.

Emerging evidence show that medical interventions for gender affirmation can improve mental health, though studies of youth are extremely limited. Use of gonadotropin-releasing hormone (GnRH) agonist therapy to suppress puberty has been associated with improvement of mental health measures, including depression and global functioning measures [27, 42]. Though rates of gender dysphoria are not significantly decreased with GnRH therapy [42], this is unsurprising given that pubertal suppression prevents additional pubertal changes, but does not eliminate secondary sex characteristics that have already developed. Studies of the specific effect of gender-affirming hormones (GAH) on mental health outcomes in youth are not yet available. However, assessment of youth after GAH *and* surgical intervention showed decreased gender dysphoria, increased body satisfaction, and quality of life (QOL), happiness, and mental health measures similar to the general population [27].

Research of GAH in TNG adults shows similar glimpses into improved outcomes, though evidence is consistently noted to be limited by cohort sizes and study designs. GAH is associated with improvement in scores for depression, anxiety, and hostility in short-term follow-up in TNG adults [43]. GAH and surgical gender affirmation in adults are also collectively associated with improvement in gender dysphoria, psychological functioning, and quality of life as well as lower suicide rates [44]. Understanding the role of gender-affirming medical and surgical therapy in the experience and mental health of TNG people can be a central component of promoting lifelong wellness.

A Word on Conversion Therapy

Conversion therapy—sometimes inappropriately labeled reparative therapy—remains a threat to the wellness of TNG youth. Conversion therapy is a term that was originally used to describe interventions to change a person's sexual orientation but now is also used to described attempts to change gender identity or expression [45]. The Obama administration denounced conversion therapy after the suicide of a transgender person that had been subjected to conversion therapy [46]. As of this writing, 10 states in the U.S. and the District of Columbia have outlawed conversion therapy [47]. Multiple professional organizations, including the American Academy of Pediatrics, the American Psychological Association, and the American Psychiatric Association, have denounced conversion therapy based on the ethical problems it presents and the potential to harm LGBTQ+ youth, as well as the absence of any demonstrated efficacy or benefit [1, 45]. Referral for conversion therapy should not be made and families should be advised of the harm in pursuing such services.

Mental Health Referrals

Standard guidelines generally recommend that TNG youth have the support of a mental health provider with training in both child and adolescent development and gender-affirming care. While this can be a critical tool for many youth, particularly those coping with depression, anxiety, or self-harm, the decision to pursue therapy should take into account the larger clinical picture, services available, and social context. For example, prepubertal youth that are thriving with or without social transition and that do not have signs of mental health concerns may not require urgent connection with a mental health provider, particularly if there are few providers with appropriate experience accessible to that family. With the central tenant of "First, do no harm," a PCP should consider whether, when, and which available mental health resources available would benefit the child and the family.

Sexual Health

PCPs can play a central role in promoting the development of healthy relationships and sexuality in all adolescents, and TNG youth are no exception. A confidential interview with a complete social history to both establish rapport over time and identify risk factors should be a part of routine health supervision visits.

To obtain an accurate assessment of risk factors associated with sexual activity, concrete and specific language is key. "Sexual activity" should be avoided as a broad term without specific follow-up to clarify what specific activities and contact are involved. When asking about partners, clarifying gender identity of partners may be helpful, as may specific questions about what body parts are involved. For example, a transman could have penetrative vaginal sex with a transgender woman that still has a penis, a cisgender man, or a person of any gender using sex toys for penetration. Asking about safety in relationships, consent, and exchange of sex for money or drugs is particularly important to identify histories of violence, sexual assault, or behaviors that are high risk for pregnancy or acquiring sexually transmitted infections (STIs), such as HIV.

The accuracy of the social history is critical in counseling about interventions to support safe sexual activity.

Contraception

Any person with a uterus and ovaries is at risk for pregnancy if they have penetrative penile–vaginal sex. Transgender men have experienced both intentional and unintentional pregnancy during or after cessation of testosterone therapy [48]. Testosterone is not and should not be considered contraception. For TNG youth at risk of pregnancy and not on testosterone therapy, a full range of contraception options should be discussed. Some TNG youth may wish to avoid combined oral contraceptives, given the potential side effects of medications containing estrogens. For TNG youth on testosterone, contraceptive counseling should be provided about barrier contraception as well as contraceptive options that do not contain estrogen, such as progestin-only pills, medroxyprogesterone injections, intrauterine devices, or etonogestrel subcutaneous implants.

Pregnancy prevention counseling can also be important for TNG youth assigned a male sex. Both spironolactone and estrogen therapy are likely to reduce sperm count but should not be considered a method of contraception. If an individual is having penetrative penile–vaginal sex, it is important to discuss the potential for partner pregnancy and use of barrier protection.

Sexually Transmitted Infections (STIs)

Information about risk of STIs in TNG youth is limited and there are few specific screening recommendations in this population. Limited studies suggest that the burden of HIV amongst transgender women is disproportionately high, particularly among black transgender women [49], and there is very little data available on STIs in transgender men. One reason for limited data is that many agencies from the local to federal level do not collect data on gender identity [50], so transgender people may be pulled into other categories (such as transgender women being categorized historically as men who have sex with men).

Screening for STIs in TNG youth should be based on body parts present, sexual activity, and routine screening recommendations for their sex assigned at birth. If a transgender man has a cervix, for example, then screening for cervical cancer should be based on routine guidelines for as long as that person continues to have a cervix. The Center for Disease Control (CDC) acknowledges TNG people as special populations in their most recent recommendations. However, specific recommendations are limited: this report states that "[c]linicians should assess STD- and HIV-related risks for their transgender patients based on current anatomy and sexual behaviors" and should make clinical decisions for evaluation based on symptoms that can be associated with STI [49].

An approach to STI and pregnancy prevention counseling that centers on risk behaviors and is organized by anatomy is suggested in Table 5.2.

As for any adolescent, guidelines and algorithms will not cover every clinical situation, and clinical judgement is important in determining actual risk to inform counseling and frequency of STI screenings.

Gender-Affirming Medical Care in Primary Care

While not all TNG youth engage medical therapies in their gender affirmation, consideration of pubertal suppression and GAH are recommended in TNG that experience gender dysphoria [9, 26]. In addition, pubertal suppression as a fully reversible intervention may be used in youth that question their gender identity to allow more time for exploration and understanding before irreversible pubertal changes occur. If appropriate criteria are met, recommendations state that GAH may be started in youth ages 14–16 years old, though some centers may start GAH

Table 5.2 Safer sex screening and counseling for asymptomatic TNG youth without other health conditions*

Anatomic location	Used in sexual activity?	Screening or counseling recommendations (preferred test)
Vagina	Yes	Chlamydia and gonorrhea screening annually under age 25 (vaginal or urine NAAT testing**)
Cervix/ uterus	N/A	Cervical cancer screening starting at age 21
	N/A	HPV vaccination to complete series up to through age 26***
	Yes or planning to be	Contraceptive counseling and prescription as appropriate
Anus	Yes	At least annual syphilis screening (Syphilis serology)
		Hepatitis B screening (Hepatitis B Surface Antigen)
		HPV vaccination to complete series up to through age 26 regardless of sex assigned at birth***
		At least annual rectal gonorrhea and chlamydia screening (Rectal NAAT testing)
		At least annual HIV testing (HIV Serology) if with new partner (or partner with new partner) since last HIV test
Penis	Yes, penetrative vaginal sex	Counseling about risk of pregnancy in partner
	Yes, penetrative anal sex	At least annual screening for urethral gonorrhea and chlamydia infection (Urine NAAT testing)
		Hepatitis B Antigen Screening
		At least annual HIV testing (HIV Serology) if with new partner (or partner with new partner) since last HIV test
		At least annual syphilis screening (syphilis serology)
Mouth	Yes, receptive oral sex with partner with penis in the last year	Annual pharyngeal gonorrhea testing (Pharyngeal NAAT testing)
All	N/A	HIV testing (HIV Serology) should be discussed and offered to all adolescents and all people that seek evaluation and treatment for STIs
		HPV***, Hepatitis A, and Hepatitis B vaccination

*Recommendations are different for youth with certain medical conditions, such as immunocompromised status, pregnancy, or HIV

**Vaginal NAAT preferred due to increased sensitivity in people assigned a female sex at birth. Urine NAAT is preferable in people that have *had vaginoplasty

***The CDC recommends HPV vaccination to complete the series for females and men who have sex with men through age 26 and other males through age 21

Adapted from CDC 2015 Sexually Transmitted Disease Treatment Guidelines 2015, Sections on "Transgender Men and Women", "Adolescents," and "Men who have Sex with Men" [49] and the UCSF Center of Excellence for Transgender Care [51]

earlier to facilitate pubertal development at ages in concordance with the young person's peers [52].

The onset of puberty (signified by Sexual Maturity Rating 2 development) is the earliest stage at which medical intervention is recommended, as this is when pubertal blockade may be initiated. However, referral for additional support or services may be beneficial prior to the onset of puberty: as previously discussed, referral to a mental health provider experienced with children and gender identity may be beneficial, depending on the needs of the child, and referral to a specialty center or provider experienced with gender-affirming care prior to the onset of puberty may help avoid delays in care related to clinic scheduling or insurance navigation. Programs that provide gender-affirming medical care for youth vary greatly in their services and team members but may include mental health providers, pediatric endocrinologists, adolescent medicine providers, PCPs, pediatric or adult gynecologists or urologists, plastic surgeons, social workers, and even chaplains [11].

While gender-affirming medical care for TNG youth has evolved over the last decade primarily as a specialty practice, it is likely that PCPs will become increasingly involved in this care as more youth seek these services. Many of the medical aspects of gender-affirming medical care, including prescription of GAH, are not technically difficult and are clearly and concretely outlined in available guidelines [9, 26, 52]. Although PCPs may be less familiar with GnRH agonists due to limited experience and cost, these regimens are also straightforward in dose and response assessment. More challenging, perhaps, is the time needed for evaluation and care coordination to fully assess a TNG youth's physical and mental health and to understand the experience and qualifications of other members of the care team, such as mental health providers, that may inform assessments of health required prior to initiation of pubertal blockade or GAH. PCPs that know youth or families well, however, are uniquely positioned to accompany youth on this path and understand their gender identity development over time, which is a perspective that may be difficult for specialists to access and that can lend valuable context to assessing the youth's whole health.

PCPs can and should challenge themselves to become as informed as possible about gender-affirming medical care for TNG youth, and to provide as much clinical care as they are able in the primary care home. Menstrual management to decrease or eliminate periods in transmasculine or nonbinary youth draws on the same knowledge as menstrual management or contraceptive options for cisgender female youth. Options for eliminating periods include continuous use of combined or progestin-only oral contraceptives (though it should be noted that some transmasculine youth prefer to avoid medications that contain estrogen), depo-medroxyprogesterone acetate injections, a levonorgestrel intrauterine device (IUD), or etonogestrel rod implant [52].

If a PCP lacks the time, care coordination support, or experience to initiate pubertal suppression or GAH, there are still many opportunities to gain additional clinical skills and increase TNG youth access to this medical care. Even if prescribed by a specialty provider, it can be very helpful for youth to be able to receive leuprolide injections for pubertal suppression every 3 months at their primary care clinic to minimize the need for travel. Additionally, continuation and monitoring of GAH in the primary care medical home is a straightforward step once stable dosing has been achieved. This too may improve accessibility to ongoing care, particularly for youth and families that travel long distances to specialty centers. An overview of recommendations for ongoing monitoring after a stable dose of GAH is established is outlined in Table 5.3.

Table 5.3 Recommended clinical monitoring of long-term GAH therapy [26, 29]

Gender-affirming medical therapy	Long-term monitoring after dose stabilization	Frequency	Clinical concerns
Any	Clinical assessment of overall well-being, weight, blood pressure, tobacco use, depression, and side effects/risks	Every 3 months in first year and then 1–2 times per year	Weight gain, hypertension, mood changes, increased risk of thrombosis (particularly if tobacco use)
Estradiol (sublingual, transdermal, or injection)	Total estrogen. Goal: do not exceed peak range of 100–200 pg/mL Total testosterone. Goal < 50 ng/dL	Every 3 months in the first year and then 1–2 times per year after reach goal range	Concern for thrombophilia, hypertension, or liver dysfunction at higher levels
	Prolactin*	Annually during "transition period" and every 2 years thereafter	Prolactinoma
Spironolactone	Basic metabolic panel	Every 3 months in the first year and then yearly	Hyperkalemia
Testosterone (usually intramuscular or subcutaneous injection)	Total testosterone drawn mid-way between injections. Goal range of 400–700 ng/dl	Every 3 months in the first year and then 1–2 times per year after reach goal range	Aromatization of testosterone to estrogen with associated menstrual bleeding or feminizing effects may occur at high testosterone levels Clot risk may be theoretically increased at higher levels
	Hemoglobin or hematocrit	Every 3 months in the first year and then 1–2 times per year	Monitoring for polycythemia
	Fasting lipid and glucose monitoring	At regular intervals based on recommendations for age and other risk factors	Monitoring for dyslipidemia, impaired fasting glucose or diabetes

*Given that elevated prolactin levels are managed expectantly for symptoms, prolactin monitoring is not recommended in all guidelines [29]

Conclusion

TNG youth deserve high-quality, patient-centered care that promotes their well-being and allows them to thrive. PCPs may be the first or primary provider that a young person encounters and can have substantial impact on that young person's experiences in and out of the healthcare system. Every PCP should be able to provide affirming primary care for TNG youth and should challenge themselves to expand their impact through clinical care, family engagement, or community advocacy to promote the health and wellness of TNG young people.

Appendix

Creating Affirming Spaces
"Office-Based Care for Lesbian, Gay, Bisexual, Transgender, and Questioning Youth" (2013). This American Academy of Pediatrics guideline and the accompanying technical report offers specific recommendations and standards around affirming spaces and provision of primary care for LGBTQ+ youth.
"Advancing Effective Communication, Cultural Competence, and Patient- and Family-Centered Care for the Lesbian, Gay, Bisexual, and Transgender (LGBT) Community: A Field Guide" (2011). This comprehensive resource published by the Joint Commission is available for free online and provides in-depth guidance and best practices related to the care of LGBT patients and families.

- Website: https://www.jointcommission.org/lgbt/

Health Equality Index (Human Rights Campaign (HRC)): The HRC has developed a benchmarking tool titled the Health Equality Index to evaluate healthcare facilities' policies and practices related to the care of LGBTQ+ patients as well as the experiences of visitors and employees. More information about how to apply for HEI designation and resources to help facilities meet HEI criteria are found online.

- Website: http://www.hrc.org/hei/resource-guide

Electronic Medical Record Resources
"Do Ask, Do Tell." This toolkit from The Fenway Institute and the Center for American Progress outlines rationale and recommendations for appropriate data collection and documentation as well as information to help train providers and staff.

- Website: http://doaskdotell.org/ehr/toolkit/

Resources for Families
PFLAG (Parents and Families of Lesbians and Gays). PFLAG is the nation's largest family and ally organization. PFLAG is committed to advancing equality through

its mission of support, education, and advocacy. PFLAG has chapters across the United States in locations ranging from rural areas to large urban centers.

- Website: https://www.pflag.org/
- Address (National Headquarters): 1828 L Street, NW, Suite 660, Washington, DC, 20036, U.S.A.
- Phone (National Headquarters): (202) 467-8180

Gender Spectrum. Gender Spectrum's mission is to create a gender-inclusive world for all children and youth by working with families, organizations, and institutions to increase understandings of gender.

- Website: https://www.genderspectrum.org/
- Email (General information): info@genderspectrum.org

School Resources

Welcoming Schools. The Human Rights Campaign's Welcoming Schools program is a national professional development program in the United States with a mission of creating safe and welcoming schools for all children and families. Welcoming Schools provides "training and resources to elementary school educators to welcome diverse families, create LGBTQ and gender inclusive schools, prevent bias-based bullying, and support transgender and non-binary students."

- Website: http://www.welcomingschools.org/
- Address: Welcoming Schools, c/o Human Rights Campaign 1640 Rhode Island Ave. N.W. Washington, DC 20036-3278, U.S.A.

GSA Network. GSA Network is a "next-generation LGBTQ racial and gender justice organization in the United States that empowers and trains queer, trans and allied youth leaders to advocate, organize, and mobilize an intersectional movement for safer schools and healthier communities."

- Website: https://gsanetwork.org/
- Phone: 415-552-4229; Fax: 415-552-4729 (U.S. Phone Numbers; country code +1)
- Email Address: info@gsanetwork.org
- Located in Oakland, California, U.S.A.

Gender Spectrum. Gender Spectrum "helps to create gender sensitive and inclusive environments for all children and teens." To accomplish this, Gender Spectrum provides in-person and online trainings, support and education to help families, organizations, and institutions increase understandings of gender, gender identity, and expression.

- Website: https://www.genderspectrum.org/
- Phone: 510-788-4412 (U.S. Phone Number; country code +1)
- Email Address: info@genderspectrum.org

GLSEN (Gay, Lesbian, Straight Education Network). GLSEN is a national organization in the U.S. dedicated to creating safe and affirming schools for all, regardless of sexual orientation, gender identity, or gender expression.

- Website: https://www.glsen.org/
- Phone: 212-727-0135 (U.S. Phone Number; country code +1)
- Email Address: info@glsen.org
- Address: 110 William Street, 30th Floor, New York, NY 10038, U.S.A.

Resources for TNG Athletes
Transathlete.com: This website serves as a resource for TNG athletes and those looking to support their participation in athletics. Included is a frequently updated list of policies from organizations in the United States and Canada for athletic organizations at the K-12, high school, collegiate, and professional levels.

- Website: https://www.transathlete.com/

References

1. Committee on Adolescence. Office-based care for lesbian, gay, bisexual, transgender, and questioning youth. Pediatrics. 2013;132(1):198–203.
2. AAFP. Recommended curriculum guidelines for family medicine residents: lesbian, gay, bisexual, transgender health. American Academy of Family Physicians.
3. The Fenway guide to lesbian, gay, bisexual, and transgender health. Philadelphia: American College of Physicians; 2015.
4. Health care for transgender individuals. In: American College of Obstetricians and Gynecologists, editor. Obstetrics & Gynecology. 2011. p. 1454–8.
5. Cohen-Kettenis P, Delemarre-van de Waal HA, Gooren LJG. The treatment of adolescent transsexuals: changing insights. J Sex Med. 2008;5:1892–7.
6. Di Ceglie DD, Sturge C, Sutton A, Executive Committee of the Child and Adolescent Psychiatry Section, editors. Gender identity disorders in children and adolescents: guidance for management. London: Royal College of Psychiatrists; 1998.
7. Spack NP, Edwards-Leeper L, Feldman HA, Leibowitz S, Mandel F, Diamond DA, et al. Children and adolescents with gender identity disorder referred to a pediatric medical center. Pediatrics. 2012;129:418–25.
8. Hembree WC, Cohen-Kettenis PT, Delemarre-van de Waal HA, Gooren LJ, Meyer WJ III, Spack NP, et al. Endocrine treatment of transsexual persons: an endocrine society clinical practice guideline. J Clin Endocrinol Metab. 2009;94(9):3132–54.
9. Coleman E, Bockting W, Botzer M, Cohen-Kettenis P, DeCuypere G, Feldman J, et al. Standards of care for the health of transsexual, transgender, and gender-nonconforming people. Version 7 ed. World Professional Association for Transgender Health (WPATH); 2012.
10. Human Rights Campaign. Interactive map: clinical care programs for gender-expansive children and adolescents 2018 [cited 2018 Mar 21]. Available from: https://www.hrc.org/resources/interactive-map-clinical-care-programs-for-gender-nonconforming-childr.
11. Hsieh S, Leininger J. Resource list: clinical care programs for gender-nonconforming children and adolescents. Pediatr Ann. 2014;43(6):238–44.
12. Russo F. Where transgender is no longer a diagnosis. Scientific American. 2017 Jan 6.

13. James SE, Herman JL, Rankin S, Keisling M, Mottet LA, Anafi M. The report of the 2015 U. S. transgender survey. Washington, DC: National Center for Transgender Equality; 2016.
14. Botsford J, Allen B, Andert B, Budge S, Rehm J. Meeting the healthcare needs of transgender, nonbinary, and gender expansive/nonconforming youth in Wisconsin: a report of the 2017 Wisconsin transgender youth community needs assessment. 2018.
15. Lambda Legal. When health care isn't caring: Lambda Legal's survey of discrimination against LGBT people and people with HIV. New York: Lambda Legal; 2010.
16. Grant JM, Mottet LA, Tanis J, Herman JL, Harrison J, Keisling M. National transgender discrimination survey report on health and health care: findings of a study by the national center for transgender equality and the national gay and lesbian task force. 2010.
17. The Joint Commission. Advancing effective communication, cultural competence, and patient- and family-centered care for the lesbian, gay, bisexual, and transgender (LGBT) community: a field guide. Oak Brook, IL: 2011 Oct. Report No.
18. Centers for Medicare & Medicaid Services. Medicare and Medicaid programs; electronic health record incentive program–stage 3 and modifications to meaningful use in 2015 through 2017. Department of Health and Human Services, 2015 42 CFR Parts 412 and 495 [CMS-3310-FC and CMS-3311-FC], RINs 0938-AS26 and 0938-AS58.
19. Deutsch MB, Green J, Keatley J, Mayer G, Hastings J, Hall AM. Electronic medical records and the transgender patient: recommendations from the World Professional Association for Transgender Health EMR Working Group. J Am Med Inform Assoc. 2013;20:700–3.
20. Blakemore JEO, Berenbaum SA, Liben LS. Gender development. New York: Psychology Press, Taylor & Francis Group; 2009. p. 516.
21. Wallien MSC, Cohen-Kettenis PT. Psychosexual outcome of gender-dysphoric children. J Am Acad Child Adolesc Psychiatry. 2008;47(12):1413–23.
22. Steensma TD, McGuire JK, Kreukels BPC, Beekman AJ, Cohen-Kettenis PT. Factors associated with desistence and persistence of childhood gender dysphoria: a quantitative follow-up study. J Am Acad Child Adolesc Psychiatry. 2013;52(6):582–90.
23. Connolly MD, Zervos MJ, Barone CJ II, Johnson CC, Joseph CLM. The mental health of transgender youth: advances in understanding. J Adolesc Health. 2016;59:489–95.
24. Peterson CM, Matthews A, Copps-Smith E, Conard LA. Suicidality, self-harm, and body dissatisfaction in transgender adolescents and emerging adults with gender dysphoria. Suicide Life Threat Behav. 2016;47(4):475–82. Epub 2016 Aug 19.
25. Garofalo R, Deleon J, Osmer E, Doll M, Harper GW. Overlooked, misunderstood and at-risk: exploring the lives and HIV risk of ethnic minority male-to-female transgender youth. J Adolesc Health. 2006;38:230–6.
26. Hembree WC, Cohen-Kettenis PT, Gooren L, Hannema SE, Meyer WJ, Hassan Murad M, et al. Endocrine treatment of gender-dysphoric/gender-incongruent persons: an endocrine society* clinical practice guideline. J Clin Endocrinol Metab. 2017;102(11):1–35.
27. de Vries AL, McGuire JK, Steensma TD, Wagenaar EC, Doreleijers TA, Cohen-Kettenis PT. Young adult psychological outcome after puberty suppression and gender reassignment. Pediatrics. 2014;134(4):696–704.
28. Ryan C, Russell ST, Huebner D, Diaz R, Sanchez J. Family acceptance in adolescence and the health of LGBT young adults. J Child Adolesc Psychiatr Nurs. 2010;23:205–13.
29. Guidelines for the primary and gender-affirming care of transgender and gender nonbinary people. San Francisco: Center of Excellence for Transgender Health, Department of Family & Community Medicine, University of California; 2016.
30. Ehrensaft D. Found in transition: our littlest transgender people. Comtemp Psychoanal. 2014;50(4):571–92.
31. Durwood L, McLaughlin KA, Olson KR. Mental health and self-worth in socially transitioned transgender youth. J Am Acad Child Adolesc Psychiatry. 2017;56(2):116–23.
32. Olson KR, Durwood L, DeMeules M, McLaughlin KA. Mental health of transgender children who are supported in their identities. Pediatrics. 2016;137(3).

33. Kosciw JG, Greytak EA, Diaz EM. Who, what, where, when, and why: demographic and ecological factors contributing to hostile school climate for lesbian, gay, bisexual, and transgender youth. J Youth Adolesc. 2009;38:976–88. Epub 2009 May 7.
34. Kosciw JG, Greytak EA, Giga NM, Villenas C, Danischewski DJ. The 2015 National School Climate Survey: the experiences of lesbian, gay, bisexual, transgender, and queer youth in our nation's schools. New York: 2016. Report No.
35. IOC. IOC consensus meeting on sex reassignment and hyperandrogenism. Lausanne, Switzerland: International Olympic Committee; 2015 Nov. Report No.
36. Associated Press. Transgender athletes can now compete in olympics without surgery. The New York Times. 2016 Jan 25; Sect. Olympics.
37. NCAA inclusion of transgender student-athletes. 2011.
38. Diemer EW, Grant JD, Munn-Chernoff MA, Patterson DA, Duncan AE. Gender identity, sexual orientation, and eating-related pathology in a national sample of college students. J Adolesc Health. 2015;57:144–9. Epub 2015 Apr 28.
39. Final recommendation statement: depression in children and adolescents: screening 2016 [2018 Mar 29]. Available from: https://www.uspreventiveservicestaskforce.org/Page/Document/RecommendationStatementFinal/depression-in-children-and-adolescents-screening1.
40. Virupaksha HG, Muralidhar D, Ramakrishna J. Suicide and suicide behavior among transgender persons. Indian J Psychol Med. 2016;38(6):505–9.
41. Rosen DS, The Committee on Adolescence. Identification and management of eating disorders in children and adolescents. Pediatrics. 2010;126(6):1240–53.
42. Chew D, Anderson J, Williams K, May T, Pang K. Hormonal treatment in young people with gender dysphoria: a systematic review. Pediatrics. 2018;141(4).
43. White Hughto JM, Reisner SL. A systematic review of the effects of hormone therapy on psychological functioning and quality of life in transgender individuals. Transgender Health. 2016;1(1):21–31.
44. Murad MH, Elamin MB, Garcia MZ, Mullan RJ, Murad A, Erwin PJ, et al. Hormonal therapy and sex reassignment: a systematic review and meta-analysis of quality of life and psychosocial outcomes. Clin Endocrinol. 2010;72:214–31.
45. Byne W. Regulations restrict practice of conversion therapy. LGBT Health. 2016;3(2):97–9.
46. Shear MD. Obama calls for end to 'conversion' therapies for gay and transgender youth. The New York Times. 2015 Apr 8.
47. Movement Advancement Project. Equality maps: conversion therapy laws 2018 [cited 2018 Mar 30]. Available from: http://www.lgbtmap.org/equality-maps/conversion_therapy.
48. Light AD, Obedin-Maliver J, Sevelius JM, Kerns JL. Transgender men who experienced pregnancy after female-to-male gender transitioning. Obstet Gynecol. 2014;124(6):1120–7.
49. Workowski KA, Bolan GA. Sexually transmitted diseases treatment guidelines, 2015. MMWR Recomm Rep. 2015;64(3).
50. HIV among transgender people: division of HIV/AIDS prevention. National Center for HIV/AIDS, Viral Hepatitis, STD, and TB Prevention, Centers for Disease Control and Prevention 2017 [2018 Apr 2]. Available from: https://www.cdc.gov/hiv/group/gender/transgender/index.html.
51. Poteat T. Transgender people and sexually transmitted infections (STIs). In: Deutsch MB, editor. Guidelines for the primary and gender-affirming care of transgender and gender nonbinary people, 2nd ed. San Francisco: Center of Excellence for Transgender Health, Department of Family and Community Medicine, University of California; 2016.
52. Olson-Kennedy J, Rosenthal SM, Hastings J, Wesp L. Health considerations for gender non-conforming children and transgender adolescents. In: Deutsch MB, editor. Guidelines for the primary and gender-affirming care of transgender and gender nonbinary people. San Francisco: Center of Excellence for Transgender Health, Department of Family & Community Medicine, University of California; 2016.

Chapter 6
Geriatric Transgender Care

Noelle Marie Javier

Introduction

As society ages over time, people who identify as transgender and non-conforming (TGNC) are an intrinsic part of the growing geriatric population. While the verdict is not out on the actual population size, the fact remains that TGNC individuals are subject to victimization and discrimination, including areas in health care, education, employment, housing, finances, social supports, and access to public resources to name a few [1–3] The personal journey of a transgender person in relation to discrimination across his or her lifetime is associated with negative health and well-being outcomes [4]. This is further supported by a 2013 study by Fredriksen-Goldsen that highlighted the significant risks experienced by older TGNC adults regarding physical health, depression, and stress [5]. Hence, there is a burgeoning need to bring high-quality geriatric care to the forefront so that this population will be treated with dignity and respect. By doing so, we in the healthcare profession can help minimize further marginalization and invisibility of this already vulnerable and underserved population. There is an ongoing need for education and standardization of best practices that will afford universal care for all. Much of the discussion will revolve around specific geriatric care approach to the older transgender adult patient. Unfortunately, there are very scant data for gender non-conforming individuals in general and very little for TGNC older adults. Representative sampling of the TGNC individuals remains a challenge because of the diversity of labels across cultures and age cohorts and the desire to remain under the radar [6]. This is, therefore, an area of greatest need for future research and best healthcare practices development. Furthermore, as gender identity continues to

N. M. Javier (✉)
Department of Geriatrics and Palliative Medicine, Icahn School of Medicine
at Mount Sinai, New York, NY, USA
e-mail: noelle.javier@mssm.edu

L. Poretsky and W. C. Hembree (eds.), *Transgender Medicine*, Contemporary
Endocrinology, https://doi.org/10.1007/978-3-030-05683-4_6

expand in scope, we should be mindful of future identities such as gender blending, gender bending, and gender-independent, all of which might have evolutionary and dynamic needs over time.

Epidemiology

As of 2014, older adults account for about 14.5% of the population in the United States of America. This translates to about 46.2 million of adults 65 years of age and older [7]. With advancing technology and better health care, it is expected that the older adult population will continue to rise and by 2060, about 98 million people will be aged 65 years old and over. Included in this cohort are individuals who identify as transgender and gender non-confirming (TGNC). As of 2010, the US Census reports an estimate between 1.2 million and 2.8 million [8]. The Williams Institute estimates about 1.4 million (0.58%) of the US population [9] (Fig. 6.1). A national survey conducted by the services and advocacy for GLBT elders (SAGE) in 2014 estimated that about 0.7% identify as transgender in the 45–75 age bracket in a sample of over 2000 respondents [10]. There is probably underreporting because of a lack of standardized sexual orientation and gender identity information questions on intake forms, population surveys, and demographic assessments. Furthermore, the TGNC older adult population is expected to grow and diversify as younger individuals emerge and age over time with their own unique experiences as gender variant. Notwithstanding this fact is the reality that aging baby boomers will also contribute to this population as they transition later in life.

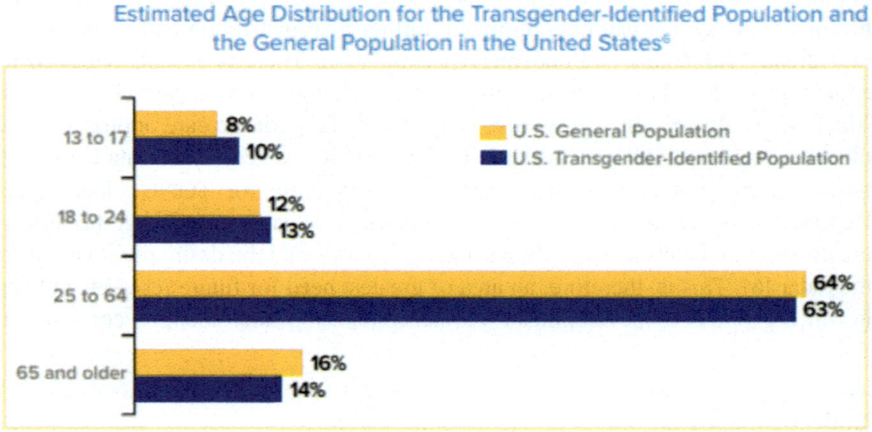

Fig. 6.1 Demographic distribution of transgender-identified individuals in the United States [9]

Overview of Relevant Constructs

Being a minority, TGNC individuals have experienced multiple societal barriers to aging gracefully and successfully. These have been rooted in the unique historical context that this population has undergone over the course of many years. There has been a long-standing history of oppression and discrimination toward the TGNC population [11]. These included but are not limited to age, race, ethnicity, class, education, disability status, and sexual orientation among others [11]. After all, aging takes place in four major domains: biomedical, psychological, socioeconomic, and political/institutional [6]. The concept of *Intersectionality* has gained momentum in the social science literature. This pertains to the confluence of multiple factors that must be considered when attending to the unique needs of the TGNC individual. The multiple forms of the stigma that arise cannot be examined separately or ranked in terms of the degree of oppression [12]. An older woman who identifies as transgender is faced with numerous polarizing factors such as ageism, sexism, racism, and transphobia among others (Fig. 6.2). As a result, the TGNC population has experienced and continues to be affected by high levels of emotional, physical, and psychological stress. The *minority stress model* plays an important role in understanding the lived experiences of the TGNC patient [13] (Table 6.1). Two operational theories are worth thinking about. Aldwin and Gilmer attempted to relate the *Life Course Theory* with how older adults age over time. It essentially presupposes that a series of transitions and choice points are influenced both by the immediate social context and the larger sociohistorical period as well as gender and social roles [14]. *Goal-oriented theories* on the other hand regard adulthood and late-life development as a balance between gains and losses, pursuit of goals, and the development and maintenance of the self [15]. For instance, many trans-elders describe "hitting a wall" when living in their birth gender, and subsequently decide to transition hoping that the losses incurred will be balanced by the personal gain of attaining the true self before they die. The integration of both

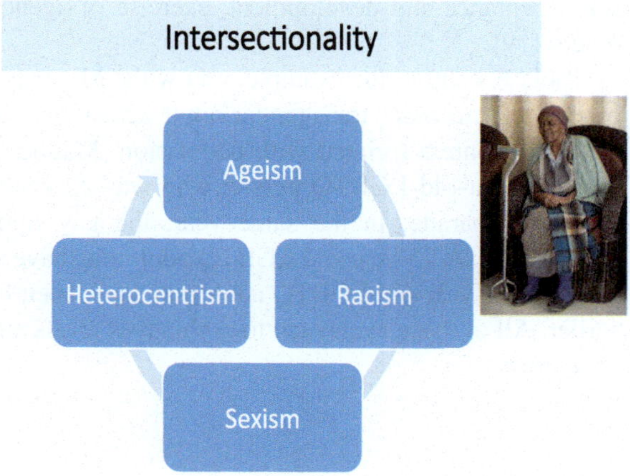

Fig. 6.2 Intersectionality in the older transgender adult

Table 6.1 Minority stress model example

	65 YO b. 1952	75 YO b. 1942	85 YO b. 1932
20 YO	1972 Stone Wall. Anita Bryant. Religious right. Harvey Milk assassinated. Gay Olympics. Watergate (cracks in US govt.) The first pride parade	1962 Arrests. Bar Raids. Don't stand too close (solicitation.) Women's Movt. No word for "gay." Sick! Things start to change. Compton riots. Society for individual rights. *The Transexual Phenomenon*	1952 Lose job. Lose custody. Prison. Forced ECT. Police raids. Mattachine society. Lose a scholarship. Bilitis. Institutionalized. ONE Inc. versus Oleson. Coopers Donuts. Executive order 10450
30 YO	1982 GRID. Act Up. Larry Kramer. White Night Riots. Gerry Studds. Rock Hudson dies. Bowers versus Hardwick	1972 Stonewall. Community Centers. APA removes from DSM. Michigan women's festival. Studio 54 (gay is chic.) The Castro 14	1962 MLK. Hippies. Arrests. Vietnam. FBI investigates "subversive groups." Berkeley freedom of speech. JFK. Bar raids. The Advocate
40 YO	1992 DOMA. Protease inhibitors. DADT. 1st Lesbian Kiss on television. Ellen. March on Washington. Col. M. Cammermeyer. Red Ribbon. Althea Garrison	1982 HIV AIDS. Cleve Jones. The Names Mem Quilt. Reagan. AZT. Domestic partnership in Berkeley. Barney Frank	1972 Youth led movement. A symbol. Salsa soul sisters. Being out = activism. Community centers

theories results in the construct of *Resilience*. This is described as a complex transaction among sociocultural, contextual, and individual resources, all of which can affect and can be affected by the individual's coping strategies in stressful situations [16]. Resilience can, therefore, be defined as the ability of the system when perturbed to return to its original state of operation [17, 18]. This is in contradistinction to the construct of *Robustness* which is the ability of the system to resist perturbation [6]. The components of resilience vary and could include nurturing the spiritual self, caring relations, advocacy, activism/volunteerism, self-acceptance and development, exercise of agency, and religiosity/faith among others [19].

Table 6.1 shows the example of how the Minority Stress Model affects the aging process for an older transgender adult across various decades and shaped by the historical context (printed with permission, Matthew Gayton NP).

A 65-year-old LGBTQ person who was 20 years old in 1972 experienced the first pride parade. In the same year, the gay rights activist Harvey Milk was assassinated. A 75-year-old LGBTQ adult may have witnessed the bar raids in 1962 while an 85-year-old LGBTQ adult may have been forced to receive ECT 10 years earlier. All of these events led to high-stress levels affecting the LGBTQ population over time.

Overview of the Healthcare Needs and Disparities

Throughout a lifetime of discrimination, prejudice, oppression, victimization, and prosecution, TGNC individuals have been significantly impacted in various aspects of life including health care. Historically, the transgender community has been quite invisible until recently. Witten identified a link between discrimination and the biopsychosocial dimensions affecting a TGNC person [20]. It could be inferred that this linkage could also be responsible for how TGNCs health will be shaped over time to include successful aging [20]. Historically, there has been a negative relationship between healthcare providers and TGNC patients [20, 21]. Previous studies have pointed out that disclosing information on sexual orientation and gender identity (SOGI) might lead to more discrimination and more mistrust toward the healthcare providers [21]. A 2015 US Transgender survey highlighted that 33% in a sample of 27,715 transgender persons had negative experiences in healthcare settings [2] (Fig. 6.3a, b).

Additionally, about a quarter needed to educate the providers about being transgender while 8% had been refused care related to gender transitioning. A good 5% noted that healthcare providers used abusive language toward them. As a result, there is consequential delay and maybe even an avoidance in seeking medical care for fear of mistreatment and disrespect further propagating the cycle of oppression. The data on healthcare outcomes is staggering as seen on this table (Table 6.2).

A 2010 survey by Lambda Legal highlighted the variability in the types of health service LGBTQ patients receive [22]. It is obvious that the barriers to health care are much more prevalent in TGNC individuals as opposed to gays and lesbians. About 70% of transgender respondents (sample of 5000) reported having had at least one of the following experiences: being refused needed care, not being touched by medical providers, subjected to harsh verbal language, rough physical care, and being blamed for their health status (Fig. 6.4a, b).

Health disparities among TGNC older adults are compounded by the barriers encountered specifically with access to health care, especially around financial resources. These economic disparities contributed to lower rates of health insurance or insurance that did not include coverage for appropriate medical treatment. Although the Older Americans Act (OAA) initially enacted in 1965 is supposed to provide support and resources for the aging older adult, there is uncertainty especially for the most vulnerable members, the LGBT at large [23]. With the ongoing debate to include sexual orientation and gender identity (SOGI) information in population-based surveys, the state of the LGBT older adult remains visibly tenuous. Although the Affordable Care Act (ACA) serves to allow for health care without discrimination, it is not clear whether medico-surgical interventions pertaining to transitioning are covered. This remains to be a work in progress. On the other hand, the Veterans Health Administration has taken steps for gender-affirming medical care [24].

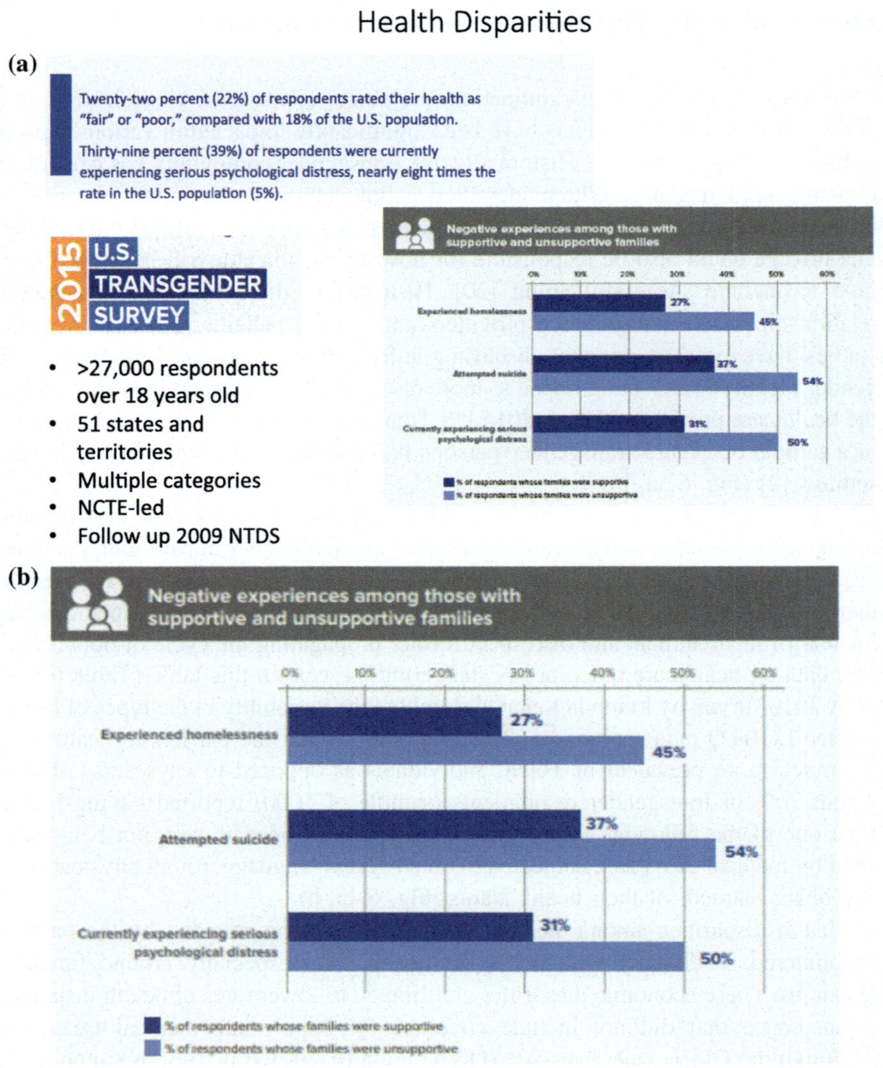

Fig. 6.3 **a** Health disparities affecting the transgender population. **b** Health disparities affecting the transgender population

Unique Healthcare Issues

In general, the health care needs of the older TGNC adults mirror that of their cisgender counterparts. However, there are unique aspects in this population that need more attention. It is essential to provide standardized nonjudgmental care for this population carefully considering some barriers to healthcare provision and access. TGNC individuals (as previously described) are subject to discrimination

Table 6.2 Health disparities comparing transgender with the general population (adapted, Hansel Arroyo MD)

Health disparities		
Risk	General population (NIH data)	Transgender
HIV infection rate	0.6%	2.64%
Incarceration	(4.9%/0.5%)	(21%/10%)
(Ever) homeless (Current) homeless	0.76% (NYC)	19% 1.7%
Alcohol or Illicit drug abuse	8–30%	8–71%
(Ever) suicide attempt	1.6%	41%

The national transgender discrimination survey 2015
National survey on drug use and health 2013
National institute of drug abuse 2016

and prejudice in related areas of education and employment thereby affecting their ability to obtain health insurance necessary for both physical and mental health services [25].

In interfacing with the older TGNC patients for the first time, it is important to bear in mind that individuals may be in various stages of transition. Therefore, "no one size fits all" in terms of how they may present or express themselves. It is helpful to begin the encounter with allowing the patient to take the lead in terms of disclosure of gender identity and sexual orientation. Address them using their preferred names and pronouns. Use open-ended questions such as (for a thorough history taking, as a provider): "I would like to ask personal questions pertaining to your sexual health. You may or may not be comfortable discussing this topic. However, I am fully committed to learning about you as a multidimensional person. Let me ask you about your gender identity, relationship status, sexual orientation, sexual practices among other things." It is also helpful to standardize eliciting this information through intake forms that will allow options for disclosure and nondisclosure. To enhance the experience of the patient in a clinical care setting, materials that pertain to the LGBTQ population, in general, may signify the institution's welcoming spirit and universal message of acceptance and commitment to serve this population. During the history taking, it is advisable to allow the patient to share their health concerns that may or may not be related to their SOGI information. In an ED study, patients actually wanted providers to ask them questions about their SOGI information. The EQUALITY study by Haider highlighted this point. In a sample of over 1500 patients and 400 ED providers, only 10% of patients reported the refusal to have SOGI information elicited. More than 2/3 of the providers assumed that patients will refuse disclosure of SOGI information [26]. In a similar study by Maragh-Bass looking at transgender patients, close to 90% felt that gender identity was more important to disclose than sexual orientation. Both males and females who identified as transgender reported that as long as there was medical relevance, they were both willing to disclose SOGI information [27].

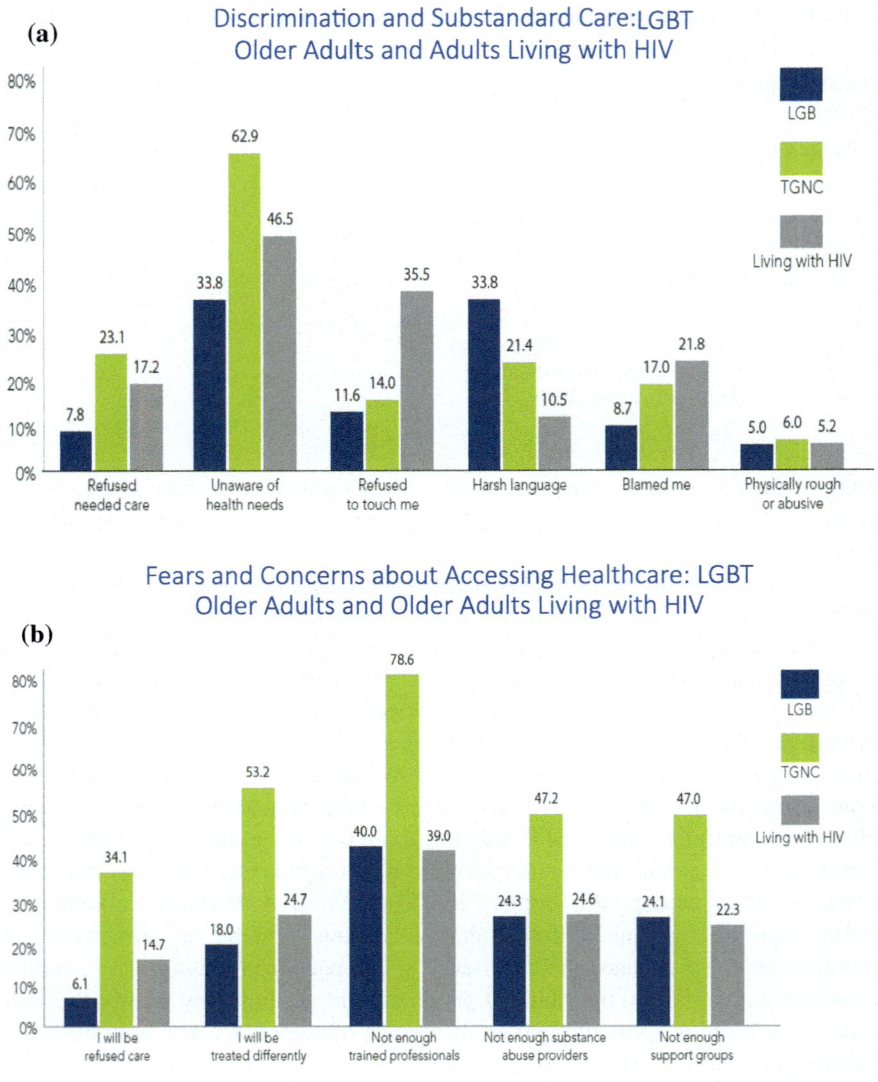

Fig. 6.4 **a** Barriers to health care for older LGBT people. **b** Health disparities toward older LGBT people

Another effective strategy in eliciting SOGI information during history taking is asking this open-ended question: "What would you like me to know about you so I can provide holistic and efficient care?" This is the dignity question phrased by Chochinov [28].

For the physical examination, one compassionate strategy to keep in mind is explaining to the patient why a specific organ system or body part needs to be examined. Additionally, for anatomical parts pertaining to their genitalia, one might consider allowing the patient to name the parts as they see fit. For example, a transgender female might refer to the penis as a bigger clitoris. Transgender males and females might refer to their vaginas and neo-vaginas as "front door". The recto-anal region is considered a sexual organ and is referred to as "back door" by both genders. A summary of these strategies is shown in Table 6.3.

Table 6.3 Culturally competent, inclusive, and affirmative strategies

Provider level (doctors, nurses, physician assistants, nurse practitioners, social workers, and medical assistants)	**Staff level** (clerks, administrators, front desk personnel, custodians, etc.)	**Institutional level**
Education and in-service training	In-service training	Creation of policies to foster respect in the workplace such as antidiscrimination, visitation, etc.
Proper greeting toward patients; use of preferred names and pronouns; use of gender-neutral language	Proper greeting toward patients; use of preferred names and pronouns; use of gender-neutral language	Operationalize forms to be transgender inclusive of SOGI information
Allow patients to share their story during history taking; ask open-ended questions Avoid assumptions and misconceptions; avoid inappropriate "outing" of patients and caregivers	As first point of contact with patients, ensure proper body language	Creation of a welcoming environment using flyers, brochures pertaining to LGBTQ
Be careful not to "out" patients who have a different mindset compared to young generation	Avoid misconceptions and prejudgments toward patients and their caregivers	Provision of gender-neutral bathrooms
Allow patients to name body parts during physical exam	Zero tolerance toward transgender patients by others; calling out people and advocating for this vulnerable population if prejudice were to happen	Zero tolerance for gender identity and sexual orientation discrimination
Ensure appropriate privacy in the exam room	Ensure proper record keeping with appropriate identifiers	Resources for transgender support within the medical system and outside communities whether online or on print
Provide appropriate resources for mental health, support groups, others …	Feedback opportunities on how well staff are treating patients	Provision of available medical and mental health services and resources within the institution
Offer to involve partner, significant other, spouse, "room-mate" in the clinical encounter if patient so chooses	Continuing education for all providers	
Open feedback opportunities on how staff will treat patients		
Continuing education for all providers		

Hormone Use in the Aging Transgender Patient

There are no set guidelines focused on transgender hormonal therapy for patients 50 years old and above [29]. As humans age, whether cisgender or transgender, there are normal and natural physiologic changes to one's biological hormones. It can be inferred that changes in hormone levels can alter the dysphoric response of transgender individuals. Depending on the stage of transition, the changes in hormone levels could either augment the dysphoria or improve its effect on the patient. For example, among transgender males, once menopause is reached either surgically or naturally, there is an expected decline in the estrogen level. These patients may have already started testosterone supplementation or just about to start this hormone if they transition earlier or later. If this were the case, then the patient might not need as much testosterone as opposed to the younger cohort. Significant monitoring for adverse effects such as polycythemia, liver dysfunction, and cardiovascular disease to name a few is integral. On the contrary, for biological men and transgender women who have not initiated testosterone blockers and estrogen it is known that by the age of 30 years and over, there is a decrease in hypothalamic–pituitary–gonadal function. Hence, there is a consequent 1% reduction per year in free testosterone levels [30]. The deficit in this hormone could lead to depression and cardiovascular dysfunction. At 70 years of age, adults (both transgender and cisgender/biological adults) have 10% of the dehydroepiandrosterone (DHEA) level produced compared to when they were 20 years old. The effect on the sex hormone production is also exacerbated by higher levels of cortisol in the older adult. A 2012 study by Tazaiux et al. showed sex differences in the infundibular nuclear structure for postmortem cisgender and transgender individuals [31]. Transgender females, for instance, exhibited female-typical structural difference in the neurokinin B (NKB) immunoreactivity system compared with cisgender males [30]. The authors concluded that as people age there is a robust female-dominant sexual dimorphism in the infundibular nucleus that in turn is thought to have an involvement in the feedback system of estrogen on GnRH secretion [30]. Although there is no set maximum dose for hormonal treatment, caution must be exercised, and therapy must be individualized. Moreover, patients who start therapy after age 40 will progress more slowly in terms of desired physical and physiological effects. Clinicians must be aware of the heightened risks for cardiovascular disease, bone demineralization, and venous thromboembolism (VTE). At a minimum, monitoring of blood work should include complete blood count, glucose, glycosylated hemoglobin, lipid panel, electrolytes, liver, and kidney function tests. Bone densitometry should be considered when patients reach 50 years old and if significant risk factors and family history are known [32]. Transgender men have a relatively preserved bone mineral density compared to transgender women. Nonetheless, bone density studies are still warranted in the former as the long-term effects of testosterone therapy are not definitely known [32].

Table 6.4 Risks associated with hormone therapy

Risk level	Feminizing hormones	Masculinizing hormones
Likely increased risk	Venous thromboembolic disease (VTE) Gallstones Elevated liver enzymes Weight gain Hypertriglyceridemia	Polycythemia Weight gain Acne Androgenic alopecia Sleep apnea
Likely increased risk with presence of additional risk factors such as age	Cardiovascular disease	
Possible increased risk	Hypertension Hyperprolactinemia or prolactinoma	Elevated liver enzymes Hyperlipidemia
Possible increased risk with presence of additional risk factors	Type 2 diabetes	Destabilization of certain psychiatric disorders Cardiovascular disease Hypertension Type 2 diabetes
No increased risk or inconclusive	Breast cancer	Loss of bone density Breast cancer Cervical cancer Ovarian cancer Uterine cancer

See table below for the expected adverse effects of feminizing and masculinizing hormones (Table 6.4).

The considerations for preventive and healthcare maintenance for the older transgender adult are depicted in the table below. These general guidelines mirror their cisgender counterparts with some exceptions (Table 6.5).

For more information regarding more specific details of medical management, refer to resources such as the World Professional Association for Transgender Health (WPATH) [33] and the UCSF Center of Excellence for Transgender Health [34] which have helpful guidelines to assist medical providers take better care of their TGNC patients.

Sexuality and Aging

Sexuality and intimacy are intrinsically important components on the full breadth of human experience. This is carried through aging regardless of gender identity and sexual orientation. Sexual health is an important personal goal for many individuals even at the point of facing a life-limiting illness. Patients with palliative care needs face unique challenges trying to balance sexual health needs and desire for sexual

Table 6.5 Preventive and healthcare maintenance general considerations

Healthcare maintenance	MTF patients, no surgery and no hormones	MTF patients, no surgery and on hormones	MTF patients, with surgery and on hormones	FTM patients, no surgery and no hormones	FTM patients, no surgery and on hormones	FTM patients, with surgery and on hormones
Vaccinations (Hepatitis B, Tdap, Pneumovax, Flu vaccine)	✓	✓	✓	✓	✓	✓
Breast cancer screening (mammography)	✓	✓	✓	✓	✓	✓ if with residual breast buds
Cervical cancer screening (PAP smear)	✓	✓	✓	✓	✓	✓ if with total hysterectomy
Prostate cancer screening (?psa and rectal exam)	✓	✓	✓	✓	✓	✓
Ovarian cancer	✓	✓	✓	✓	✓	✓ if with total oophorectomy
Colon cancer (colonoscopy, FOB etc)	✓	✓	✓	✓	✓	✓
Anal cancer screening (anal pap smears)	✓	✓	✓	✓✠	✓	✓
Cardiovascular disease (lipid testing, risk stratification, blood pressure checks, aspirin prophylaxis	✓	✓	✓✠	✓	✓	✓
Endocrine (diabetes, thyroid)	✓	✓	✓	✓	✓	✓
Hyperprolactinemia	✓	✓	✓	✓	✓	✓
VTE	✓	✓	✓	✓	✓	✓
Smoking cessation	✓	✓	✓	✓	✓	✓
Osteoporosis	✓	✓	✓	✓	✓	✓
Sexual health	✓	✓	✓	✓	✓	✓

expression with other underlying medical illnesses and disease progression. The aging transgender patient will have the same needs as the general population. Sex and sexuality are closely linked to societal role, self-esteem, pleasure, mood, and other components that affect the quality of life [35]. Much of the information pertaining to best practices in sexual health among older transgender adults are derived from the literature focusing on other sexual and gender minorities.

As one ages, the chances of having and developing multiple medical problems increase. The individual will also have to contend with taking numerous medications and complications from multiple diseases that will further affect the sexual drive of the patient. Natural hormonal changes as a consequence of aging as well as diseases such as hypertension, diabetes, peripheral vascular disease, cancer, urogynecologic problems, kidney disease on hemodialysis, and rheumatologic conditions are just some of the medical conditions that can have an overall impact on the sexual health of the patient. The anatomic and physiologic changes that come with these problems will have a bearing on the perception of body image and sexual function in various capacities [36, 37]. Consequent mental health concerns such as depression, anxiety, grief, and stress could lead to more sexual health issues for the TGNC patient. Complicating these issues will be changes to the relationship status of partners and/or caregiving ability toward patients. Relationship factors may include partner silence, emotional distance, and even actual abuse (verbal, physical, or emotional) [38]. It is therefore imperative for the healthcare professional not to overlook these issues as these may well affect the overall well-being of patients. Furthermore, clinicians may be able to give specific suggestions to palliative care patients and their partners on ways to facilitate sexual intimacy such as referral to appropriate sex therapists and other counselors. The details pertaining to sexual function and enhancement for TGNC patients who have undergone gender-affirming surgeries are beyond the scope of this chapter. One would need the expertise of plastic surgeons, urologists, sex therapists, and gynecologists in providing appropriate sexual health care.

When patients' diseases advance, sexual health is one dimension that should be considered in providing high-quality palliative and end-of-life care for as long as this continues to be of importance to the patient and the partner. Lawton and colleagues reviewed recommendations for best practice and techniques to enhance communication between patients and providers, engage patients and their loved ones in this process, and include considerations of sexual orientation in sexual health care [39]. In a supporting study by Stausmire, the approach to communication should be open and nonjudgmental and that selected language should be appropriate to any sexual dynamic including gay and straight relationships [40].

Clinicians can help limit barriers by maintaining a compassionate, open-minded, and affirming approach with all patients at all times and ensuring confidentiality, privacy, and high degree of professionalism in various areas of health care.

Aging Across Care Settings

The aging health concerns of the transgender population are not different from their cisgender counterparts. Their worries pertaining to illness and disability go beyond the management of their physical needs. Equally important is the accessibility and eligibility for higher levels of care including transitional care plans. Other determining factors to post-hospitalization plan of care include safety in the home environment, ability to perform activities of daily living (ADLs), and social supports at home and in the community. In a 2014 Transgender Metlife Survey

(TMLS) in which close to 2000 transgender individuals were surveyed, twenty-five percent (25%) of the respondents stated that they were extremely concerned or very concerned that, at some age, they would be unable to function independently because there was nobody to take care of them [20]. On the other hand, about thirty-six percent (36%) were concerned that functioning independently would be tied to the availability of financial resources [20]. Respondents in this survey ranked their list of concerns in order of importance, namely inability to care for oneself, becoming sick or disabled, becoming dependent on others, and becoming confused or demented [20]. After an acute illness has resolved or stabilized, there might be a consequential need for further functional recovery. This usually includes placement either in subacute rehabilitation or long-term care facilities. If patients are deemed safe to go home with enough support, this typically is the preferred plan for discharge. If not the former two will be considered as viable options to further optimize care.

When home is the first disposition plan, often times these individuals may or may not have adequate supports. If they do, their families of choice will serve as caregivers. Otherwise, they will rely on themselves primarily to stay in the home for as long as they are able to. The placement of additional services such as home care is a good strategy to mitigate gaps in care immediately post-discharge and their follow-up with primary care. Home care will provide nursing and rehabilitation therapist's visit to ensure that care needs are addressed accordingly.

Many older transgender adults who receive further care in facilities such as rehabilitation units and long-term care residences express concerns related to how they might be treated in those environments. The concern about mistreatment by staff and other residents is very real. It starts with their visibility as older patients who might physically present differently depending on their stage of transition and/or whether or not there has been hormonal or surgical manipulation. In addition, the sexual orientation of these individuals is variable. Therefore, these patients could attract outright discrimination and prejudice to include blatant mis-gendering, verbal ridicule, and physical abuse. Furthermore, the medical staff might not be equipped with the training and resources to provide the best care for these patients to include ensuring their safety and security. Transgender females might be roomed in with cisgender males while transgender males might be roomed in with cisgender females. Other factors that could come into play that affect both staff and other residents include cultural, religious, and economic preferences and considerations. Hence, if there are no policies or guidelines on the provision of a safe landscape for the older transgender adult, then there will certainly be gaps in the care with enormous impact on the well-being of the transgender patient. It is also essential to ascertain that this vulnerable population develops allies during their stay and/or be connected to individuals with the same interests who can, in turn, serve as a support group. After subacute rehabilitation, patients usually go back home or are transitioned to a more stable environment such as long-term care residences. If patients have the means to afford assisted living facilities, they continue to be governed by the same concerns that exist within any institutional setting. Much of the logistical aspect for post-acute care also has to do with the type of medical insurance the patient has as this becomes the driving force in terms of where they could be placed. A 2011 national survey on LGBT older adults in long-term care settings reported instances of abuse, namely harassment by other residents and staff, staff refusal to acknowledge a healthcare proxy form, staff refusal to use preferred name and gender, refusal to provide appropriate medical care, and wrongful transfer and discharge [41]. Furthermore, there are definite concerns for TGNC older adults to be subjected to heteronormative assumptions leading to bias and discrimination. TGNC older adults often feel compelled to de-transition and "going back to the closet" for fear of further victimization, oppression, isolation, and abuse [42]. In this 2011 survey, strategies were proposed to implement changes to the care of the TGNC residents in long-term care facilities. These include staff training, creation of institutional model policies to protect this vulnerable population, stronger advocacy ombudsman programs against bullying and prejudice, and better research studies on the needs and struggles of the population.

Advance Care Planning

It is a natural process for the aging patient that the type of care he or she prefers in the event that a chronic and/or a life-limiting illness happens, be known to the medical providers. Unfortunately, not everyone prioritizes advance care planning in their overall health care. In light of a paucity of robust family or friends, the LGBTQ population at large is making strides to make this a primordial goal in their health care. Much of this conversation should occur when patients are healthier. Primary care providers can certainly facilitate and coordinate this type of discussion in the outpatient clinics. By so doing, an individual's autonomy will be protected in the process. A 2012 study by Rawlings [43] reported that sexual minorities who live authentically are prone to much discrimination and prosecution, thereby calling to action a need to pursue advance care planning. Whom to appoint as advocates could depend on the availability of families of choice versus biological families. The MetLife study in 2006 cited that in general, one in four sexual minority participants served the role of informal caregiver to a sexual minority patient [44]. It is not known how many of them identified as transgender. Cartwright's study in 2012 identified some barriers to fulfilling advance care planning. These included a lack of knowledge of legal rights relating to end-of-life care, time constraints for advance care planning, patients' overall good health status, and the lack of recognition by the provider of the patient's gender identity or sexual orientation as a result of assumed heteronormative role [45]. Furthermore, an Australian study led by Hughes and Cartwright found that younger patients, people who were in the closet, transgender-identified participants, and gender non-conforming individuals were less comfortable in discussing end-of-life (EOL) issues with healthcare providers [46]. This area of importance could not be overemphasized.

Advance care planning pertains to the planning process of verbally and legally expressing and documenting an individual's preferences for care should he or she is

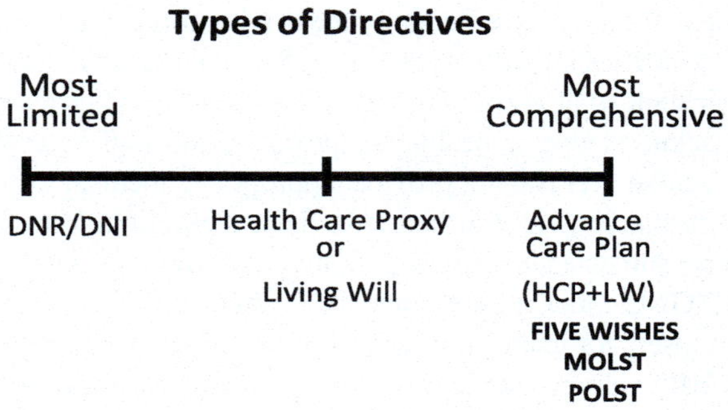

Fig. 6.5 Types of advance care planning documents

unable to speak for himself or herself and is facing a life-limiting or life-threatening illness. When translated into writing, this becomes an advance directive that could take the form of a living will or a healthcare proxy document or maybe even both or some variation of them (see Fig. 6.5). FIVE Wishes is a portable document that combines both and is honored in numerous states [47]. The medical orders for life-sustaining treatment or MOLST (also known as provider order for life-sustaining treatment in other states/POLST) are another portable documentation of wishes and preferences for care when faced with a terminal or life-limiting illness [48, 49] (see Fig. 6.6a, b). Both of these documents reflect preferences for specific interventions such as antibiotic use, blood transfusions, artificial nutrition/hydration, and resuscitation status. The healthcare proxy form or durable power of attorney form for health is a specific document that names an individual or two as designated decision maker(s) should the patient not have the capacity nor the ability to speak for himself or herself in the event that an irreversible illness ensues. These forms vary from state to state.

As is mentioned above, one of the challenges in completing this form is identifying an advocate or decision maker who knows the patient well. TGNC individuals are often ostracized from their own biological families inasmuch as there is now a secondary reliance on families of choice who are typically friends they have formed an alliance with over time. Additionally, the motivation to complete such forms also depends on how the primary care provider prioritizes this type of conversation. If the TGNC older adult does not have a primary care provider for various reasons, then this becomes a moot point. The ideal situation would be that both parties be proactive and held accountable for discussions around future healthcare planning to include end-of-life care. A study by Stein in 2001 noted that the majority of cisgender gays and lesbians had the knowledge of advance directives but that over 50% of them did not fill out a healthcare proxy form or complete a living will [50]. Although this study was targeted at cisgender sexual minorities, it would be safe to assume that the findings also apply to their transgender counterparts and more so because of a lack of disclosure of their SOGI information. Another challenge in these types of discussions is the lack of standardization. Some providers might be more detailed than others when discussing future care plans. Some will delegate the work to their social workers. Still, some will have the patient

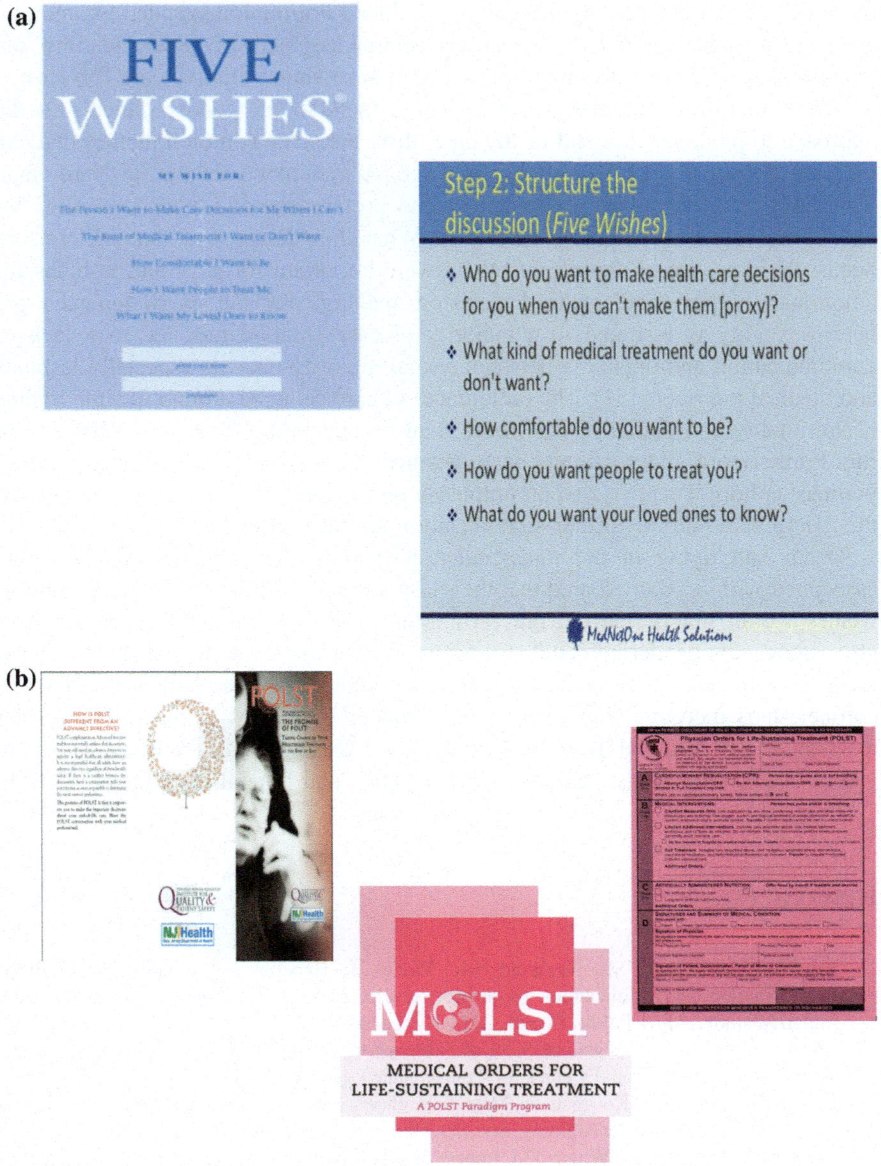

Fig. 6.6 **a** Advance care planning documents are depicted below. **b** MOLST forms are as follows

fill out the form with or without guidance from a medical professional and have these forms signed and submitted for record keeping. These can create uncertainty and insecurity from either party.

Cartwright in 2012 also highlighted complicated grief and survival gift for remaining partners [45]. In this way, the bereavement process is not acknowledged or perceived as legitimate by healthcare providers. For the transgender community, the lack of understanding or appropriate acknowledgment of gender identity and expression may cause substantial difficulty in accessing palliative care services.

While there are not many studies which include transgender patients in the approach to palliative and end-of-life care, there are some common themes that can be learned from the LGBT surveys at large. A systematic review by Harding in 2012 looked at the needs, experiences, and preferences of sexual minorities for end-of-life care and palliative care [51]. What they found was that in terms of needs, the presence of significant others were important for gays and lesbians for emotional support and medical decision making. As far as preferences go, heterosexuality is assumed in a majority of cases that in turn led to a lack of communication and openness between sexual minority patients especially lesbians and medical providers [51]. The preferences of care centered around the importance of spirituality and palliative care more than life-extending therapies at the end of life. Furthermore, older patients have advance directives in place compared to the younger cohort. There is also an emphasis on the avoidance of long-term care as this could be a site for further stigmatization and discrimination [51].

Death and dying in the transgender community has only anecdotal stories associated with it. Many feared that their last few days will be disrespected and last wishes would not be carried out [20]. Many are concerned that even on their gravestones mis-gendering could still occur. Furthermore, when a patient dies, what appears on the death certificate is in large part decided by the medical examiner or coroner. It is therefore important to have funeral directives in place. For further assistance, the National Resource Center on LGBT Aging has documents and videos that explain wills, social security benefits, and funeral directives [52].

References

1. Bradford J, Reisner SL, Honnold JA, Xavier J. Experiences of transgender-related discrimination and implications for health: results from the Virginia transgender health initiative study. Am J Public Health. 2013;103:1820–9.
2. James SE, Herman JL, Rankin S, et al. The report of the 2015 US transgender survey. Washington, DC: National Center for Transgender Equality; 2016.
3. Poteat T, German D, Kerrigan D. Managing uncertainty: a grounded theory of stigma in transgender health care encounters. Soc Sci Med. 2013;84:22–9.
4. Walker RV, Powers SM, Witten TM. Impact of anticipated bias from health care professionals on perceived successful aging among transgender and gender non-conforming adults. LGBT Health. 2017;4(6):427–33.
5. Fredriksen-Goldsen KI, Cook-Daniels L, Kim HJ, et al. Physical and mental health of transgender older adults: an at-risk and underserved population. Gerontologist. 2013;54 (3):488–500.
6. Witten TM. It's not all darkness: robustness, resilience, and successful transgender aging. LGBT Health. 2014;1(1):24–33.
7. United States Census Bureau. Population estimates. https://www.census.gov/newsroom/facts-for-features/2016/cb16-ff08.html (2014). Last accessed Apr 2018.

8. Porer KE, Brennan-Ing M, Chang S, et al. Providing competent and affirming services for transgender and gender non-conforming older adults. Clin Gerontol. 2016;39(5):366–88.
9. Flores AR, Herman JL, Gates GJ, Brown TNT. How any adults identify as transgender in the United States? Los Angeles. The Williams Institute: CA; 2016.
10. Espinoza R. Out and visible: the experiences and attitudes of lesbian, gay, bisexual, and transgender older adults, ages 45–75. Services and Advocacy for Gay Lesbian Bisexual Transgender (SAGE) 2014.
11. Parent MC, DeBlaere C, Moradi B. Approaches to research on intersectionality: perspectives on gender, LGBT, and racial/ethnic identities. Sex Roles. 2013;68:639–45.
12. Nadal KL, Davidoff KC, Davis LS. A qualitative approach to intersectional microaggressions: understanding influences of race, ethnicity, gender, sexuality, and religion. Qual Psychol. 2015;2(2):147–63.
13. Carroll L. Therapeutic issues with transgender elders. Psychiatr Clin N Am. 2017;40:127–40.
14. Aldwin CM, Igarashi H, Gilmer DF, Levenson MR (2013) Health, illness, and optimal aging: biological and psychological perspectives, 2nd ed. New York: Springer Publishing Company; 2013.
15. Van Wagenen A, Driskell J, Bradford J. I'm still raring to go: successful aging among lesbian, gay, bisexual, and transgender older adults. J Aging Stud. 2013;27:1–14.
16. Diewald M, Mayer KU. The sociology of the life course and life span psychology: integrated paradigm or complementing pathways? Adv Life Course Res. 2009;14:5–14.
17. Bonanno GA, Westphal M, Mancini AD. Resilience to loss and potential trauma. Annu Rev Clin Psychol. 2011;7:511–35.
18. Smith BW, Tooley EM, Christopher PJ, Kay VS. Resilience as the ability to bounce back from stress: a neglected personal resource? J Posit Psychol. 2010;5(3):166–76.
19. Porter KE, Oala CR, Witten TM. Transgender spirituality, religion, and successful aging: findings from the Trans Metlife Survey. J Relig Spirit Aging. 2012;25:112–38.
20. Witten TM. End of life, chronic illness, and trans-identities. J Soc Work End Life Palliat Care. 2014;10:34–58.
21. Grant JM, Mottet LA, Tanis J, et al. Injustice at every turn: a report of the national transgender discrimination survey. Washington: National Center for Transgender Equality and National Gay and Lesbian Task Force; 2011.
22. When health care isn't caring? Lambda legal survey on LGBT people and people living with HIV; 2010.
23. Adams M, Tax AD. Assessing and meeting the needs of LGBT older adults via the Older Americans Act. LGBT Health. 2017;4(6):389–93.
24. Johnson L, Shipperd JC, Walton H. The psychologist's role in transgender specific care with US veterans. Psychol Serv. 2016;13(1):69–76.
25. Puckett JA, Cleary P, Kinton R, Mustanski B, Newcomb ME. Barriers to gender affirming care for transgender and gender non-conforming individuals. Sex Res Soc Policy. 2018;15:48–59.
26. Haider AH, Schneider EB, Kodalek LM, Adler RR, Ranjit A, et al. Emergency departmental query for patient-centered approaches to sexual orientation and gender identity: the EQUALITY study. JAMA Intern Med. 2017;177(6):819–28.
27. Maragh-Bass AC, Torain M, Adler R, Ranjit A, Schneider E, et al. Is it okay to ask: transgender patient perspectives on sexual orientation and gender identity collection in healthcare. Acad Emerg Med. 2017;24:1–13.
28. Chochinov HM, McClement S, Hack T, Thompson G, Dufault B, Harlos M. Eliciting personhood within clinical practice: effects on patients, families, and health care providers. J Pain Symptom Manag. 2015;49(6):974–80.
29. Mahan RJ, Bailey TA, Bibb TJ, Fenney M, Williams T. Drug therapy for gender transitions and health screenings in transgender older adults. JAGS. 2016;64:2554–9.
30. Ettner R. Care of the elderly transgender patient. Curr Opin Endocrinol Diabetes Obes. 2013;20:580–4.

31. Tazaiux M, Swaab DF, Bakker J. Sex differences in the neurokinin B system in the human infundibular nucleus. J Clin Endocrinol Metab. 2012;97:2210–20.
32. Sherbourne Health Centre. Guidelines and protocols for comprehensive primary health care for trans clients. http://sherbourne.on.ca/guidelines-protocols-for-trans-care/. Last accessed 3 May 2018.
33. The World Professional Association for Transgender Health (WPATH). https://www.wpath.org/publications/soc. Last accessed 3 May 2018.
34. The University of California San Francisco (UCSF) Center of Excellence for Transgender Health. http://www.transhealth.ucsf.edu/trans?page=guidelines-home. Last accessed 3 May 2018.
35. Shell JA. Sexual issues in the palliative care population. Semin Oncol Nurs. 2008;24:131–4.
36. Bober SL, Recklitis CJ, Bakan J, et al. Addressing sexual dysfunction after risk-reducing salpingo-oophorectomy: effects of a brief, psychosexual intervention. J Sex Med. 2015;12: 189–97.
37. Chung E, Brock G. Sexual rehabilitation and cancer survivorship: a state of art review of current literature and management strategies in male sexual dysfunction among prostate cancer survivors. J Sex Med. 2013;10(Suppl1):102–11.
38. Griebling TL. Sexuality and aging: a focus on lesbian, gay, bisexual, and transgender (LGBT) needs in palliative and end of life care. Curr Opin Support Palliat Care. 2016;10:95–101.
39. Lawton A, White J, Fromme EK. End of life and advance care planning considerations for lesbian, gay, bisexual, and transgender patients. J Palliat Med. 2014;17:106–8.
40. Stausmire JM. Sexuality at the end of life. Am J Hospice Palliat Care. 2004;21:33–9.
41. LGBT older adults in long term care facilities: stories from the field. SAGE, Lambda Legal, and National Senior Citizens Law Center collaboration. https://www.diverseelders.org/resource/lgbt-older-adults-in-long-term-care-facilities-stories-from-the-field/ (2011). Last accessed 3 May 2018.
42. Arthur DP. Social work practice with LGBT elders at the end of life: developing practice evaluation and clinical skills through a cultural perspective. J Soc Work End Life Palliat Care. 2015;11(2):178–201.
43. Rawlings D. End-of-life care considerations for gay, lesbian, bisexual, and transgender individuals: case study. Int J Palliat Nurs. 2012;1(18):29–34.
44. Metlife Mature Market Institute. Still out, still aging: the Metlife study of lesbian and gay baby boomers. https://www.tandfonline.com/doi/full/10.1080/15504280903472949?scroll=top&needAccess=true (2010). Last accessed 3 May 2018.
45. Cartwright C, Hughes M, Lienert T. End-of-life care for gay, lesbian, bisexual, and transgender people. Cult Health Sex. 2012;14(5):537–48.
46. Hughes M, Cartwright C. LGBT people's knowledge of and preparedness to discuss end-of-life care planning options. Health Soc Care Community. 2014;22:545–52.
47. Aging with dignity: five wishes. https://agingwithdignity.org/docs/default-source/default-document-library/product-samples/fwsample.pdf?sfvrsn=2. Last accessed 3 May 2018.
48. POLST: advance care planning for the seriously ill. http://polst.org/wp-content/uploads/2018/01/2013.09.26_Final-POLST-Article.pdf. Last accessed 3 May 2018.
49. MOLST: medical orders for life sustaining treatment. https://www.health.ny.gov/forms/doh-5003.pdf. Last accessed 3 May 2018.
50. Stein GL, Bonuck KA. Attitudes on end-of-life care and advance care planning in the lesbian and gay community. J Palliat Med. 2001;4(2):173–91.
51. Harding R, Epiphaniou E, Chidgey-Clark J. Needs, experiences, and preferences of sexual minorities for end-of-life care and palliative care: a systematic review. J Palliat Med. 2012; 15(5):602–11.
52. National Resource Center on LGBT aging. https://lgbtagingcenter.org/resources/resource.cfm?r=569. Last accessed 3 May 2018.

Chapter 7
Mental Health Issues in Caring for the Transgender Population

Shervin Shadianloo and Richard R. Pleak

Introduction

Psychiatrists and mental health providers have been closely involved with the care of transgender and gender variant/nonconforming individuals. Gender development and sexuality are closely intertwined with one's core identity, course of development, individuation, and relationships with family and society. Any interruption or conflict in this dynamic can potentially result in emotional and familial dynamic changes which eventually impact one's mental health and can either be overcome by use of the individual's resilience or lead to psychiatric symptoms of distress. The rates of psychiatric and substance use disorders are higher in transgender and gender variant/nonconforming individuals than in the general population [1]. The course of transitioning requires in-depth evaluation of emotional health to assist with improved outcomes. In this chapter, we focus on the role of psychiatrists and mental health providers in caring for the transgender population.

S. Shadianloo
Division of Child and Adolescent Psychiatry, Zucker Hillside Hospital, Glen Oaks, NY, USA

R. R. Pleak (✉)
Division of Child and Adolescent Psychiatry, Donald and Barbara Zucker School of Medicine at Hofstra/Northwell, Glen Oaks, NY, USA
e-mail: rpleak@northwell.edu

L. Poretsky and W. C. Hembree (eds.), *Transgender Medicine*, Contemporary Endocrinology, https://doi.org/10.1007/978-3-030-05683-4_7

Understanding Basics of Gender and Sexuality

Terminology

Terminology related to gender and sexuality has been rapidly evolving over the last few decades [2]. What follows is a brief review of the basic terms and the differences in regards to gender and sexuality. Newborns are assigned a gender at birth often based on their external genitalia. The term *gender assigned at birth or natal gender* is commonly used and is preferred over *biological gender or anatomical gender*. The term *gender assigned at birth* is different from someone's *gender identity*, which refers to a person's internal feeling about their gender. Individuals may express their *gender identity* beyond the traditional binary of female or male and includes transfemale, transmale, agender (no gender), gender nonbinary (in-between female and male), or gender fluid (changing within a spectrum of genders). *Transgender* is often used as an umbrella term to encompass all gender identities besides binary male or female, and *cisgender* refers to having the same gender identity as the gender assigned at birth. *Gender role* refers to a set of actions (behaviors, clothing, and expressions) that society considers typical for a particular gender; these change as a culture changes. *Gender variant* or *gender nonconforming* refers to a person whose behavior and expression is not typical for a male or female in their society—for children, this often includes favorite types of toys, choice in role play, dress-up clothing preferences, and statements about their gender. *Sexual orientation* refers to who a person is romantically or sexually attracted to. This may be confused with *gender identity* and assumed based on a person's social *gender role*. Terms such as *heterosexual, homosexual, or bisexual* are commonly used but can be misleading and may be gradually replaced by terms such as gynephilia (attracted to females), androphilia (attracted to males), or others. It is important to clarify with patients what they mean if they use a term to describe their gender identity or sexual orientation such as "I am a birth-assigned female, identifying as gender fluid and interested in males (cis and trans)."

Gender Development

Children begin having an understanding of their gender around the age of 18 months old. This is often evidenced by the child showing choices of clothes, play, fantasies, or peers. These choices may be conforming fully, partially, or not at all with what a culture considers typical for the gender to which a child is assigned at birth. Young children develop gender identity and have an inner representation of its concept. The concept of gender evolves with a child's mental development, such as moving from a primitive and concrete concept in preschool- and school-age years to more complex understanding of cultural gender roles during adolescence with the formal operations of abstract thinking. Preschool- and school-age children often make friends with their birth-assigned gender peers and play with these peers including imaginary playing where they choose roles and activities generally matching their birth-assigned gender. However, some children may not follow this path and are known as gender nonconforming (similar terms include gender variant). The use of the term *transgender* for prepubertal children is problematic and avoided by many in the field, as gender nonconforming children may not grow up to be transgender adolescents. Among gender nonconforming children, some may strongly and/or persistently identify with the gender opposite to their birth-assigned gender.

The transition from prepuberty to puberty is an important milestone in the course of gender development physiologically, socially, and mentally. The body is developing secondary sexual characteristics and growing to adult size. Society often expects youth to take specific and binary gender roles as the brain goes through its stages of development to reach full maturity and abstract thinking. Gender identity consolidates throughout puberty into adulthood. Some children who never experienced gender nonconformity nor were gender variant will develop cross-gender identification and perhaps gender dysphoria during their puberty. Some gender nonconforming children will identify as transgender in adolescence, while others will identify as their assigned gender at birth (cisgender).

Gender nonconforming children who maintain (or persist in) their cross-gender identity as the other gender into their adolescence and adulthood are known as "*persisters,*" and the ones who at some point reverse (desist) to cisgender identification are known "*desisters.*" The studies of these children are limited and criticized for their sample size and methods, but a recent review of available published studies in transgender children shows that the outcomes range between 2 and 39% being *persisters* [3]. Most nonconforming children identified later as cisgender gay, lesbian, or bisexual, and approximately 30% identified as cisgender heterosexual. One criticism of such studies is that they included children who did not meet the DSM criteria for gender dysphoria or gender identity disorder and were gender variant with subthreshold symptoms. Adolescents, by Tanner stage 2 (the first physical signs of puberty), are more likely than prepubertal children to maintain their gender identity, and gender identity generally remains stable through their adulthood [3]. This should not be confused with "coming out," in which a person discloses their gender identity to others. Some transgender people may have suppressed their gender identity for several or many years for the fear of rejection, and may not come out until later in life.

The development of gender identity can be impacted or disrupted by incidents and issues related to one's mental health and developmental differences. Trauma, major mental health disorders, and medical illnesses can alter the normal course of gender development. Intellectual disability may leave a person in a younger mental age and can impact their conceptualization of their gender. Recent studies are showing that individuals diagnosed with autism spectrum disorder are around seven times more likely to report gender variance. However, the currently available data have not established an increased rate of gender dysphoria in autism spectrum disorder.

History of Diagnosis of Gender Variance in Psychiatry

Psychiatric Diagnoses for Transgender and Gender Nonconforming People

Magnus Hirschfeld, the German physician and sexologist active in the late 1800s to 1935, saw and worked with people who are now regarded as transgender and gender nonconforming (TGNC), and in 1919, he opened the Institute of Sexual Research in Berlin. He developed the terms *transvestite* (in 1910) and *transexualismus* (in 1923) for people who identified as the other sex. David Caudwell, an American physician and sexologist, was the first to use the term *transsexual* in English, in a 1949 publication, for people who desired to change their sex. Harry Benjamin, a German–American physician and sexologist, used the term *transsexual* in a 1953 public lecture. Benjamin worked with people who wished to transition to the other sex, from male to female or female to male, primarily in New York City. His expertise in this area led to his name being on an organization founded in 1979, the Harry Benjamin International Gender Dysphoria Association, which was renamed in 2006 to the World Professional Association for Transgender Health (WPATH). The term *transgender* was first established by the American psychiatrist John Oliven in 1965, due to the term *transsexual* being confused with sexuality rather than gender. *Transgender* became an umbrella term, especially in the 1990s, generally used for people whose gender identity did not match their assigned sex at birth, and who did or did not wish to or did fully or partially transition to another gender. However, the umbrella coverage for this term has been variably extended—for some, transsexual people are not included, nor are gender nonconforming or agender people. The use of *transgender* for children has also been controversial, due to the unpredictability of continuation of cross-gender identification from early childhood through later adolescence. The medical field did not embrace the term *transgender* until the late 1990s to early 2000s.

DSM (the Diagnostic and Statistical Manual of Mental Disorders) is developed and issued by the American Psychiatric Association (APA), giving criteria for psychiatric disorders. Prior to the publication in 1980 of *DSM-III* (the *Third Edition*), there were no psychiatric diagnoses specific for TGNC people [4]. In the medical literature in the 1960–1980, TGNC people were generally referred to as transsexual. Gender nonconforming children were often referred to as gender-disturbed, gender-disordered, or gender dysphoric. None of these categories had agreed upon criteria, and could be used quite broadly. DSM-III established two diagnoses primarily related to gender identity: *transsexualism (TS)* and *gender identity disorder of childhood (GIDC)* [5]. The revised revision, DSM-III-R, was published in 1987, and added a third diagnosis, *gender identity disorder of adolescence or adulthood, non-transsexual type (GIDAANT)*. Some changes to the criteria of TS and GIDC were also made.

The criteria for TS in DSM-III included the following (DSM-III-R changes are in brackets) [5]:

- Sense of [persistent] discomfort and [sense of] inappropriateness about one's anatomic [assigned] sex.
- Wish [persistent preoccupation for at least 2 years] to be rid of one's genitals (primary and secondary sex characteristics) and live as the other sex [acquiring the primary and secondary sex characteristics of the other sex].
- Disturbance present for at least 2 years [the person has reached puberty].

The DSM-III criteria for GIDC, with onset before puberty, included the following (DSM-III-R changes are in brackets) [6]:

- Strongly and persistently stated desire or insistence being the other sex [persistent and intense distress about being a boy and an intense desire to be a girl or insistence that he is a girl; or persistent and intense distress about being a girl and a stated desire to be a boy or insistence that she is a boy].
- Persistent repudiation of male/female anatomic structures or, for boys only, preoccupation with female stereotypical activities.

The criteria for GIDAANT in DSM-III-R included the following [6]:

- Persistent or recurrent discomfort and sense of inappropriateness about one's assigned sex.
- Persistent or recurrent cross-dressing in the role of the other sex, in fantasy or actually (not for sexual excitement).
- No persistent preoccupation with getting rid of one's genitals.

Major changes in the diagnoses were made in the DSM-IV, published in 1994 [7]. The committee overseeing this section made the decision to lump the three previous diagnoses into one diagnosis, *gender identity disorder* (GID), which was then specified for GID in children or GID in adolescents or adults. Objections to this lumping came from adults previously classified as transsexual and now with a "disorder," and from parents whose children with GIDC now had the same major diagnosis (GID) as transsexual adults, seemingly indicating a continuity in the disorder that was not to be the case for many children (desistance). The criteria for GID in DSM-IV included the following:

- Strong and persistent cross-gender identification,
- Persistent discomfort with his or her sex or sense of inappropriateness in the gender role of that sex, and
- The disturbance causes clinically significant distress or impairment in functioning.

DSM-5, published in 2013, kept the diagnosis as one, but changed the name to *gender dysphoria* (GD), with separate specific criteria for children and for adolescents and adults [8]. The committee decided to keep the diagnosis applicable to children, despite opposition from many critics and from human rights and political organizations which questioned the need for the diagnosis when no prepubertal biological transition was possible. Recommendations from WPATH and other organizations did lead the committee to make the individual's dysphoria about gender a necessary criterion (including changing the diagnosis's name from gender identity *disorder* to gender *dysphoria*, returning to the older term also used in WPATH's original name). Additionally, several other changes became helpful to clinicians and patients: moving the diagnosis out of the previously titled *Gender and Sexual Disorders* section in DSM-5 to its own section, adding a post-transition specifier (allowing proper diagnostic coding for people continuing on exogenous hormones despite no longer having dysphoria), and no longer excluding intersex people from possibly having GD.

The DSM-5 criteria for GD must last at least 6 months and require significant distress or problems/impairment in functioning.

- In children, with at least six of the following:

  1. Strong desire to be of the other gender or insistence that one is the other gender.
  2. Strong preference for wearing clothes typical of the opposite gender.
  3. Strong preference for cross-gender roles in play.
  4. Strong preference for toys, games, and activities stereotypically of the other gender.
  5. Strong preference for playmates of the other gender.
  6. Strong rejection of toys, games, and activities typical of one's assigned gender.
  7. Strong dislike of one's sexual anatomy.
  8. Strong desire for the physical sex characteristics that match one's experienced gender.

- In adolescents and adults, with at least two of the following:

  1. Marked incongruence between one's experienced/expressed gender and primary and/or secondary sex characteristics.
  2. Strong desire to be rid of one's primary and/or secondary sex characteristics.
  3. Strong desire for the primary and/or secondary sex characteristics of the other gender.
  4. Strong desire to be treated as the other gender.
  5. Strong conviction that one has the typical feelings and reactions of the other gender.

DSM has had additional gender diagnoses which included *atypical gender identity disorder* or *not otherwise specified* (NOS), and in DSM-5, *unspecified* and *other specified*. Therefore, people who meet some but not all of the criteria for a gender disorder could be given the unspecified or other specified diagnoses, such as *gender dysphoria, unspecified*. DSM also has diagnoses related to cross-dressing (in heterosexual men) with sexual excitation but not with desire to transition to the opposite sex, named *transvestitism* (DSM and DSM-II), *transvestism* (DSM-III), *transvestic fetishism* (DSM-III-R and DSM-IV), and *transvestic disorder* (DSM-5) [4–9].

Whereas the DSM is developed and issued by the APA, the International Classification of Diseases (ICD) is issued by the World Health Organization of the United Nations, although the process is also by committees of professionals, but on a global basis. ICD-10 was issued in 1990, and ICD-11 is scheduled for publication in 2019 [10, 11]. ICD-10 includes the diagnoses *gender identity disorder of childhood*, *transsexualism*, and *dual-role transvestism*, as well as *other gender identity disorder*. ICD-11 will have a diagnosis named *gender incongruence* (GI), with the specifiers *in children* and *in adolescents and adults*, and will move this diagnosis from the *Mental, Behavioural, or Neurodevelopmental Disorders* section to the section *Conditions Related to Sexual Health*, i.e., no longer categorizing this as a psychiatric disorder. In ICD-11, the primary focus of the GI diagnosis is the experience of incongruence between experienced gender and assigned sex, while DSM-5 emphasizes the distress or dysphoria related to gender identity [12].

The primary utility of medical diagnoses is for communication—so that one person understands a diagnosis essentially the same as another, across disciplines, across countries, and across cultures. Diagnoses have another utility, which is for coding and billing, allowing patients, medical professionals, and medical institutions to have insurance coverage and reimbursement related to a diagnosis. This has made necessary the continuation of diagnoses for gender identity issues requiring mental health care (such as therapy) and biological transitioning (such as blockers, hormones, and surgery). Despite criticism that nonconforming or transgender identities should not be deemed as disorders or abnormal conditions, these diagnoses help ensure that the person can obtain treatments needed and desired for transitioning gender.

Importance of Mental Health Care in Transgender People

Transgender and gender nonconforming (TGNC) individuals are at higher risk of mental health problems including suicide [1]. Social discrimination, stigma, minority stress, and trauma are higher than general population among TGNC people. The social minority and stress model in general populations have shown the effect of stress on mental health with increased risk of suicide. A 2006 survey of youth across the European Union showed that LGBT youth were especially vulnerable to social exclusion including discrimination and rejection from their families [13, 14]. In contrast, a review of studies from 2011 to 2016 showed that gender-affirming medical interventions and supported social transition in youth correlated with improved psychological functioning [15], and parental support has been found to improve mental health and quality of life in transgender adolescents [16].

Given the increased risk of mental health problems including suicide and the importance of improving familial support, psychiatrists and other mental health practitioners have a critical role in promoting and helping the quality of life and addressing risks in this population. In addition to their increased mental healthcare needs, TGNC patients who wish to go through medical transitioning and legal gender marker changes need letters of support based on a comprehensive evaluation of their gender and mental history.

Role of Psychiatrists

Evaluation

Evaluation of Gender

It is important for psychiatrists to create a neutral and welcoming environment to discuss sexuality and gender. A basic screening of one's gender is part of an overall psychiatric evaluation and should be offered to everyone regardless of the presence of gender nonconformity. If the screening indicates that the patient's chief complaint is related to being TGNC, the interview requires more detailed and in-depth evaluation of gender, adjusted to the current needs of patient. For example, a 35-year-old medically transitioned transman who is presenting with anxiety after his younger son is diagnosed with cancer may need an understanding of his gender transitioning and asked for his narrative to help understand his background better, while working with him on his depression, while details of his puberty or stages of transitioning may be less relevant or less appropriate to include in the evaluation. On the other hand, a 28-year-old birth-assigned man with severe depression who is not out but internally identifies as a transwoman may only feel comfortable to talk to you if, in the initial screening, you ask about gender identity, and subsequent to the patient's response, explore more details.

The following will review gender evaluation based on age and developmental stages. It is important to remember that evaluating gender in children and youth requires in-depth training in child development and mental health. We are hoping that by reading this section you will be able to incorporate gender development in your day-to-day practice, and provide in-depth evaluation of gender identity in patients in need of it.

Preschool-age children
Typically, preschool-age children have developed language skills but have primitive capacities to conceptualize, and gender is mainly known in a binary form. In many families and cultures, it is accepted that children of this age can show some cross-gender behavior and this is addressed within the family. However, this may become an issue when the child mainly presents with another gender's characteristics or identifies with or as the opposite gender. These children are often taken to their pediatricians who can play an essential role in screening the child and referral for further in-depth evaluation to mental health providers, preferably to an experienced child psychiatrist. The child may also present with behavioral issues, which may have originated or coincided with their development of being gender

nonconforming. Parents may feel ashamed of bringing this up until a medical provider finds it out in the process of evaluating the child. Based on the chief complaint, an initial screen of the child's playing preferences, peer choices, dressing, and pretend/fantasy play should be incorporated into the initial evaluation. It should include a comprehensive developmental and psychiatric history obtained from the parents and other family members. The child also should be evaluated by observation, with use of toys and having various gendered and non-gendered choices available to them to play. It is very important that the interviewer does not lead the play and remains neutral to allow the child present their true self and fantasies. This may be more possible in a long-term play therapy to further explore the child's inner world. Depending on the child's ability to draw, you may use drawing as well, using the draw a person technique and/or asking the child to draw self and family and then asking the child to describe the people. This may facilitate the child's expression of self and gender. Evaluation of family dynamics and values is essential and is discussed further below.

School-age children (prepubertal)
School-age children have more advanced language skills, provided they are on a normal developmental trajectory. Children often present in this age group with behavioral issues and may or may not talk about their gender identity, although there is a growing understanding of gender nonconformity, and parents may bring in their children seeking advice and help in this regard [17]. The child's cognitive skills can vary based on their age and how close they are to puberty. You may ask screening questions from parents and the child about the child's history of choices of play and clothes at a younger age, as well as current preferences, and use draw a person or self and family as a tool to explore the child's image of self. Younger school-age children may find it easier to express themselves in the form of play, drawings, and fantasies. The gender evaluation can be a dynamic process when a child engages in a therapeutic relationship with you for other mental health reasons, as the child may have suppressed their gender identification due to fear of rejection. If the child is presenting or found to be on the gender spectrum or identified as gender variant or nonconforming, you will need to evaluate their gender and the family dynamics more in depth. The evaluation may start with more general and developmental questions including the child's choices of gender role, play, and dress, as well as gender identity and what the family thinks of the differences and how they approach it. You need to understand what a child is thinking in terms of their future roles and gender. Some questions may need to be asked when alone with the child, and this can be decided case by case and based on the initial visit with the parents. You may also ask a child what their preferred name is or how they think of themselves. The choices that are gendered in society and schools such as bathrooms, lining up, expected clothing, locker rooms, haircuts, etc., may come up as the child or parent talk further about differences the child experiences. The feelings and distresses around differences are important to be recognized for further interventions, such as how the child or family reacts to requests to get a short haircut, or how persistent or distressing these are for the child or parents. Future

fertility is an important topic to be included in the discussion and must include the parents. The child's developmental stage may limit their understanding or ability to explore future wishes of having offspring.

It is essential to understand how the nonconforming features or identifying with/ as another gender impact a child's life and what the child's wishes and his/her family's are. We refer you to the diagnosis section to read more about diagnosis of gender dysphoria in this age as the criteria are more than for a postpubertal person. Appropriate diagnosis as one gets close to puberty is important for discussion of the options of puberty suppression once puberty starts, which will be further discussed in the treatment section (see also [18]).

The evaluation needs to be done using a very neutral approach, and often requires several sessions to understand the family's culture, gender roles, attitudes toward gender and sexual categories, and religious and traditional/cultural values.

The social transition of a gender nonconforming prepubertal child to the other sex is a very controversial topic due to the possibility of desistance. Such social transitioning often occurs outside the home and at school, and includes: (1) having others use the child's preferred name and pronouns, (2) the child dressing and engaging in play typical of their gender identification, and (3) using gendered bathrooms consist with their gender identification or other specially arranged and convenient bathrooms. If a socially transitioned child desists and later comes to identify with their birth-assigned gender, the child must then retransition to that gender, which could be difficult and pose risks for the child at that older age. These possibilities need to be addressed and considered when the child and family are in therapy, although many families are now transitioning their children without seeking therapy or advice from therapists and medical professionals.

Puberty and adolescents

As discussed in the gender development section, puberty is an important milestone in gender development. Confidentiality is a crucial matter in any age, and, in particular, in this age group, as teenagers may not have disclosed much or anything about private aspects of themselves to their parents. Confidentiality must be fully respected as far as safety issues allow. Documentation of the discussions is also very sensitive as parents technically have legal access to the adolescent's medical record in most localities. Premature disclosure of someone's gender or sexual orientation via the medical record to their parents can be harmful to the child, their relationships, and therapy. The diagnosis code of a gender disorder also can negatively impact a child as it is revealed through insurance documents to parents.

Gender dysphoria symptoms may have existed prior to the start of puberty or only start with the beginning of puberty with development of secondary sexual characteristics. Some adolescents do not realize their transgender identity until later in adolescence. It is recommended that gender identity screening questions be asked of all patients regardless of their presenting problem. If any gender identity issues are highlighted, a more detailed history needs to be obtained. Adolescents are reaching more abstract thinking and thrive for independence while they are still highly dependent and legally under the care and authority of their parents/

guardians. In screening questions, one may ask a teen about the start of puberty, how they feel about the changes, what they think of their gender now and in the future, and how they feel in terms of other people to whom they may be romantically and/or sexually attracted. Questions can be direct, with consideration and clear acknowledgement that there is no pressure to answer any questions even before you start asking them, and always in the context of clear expectations of confidentiality. The adolescent should be able to defer answers at any point and feel comfortable discussing these with their doctor. Often the gender and sexuality questions are asked in private, and confidentiality and privacy must be respected.

We strongly suggest asking every teen for their preferred pronoun and name, and also to clarify in what settings the teenager wants you to use them. Although the teen may use known terms to you such as "gender fluid," you should further clarify in a narrative manner what the adolescent means by them. An example would be: "I have an idea what you mean by gender fluid, but my idea may be different from yours. How does gender fluid apply to you?" In obtaining a further and thorough gender identity evaluation, especially in youth presenting with a chief complaint of gender nonconformity or being transgender, you will need to get a more detailed history of gender development. If they are out to them, the parents are an essential source to understand gender development, but if the teenager is not out, you may need to defer this to later stages of therapy.

Changes in secondary sexual characteristics, such as growth of the penis, hair on the body and face, and deepening of voice in birth-assigned males, and start of menstruation and growth of breasts in birth-assigned females, should be discussed to understand the adolescent's gender identity and the impact of puberty on the teenager's life. Puberty suppression to delay the early stages of puberty can be a very important intervention for a young teenager who is presenting with gender dysphoria. Therefore, it is important that these details be asked about and identified. Sexual fantasies, masturbation, and erotic dreams may also be helpful information to ask about to better understand a teenager's gender and sexual development, but it may take time for a teenager to develop enough trust to be open to talk about this. You may tell the patient that you would like to know about them if they are able to talk about any of these things to better understand them. In this process, if the teen is ready and open, they may talk about their plans or wishes of how they want their adult body to appear or how they wish to socially present in terms of gender. They may not have a clear understanding of what they envisage their ideal future sexual development will be. The chance for biological interventions to make changes in early stages of puberty is higher than later. It is important to understand the teenager's cognitive capacity to consider the pros and cons of these changes.

Legal changes of name, gender marker on documents, need for hormonal treatment, and wishes for surgeries may all be discussed in therapy based on what the youth is bringing up and where they are in their cognitive development. TGNC teenagers may be too eager, avoidant, or anxious about the steps of transitioning. At times, the use of drawing a path (known as a road map) from now to where the teen considers their ideal endpoint in order to identify planned milestones for the future can be very helpful, as well as leaving this path open to any changes as the teen grows and changes [19]. It is very helpful for the person to realize that there is not one path to transition, but multiple ways and possibilities. For example, TGNC teenagers are often surprised to learn that many transmen do not have phalloplasty, but may limit surgery to chest reconstruction as male, and may have hysterectomy and oophorectomy. They may also be surprised that some transmen and trans-women decide on no biological transition. These realizations open much wider the possibilities of transitioning for the individual to consider and decide upon. Although desisting is rare at this age, it is still possible and should be included in evaluating an adolescent's gender identity.

When the teenager is out to their parents, the evaluation needs to include identifying parents or legal guardians and getting a detailed history of the teenager's childhood from them. This may be delayed till the teen decides to come out to the parents.

The evaluation of sexuality, interests, and activities is also a very important part of gender evaluation, as these issues are in many ways relevant as adolescents start sexual activities. Gender minority teenagers are more likely to engage in high-risk sexual behavior than cisgender teenagers. Opening the conversation up is needed about type of interests, activities, parts of the body involved, and types of protection used. Often the question of "are you sexually active?" is vague and insufficient. We recommend that you start asking about who they are interested in and what kind of emotional or physical experiences they have had or wish to have. This may lead to further open-ended and specific questions. You may hear the youth using words that are unfamiliar to you or not fully clear. As earlier discussed, asking for clear meaning and narrative of what a youth is discussing clarifies the situation and helps with further future open communications.

Coming out and how to come out including the risks and benefits of disclosure are important to discuss to help the adolescent make decisions. The teenager must be the lead in this process. Aspects of fertility and wishes to have biologically related children are always an important issue to bring up throughout therapy.

In recent years, there has been growing evidence of increased autistic spectrum diagnosis concurrence with gender dysphoria [20, 21]. The evaluation of people with autism spectrum disorder requires more attention to interpret and decide on conducting interview with the patient's differences in processing and abstract thinking [22].

Younger adults (transitional age 18–25)

As teenagers transition to early adulthood and have legal rights to consent for their own care, the approach to their care may slightly or greatly change. As recently emphasized in the field of psychiatry, young adults during this transition age have different needs than adults past this stage. There is no definite age for this transition, but it can be clearly evidenced by emotional, cultural, and financial dependence on parents after finishing high school. Needs of younger adults can be similar to an older teen and understanding these dependencies are essential in evaluating and treating young adults. For example, young adults may be attending college and may be entirely or largely financially dependent on the parents; they may not have a job or only seasonal or part-time employment; they may live at home full time or at least during college breaks; and they may remain on their parents' health insurance. Thus, involvement of the parents is critical in the therapy of the TGNC young adult. Even though their gender and sexuality are more developed than in adolescence, the young adult may still be in the exploring phase and should be evaluated and understood with that developmental lens. They still may not be fully independent or able to or wish to determine and decide everything by themselves. In most families, young adults at least in part depend on their parents, and are expected to consult with their parents on major decisions. This needs to be understood as part of evaluation and ongoing therapy.

Just as with adolescents, in any young adult we recommend that the psychiatrist ask basic questions about gender and sexuality, always with the option that the person answers to the extent that they are comfortable. The questions may start from how they feel about their sexuality and gender, or start with "tell me more about your social and intimate life," or "I would like to ask about how your teen years were, and how the transition during puberty was for you." You may then advance to more detailed questions about how one identifies their gender, who they are interested in sexually, and what kind of sexual activities they have engaged in.

In a more detailed evaluation of a young adult's gender, similar steps as with a teenager may be discussed, but at this age, patients often have better formed ideas about themselves and plans for social and biological transition. Some may also have partly transitioned or be in different stages of their transition. Identifying the purpose of the evaluation is very important. In a general evaluation of a TGNC person who has transitioned and is seen for another reason, the detailed questions have to be tailored to the need of the interview. While evaluating an adult whose issues are related to gender variance and who is seeking help in the steps of transitioning, the evaluation will need to be more goal-directed and specific. The developmental history, puberty, secondary sexual characteristics, and type of dysphoria for each social or anatomical aspect need to be evaluated. Depending on where the patient is in their transition journey, you will need to further explore their wishes and plans. Similar to adolescents, young adults' sexual histories, risks, and issues related to sex need to be explored. These are all needed to help formulate a stepwise plan for future treatment. Fertility is again an important topic to be discussed, including all the ways of having children.

Coming out remains a significant milestone in each gender and sexual minority person, and as discussed in previous age groups, needs attention and care. Documenting the person's gender dysphoria diagnosis is an important issue, as it is necessary for referral for endocrinological and surgical treatments. This documentation may have legal impact on their employment and social lives. Since transgender people have no federal protection in the U.S. or in most states, or in most countries, the diagnosis of gender dysphoria could lead to the person being fired or excluded from the military or top security positions, or prevented from owning or renting a home.

Young adults with autism spectrum disorder (primarily those with what is commonly referred to as Asperger's syndrome) need extra attention and should be evaluated by psychiatrists with knowledge of Asperger's to understand their thought process and emotional regulation, as well as how this may affect their gender identity and transitioning [22].

Adults

Evaluating persons in early adulthood may be different than for young adults. They may now live independently, be fully employed, and have formed their own families and relationships. It is essential to be mindful of the possibility of gender variance in any adult in psychiatric evaluation and include questions inquiring about their gender identity and existence of gender nonconformity. For example, a cisgender man married to a cisgender woman with children may have cross-dressing interests or fantasies with or without identifying as a woman or as a gender different than male. As always, open-ended questions about one's gender and sexuality and intimacy may be the best way to start. In further evaluating TGNC patients, it is important to initially identify where in the course of transition they are, both socially and biologically. The plans, desires, and questions of a pre-transitioned or transitioning patient who is seeking help with further steps of medical interventions will need to be more focused on the transition. With a post-transitioned adult who is presenting with other issues, the interview needs to stay on track with the patient's chief complaint which may no longer be gender dysphoria. It is still important to understand their journey of transitioning.

As some adults do not come out to self or others until after they have lived in the shell of a cisgender life, one may need to include aspects of their social life in this evaluation [23]. Coming out in a stage later than youth or early adulthood may in some ways be easier, in that the person is no longer dependent on others and has less fear of rejection, However, in contrast, this may be harder if person has formed their social identity in a gender that is not matching their gender of identity, and now has more fear of rejection at work and society. Anatomically, it might be harder to change secondary sexual characteristics the later a person transitions. Despite this, there are many examples of people successfully transitioning in their 50s, 60s, and 70s.

In a comprehensive gender evaluation, one's childhood development of gender, reaction to puberty, the beginning of dysphoric symptoms, areas of dysphoria, and how they have dealt with these need to be evaluated. Wishes, dreams, fantasies, and sexual activities all are important to explore. Sexual health and type of activities also need to be asked about and understood.

Fertility is still an important subject to discuss. Steps such as coming out, name change, gender markers, ID cards, insurance, legal grounds, or job loss if they came out are a reality of a transgender person's life and need to be explored. Grief over possible and actual losses of relationships, marriages, and employment are very relevant in transgender adults' lives.

Older adults

With the growing public presence of transgender people and their social and medical transitioning, more older adults are coming out as transgender. Their evaluation requires an understanding of one's social life, the different risks and benefits of transitioning, as well as their cognitive capacities. The process of possible grief over changes or losses in relationships needs to be further evaluated, as well as the need for social supports as one transitions or wants to transition. The discussion about hormonal treatment may need more detailed collaboration with other specialties to evaluate risks and benefits of hormonal replacement or surgeries. Transgender seniors entering assisted living facilities or nursing homes often face discrimination, hostility, refusal to use correct names and pronouns, and even withholding of treatments. Working with advocates for transgender seniors is very important.

Evaluation and Diagnosis and Treatment of Other Co-occurring Mental Health Issues

A full psychiatric evaluation and diagnosis of different mental health issues are part of a comprehensive evaluation. Any psychiatric diagnosis can be found coexisting with gender dysphoria. The risk of psychiatric disorders and suicide is much higher in the transgender population and it is thought to be related to the social marginalization and trauma associated with rejections at early stages of development.

We would like to break down the coexisting mental health issues associated with gender dysphoria or variance in different categories to better understand working with gender variant patients.

Psychiatric Disorders as a Direct Result of Gender Dysphoria

Some patients report only anxiety or mood symptoms related to gender dysphoria. As their dysphoria is treated, their anxiety/mood symptoms resolve as well. It is likely that stress and difficulties adjusting to dysphoria are contributing factors and the patient's mental health vulnerabilities in coping skills result in these types of issues. These psychiatric issues are often not serious and are relatively easy to treat. They often are mild, likely can be justified in the context of gender dysphoria stress, do not need long-term treatment, and are limited to the period that dysphoria is increasing with the patient coming to terms with their gender and resolve with transitioning.

Psychiatric Disorders Coexisting with Gender Dysphoria but not Impacting Gender Development

Psychiatric disorders in this group are often more serious and can range from affective to anxiety to psychotic disorders, or any other diagnosis. The patient often presents with a course of a mental health disorder which needs more intense levels of treatment before, during, and after transitioning. The symptoms are beyond what can be justified as related primarily to gender dysphoria; however, these symptoms may not directly complicate the gender development trajectory or current gender presentation. Many or most of the patients seen in psychiatric settings fall under this category, and a thorough evaluation of their mental health together with their gender needs is required from the beginning and throughout the course of treatment. It is important to consider when it is safe for the patient to go through each step of transitioning, and how to manage mental health complications and side effects of hormones such as depression, mood changes, or relapse of preexisting mental health disorders.

Substance use is a serious issue that is also prevalent in TGNC populations. Based upon its severity, a separate course or full program of treatment should be addressed before, after, and/or during the process of transitioning. The impact of substance use on transitioning and the patient's functioning also need to be thoroughly evaluated and addressed. This must include assessment of use of nicotine products, which may impose higher morbidity for surgical procedures.

Psychiatric Disorders Which Directly Impact or Are Thought to Impact Gender Development

There are some diagnoses that can impact the gender presentation. Autism spectrum disorders (ASD) are suspected to be more common in transgender youth. The relationship between ASD and gender dysphoria needs to be studied more thoroughly. Their coexistence requires the psychiatrist or mental health practitioner to be familiar with ASD in order to better evaluate and assist the transitioning plan and to problem solve with families [22].

Another common co-occurring psychiatric issue is trauma. Trauma, including sexual trauma, may impact the course of gender development, and adjustment disorder and PTSD symptoms complicate exploring the patient's gender development. In these situations, it is important to know that trauma is highly prevalent and that being the victim of sexual abuse, although higher in gender variant and sexual minority people, does not have causal effect. The treating mental health practitioner should be experienced in working with trauma as well as with gender issues. Medical providers should be able to contain the traumatic experiences and avoid colluding with negative thoughts and shame associated with trauma.

If an eating disorder is present in gender variant and transgender youth, it may need to be treated first, before any medical transitioning occurs.

Rarely, a person may present with gender dysphoria as the result of a psychotic or cognitive disorder or complicated with coexistence of these disorders. Taking a thorough history in order to identify time of onset of gender dysphoria and whether it predated the psychosis, mania, or cognitive decline is essential. If the condition is treatable, it is recommended that the patient be supported in forms of social accommodation, but that no biological transitioning interventions be newly started until the patient achieves a stable mental state. If the patient presents with cognitive decline or deficit, their evaluation needs to include the course of symptoms, their ability to comprehend gender in depth, and how their life is impacted by their symptoms. It is essential to monitor the persistence of these symptoms.

The brief description in this section is only an introduction to understanding the complexities of the coexistence of mental health issues with gender dysphoria. Consulting with psychiatrists experienced in areas such as eating disorders, substance use, geriatric psychiatry, child psychiatry (especially for ASD), and so on, can be extremely helpful.

Treatment

Age-Appropriate Therapy from Gender Exploration to Transition Planning

Preschool children

In the preschool-age group, appropriate interventions are always nonbiological and can only be done with the parents'/legal guardians' consent. The consultation often is mainly with parents and follows with evaluation of the child. Family therapy with the parents (without the child) is very beneficial to help them address the issues, as the parents have a key role in the treatment. Their cultural beliefs and wishes are important and need to be addressed in maintaining or restoring the parent–child relationship. The therapist may initially need to identify parental emotions, wishes, fears, projections, identifications, and reactions to the situation. Parents may have negative or positive feelings which can lead to avoidance, resistance, and shame. In play therapy, children can explore their feelings, emotional and behavioral responses, fantasies, gender identification, and more [24]. The therapist will use age-appropriate toys, including those typical for different genders and gender-neutral ones, and let the child construct the play. The purpose of play therapy is often to address the child's other presenting behavioral issues which may be related to gender nonconformity.

The therapist needs to screen for child abuse, and treat trauma in all children by use of a variety of techniques, and may also suspect abuse or trauma in the course of therapy and help parents to identify the risks. In cases of parental abuse of the child, the involvement of child protective services is mandatory, and the therapist can help to advocate for placements which can be supportive of the gender non-conforming child.

Early social transitioning of the gender nonconforming preschooler may be an option if child is persistent and insistent in the gender variance, such as stating that they are the other gender, and if the parents express a strong acceptance and desire for it. Since in this age group children are developmentally at early stages of gender differentiation, nonconformity among preschool-age children is less socially noted or ostracized. This may alleviate the need for actual social transitioning, for example, in preschool programs. These children may never present to a gender specialist or even as gender nonconforming to their pediatricians, and are often taken care of at the primary care level. Some suggest caution in social transitioning in this age group as the rate of desistance might be higher than in older children. Detransitioning at a later age can be quite difficult for the child and family.

Legal changes of name and/or gender marker on some documents (nursery school identification badges) are possible in preschoolers but have to be done with much in-depth consideration, e.g., discussing with a therapist the risks and benefits, and considering possibility of desistance.

Advocacy is one of the important elements of treatment. Society, preschools personnel, and teachers may need support and guidance on how to work with gender variant children and how to avoid punitive responses to these children's wishes and nonconforming play and behaviors.

School-age children

As children age, their ability to benefit from individual therapy increases. The treatment plan with goals and objectives of treatment need to be laid out in the beginning of therapy after a comprehensive evaluation is done. The treatment plan has to consider the child and parents/family and the impact of society and environment. Children who present with gender dysphoria in this age group experience more distress with their gender dysphoria than younger children, and may present initially with depressive symptoms, anxiety, or other psychiatric issues. They may not be able to discuss their identity and feelings with their parents. The therapist may decide to start with family therapy, individual therapy, or (most commonly) a combination of both based on the dynamic of issues between child and parents. Family therapy is almost always necessary and has to be included in the treatment. These children need to have individual time and be able to share their thoughts, feelings, and questions about sexuality and gender.

In working with families, parents may express worries and shame, such as "the treatment is to change my child or push them to change to another gender" or "no one will accept him." The parental responses, coping skills, and anxiety, as well as values, shame, and a whole host of other emotions, must be explored. The therapist may initially provide a safe environment for the parents to share their thoughts and help to reframe them and work with them through support and psychoeducation. The parents may have negative or positive views about TGNC people, and the therapist can help parents explore these negative and positive feelings. For example, parents may think that it is their fault that the child is TGNC or may be angry about it and make hurtful comments toward the child. Other parents may be extremely concerned about the child's co-occuring psychiatric problems and may avoid discussion of gender issues. Some parents may feel worried that if they show their concerns they would harm their child. To compensate for that, they may push for faster transitioning. In each of these situations, the therapist needs to understand the dynamics and address them accordingly. For example, early confrontation of defenses may lead to disruption of treatment, and the therapist can use reframing to help the parent–child relationship. Psychoeducation about gender and sexuality is often required. Therapists should use available resources, such as peer-recommended books about transgender children and adolescents, to create more open dialogue and material for discussion within family (e.g., [25]). Parent support groups can be extremely helpful, especially those in which parents of TGNC youth meet and discuss their experiences. PFLAG (Parents, Families, Friends, and Allies of LGBTQ People) has such groups across the U.S. and in many other countries, and has excellent website information and links.

School-age children are more interested in talking about their gender, but younger ones may still engage primarily in play therapy and explore their gender most comfortably in their expression of their fantasies in play. The therapist can work on presenting the problem and, when child is ready, can open the discussion about gender. The method of therapy and coexisting psychiatric issues may require different treatment types but, in all of them, the therapist needs to be aware of how to look for gender issues and explore the gender with the child. As the child gets closer to puberty, their questions may also be more relevant to puberty and possible changes; fears of their body changing may become major symptoms.

Social transitioning and puberty blockers are two major interventions relevant to this age group. Social transitioning becomes more relevant and has to include the child's and family's decisions. Social transitioning can be occasional, part time, or full time. The therapist and parents need to review the pros and cons, including local policies and obstacles and possible dangers at school and home. There are data suggesting that social transitioning may benefit some children who are more insistent about being the other sex. There is also concern about children desisting in cross-gender identification after puberty and the impact of detransitioning if the child socially transitioned before [26].

Puberty blockers can benefit a young adolescent significantly by stopping further development of secondary sexual characteristics. WPATH's Standards of Care [27] and the Endocrine Society Guidelines [28] recommend starting pubertal blockers only after the child reaches Tanner stage 2. This treatment is fully reversible and provides the child and family time as the child grows and matures mentally before deciding to go with affirming hormonal treatment or to allow the body to go through its genetically determined puberty. It can save the youth future surgeries and stressful procedures to reverse changes during puberty. Therapists and psychiatrists need to familiarize themselves with the available information to educate the family and child about their future choices. An open discussion and information about this option before puberty is important. Discussion of how puberty blockers affect fertility is necessary before referring the child to a pediatric endocrinologist.

Pubertal youth and teenagers
Working with adolescents builds on the same principles as working with younger children, but with major differences. Adolescents often need more individual therapy, while the family also needs to be involved: therapy sessions can involve the family while also providing individual time for the adolescent. Providing a safe environment for adolescents to discuss their fears, wishes, and hopes is essential. It is crucial to develop trust and demonstrate confidentiality in the sessions: confidentiality is a key point in working with youth. Premature or unwanted outing of a youth may expose them to risks for their physical safety, mental health, and relational well-being, and negatively impact alliance with the therapist.

The presenting problem may be another psychiatric issue, and working on all co-occurring mental health issues is imperative. As biological transitioning becomes an increasing request in this age group, one must learn and reference the current guidelines [27, 28]. Significant coexisting mental health problems may be a barrier to the start of biological transitioning, but the full recovery from these problems may not be achieved after treating the gender dysphoria. TGNC youth may be seen in any setting, ranging from outpatient solo therapy to a multidisciplinary team treatment in a state hospital due to complex and severe coexisting mental health issues. Gender issues need to be carefully and affirmatively incorporated to the treatment, working with the youth and family and setting regarding social transitioning, pubertal blocking, or hormonal treatments as the youth brings them up. The discussion should be lead by them, rather than the therapist leading or enforcing progression to either transitioning or not.

The co-occurring mental health issues may be found to be the leading reason for gender dysphoria, such as psychosis or mania resulting in identification with other than the birth-assigned gender. In the course of an active episode, the treatment of the primary psychiatric diagnosis becomes a prerequisite before any biological transitioning is considered. Meanwhile, the treating team should provide a supportive environment and social accommodation to the patient's requests such as using preferred name and pronouns within the treatment setting. If the gender issues persist outside of the acute psychiatric episode or are unrelated or coexisting with these psychiatric issues, the therapist should formulate a plan that includes addressing gender issues. WPATH guidelines [27] state that the person needs to be in reasonably stable mental health before biological transition is started, especially before taking steps that are known to be only partially reversible or nonreversible. Involvement of child and adolescent psychiatrists in the care of psychiatrically unstable adolescents is crucial in making these assessments and stabilizing the patient's mental health in order to promote appropriate decision-making for biological transitioning.

Parental or legal guardian consent (often more than one person, especially with joint guardianship in divorce situations) is necessary before any referrals for medical interventions is done. One should assume that all biological and adoptive parents have equal rights and need to give consent unless there is a court decision stating otherwise. Mental health practitioners have a unique role to explore child and parents/guardians comprehension and emotional complicating issues in the process of referring to another medical specialty for medical interventions. Our work can explore emotions, motives, undiscovered defenses, vulnerabilities, and strengths to formulate a safer and more successful treatment plan. Education and informed consent are part of this process. Family sessions before referral, identifying legally consenting parent(s), working with all allies, and in rare occasions including child protection services or legal systems, are needed.

The Endocrine Society Guidelines [28] clearly states that a TGNC youth has to be evaluated by a mental health practitioner trained in both child and adolescent psychiatry as well as in gender developmental issues. Puberty blocker treatment may be started at Tanner stage 2 to provide more time for exploring the course of gender development and also delaying or eventually stopping the development of undesired secondary sexual characteristics. Gender-affirming/cross-hormonal treatment may be an option for some youth after in-depth understanding of this treatment, and when the adolescent has reached level of maturity to make a reliable decision. Most adolescents reach this mental capacity by the age of 16 years; however, there may be cases in which the adolescent can be started on estrogen or testosterone earlier. In such a case, a comprehensive assessment of the course of gender dysphoria, its persistence, as well as the adolescent's behavior and ability to process at a complex level should be included. There is some evidence that earlier biological transitioning may benefit the youth with favorable outcome in teenagers. Once the youth is referred for cross-hormonal treatment, there needs to be mental health follow-up for assessment of response and potential psychiatric side effects. Youth may require remaining in intensive mental health treatment as they start medical transitioning. The decision of how to formulate their mental health treatment should be individualized and include a multidisciplinary treatment team. In complex clinical situations where a youth is noncompliant with mental health or substance use treatment, there is a risk that medical transitioning becomes a leverage or reward to engage the youth in treatment. In these situations, an honest discussion with the youth and forming an alliance with them is an important step. It is often helpful to find an advocate that the youth can trust to assist in safe engagement in treatment. In some cases, young people attempt to buy hormones online or off the street and use them unsupervised, sometimes sharing syringes and needles, creating a risk for hepatitis and HIV infection. Exploring these risks and working with the patient openly is essential, and harm-reduction strategies are helpful.

Surgery may be discussed as the youth brings up questions and desires about physical changes, but referrals are done infrequently. Chest masculinization ("top surgery") is a relatively new field for teenagers and requires more study. At times, breast reduction in a transmale teenager can be extremely beneficial years before chest reconstruction as male. Reducing the size of the breasts for a young adolescent can decrease the teenager's embarrassment, the need for hiding the breasts (crouched posture, wearing loose shirts, reluctance to engage in exercise, and not going swimming), and reduced reliance on uncomfortable and potentially unhealthy binding. Some parents will agree to reduction in breast size for their transmale teenager before they are ready to agree to chest masculinization. The experienced surgeon must examine the teenager to determine if this is feasible, or if this will prevent appropriate and optimal chest reconstruction later. More major surgeries such as vaginoplasty or hysterectomy are irreversible steps, requiring a high level of care, and are extremely rare to consider below the age of 18.

Young adults

Young adults may have gained some independence or may still be fully or partially dependent on their parents. Including families in evaluating and treating young adults should be done when possible, and improving family–youth relationships can be achieved through family therapy. Treatment goals are similar to those for older teenagers, with gradually moving to more mature stages. A young adult who may be a college student or an independent working person has often already formed their outside relationships and some financial independence. Their mental health issues are more crystallized and the need for an appropriate mental health level of care before, during, and after medical transitioning should be included in treatment planning.

Depending on where in the course of their transitioning they are, young adults may request and require referral for gender-affirming hormonal treatment or surgeries. Pubertal blocking alone is no longer an option if the person has fully developed secondary sexual characteristics; however, it is often helpful prior to cross-sex hormone treatment to reduce the endogenous testosterone or estrogen, decreasing the need for higher cross-sex hormone doses to achieve the desired results. This also allows for assessment and management of possible psychiatric side effects, such as (increased) depression. Fertility desires and discussion about these are essential, and adult patients may be more interested in this than younger patients. Sperm or egg freezing or planning for pregnancies or fertilization before or after hormonal transitioning should be discussed with patients. Transmen who are on hormonal treatment and still have their ovaries may remain fertile and become pregnant. Anecdotally, it has been reported of growing number of transmen who have delayed or stopped puberty blockers and testosterone in order to carry a baby and give birth. Contraception, sexual health, and sexual safety should be part of ongoing treatment plans. Surgeries are possible if a patient wishes to address particular areas of gender dysphoria such as the chest, gonads, and/or genitalia.

Starting hormonal treatment may impact the course of a previously stabilized mental disorder such as an affective disorder. It is important for the psychiatrist to follow these patients closely and adjust their therapy and psychiatric medications accordingly, and consult with the endocrinologist. Similar to teens, one may need for separate mental health clinicians working on coexisting psychiatric problems to liaise with the gender treating team.

Adults and older adults

Adults have reached their maximum mental capacity and maturity. Coexisting mental health issues are also mostly known by adulthood, and the prognosis or impact on one's capacity or decision-making is known. Adults may be more independent but at the same time may have fewer people involved in their lives to assist them in the course of their medical transitioning. Some gender clinics have used the informed consent model of treatment in which a consenting adult can choose to start medical transitioning without mental health involvement. Alternatively, some gender clinics believe that the complexity of mental health issues and high need for mental health care in many TGNC patients warrant mental health evaluation and ongoing psychiatric care as needed prior to biological transitioning.

After the initial evaluation, the goals of treatment and plans for transitioning should be identified. The treatment plan will vary depending upon the status on the person's path of transitioning. A patient may be in the very beginning steps and need more help and focus in coming out. Another person may wish to proceed with medical transitioning, including hormonal treatment or surgeries. Fertility, contraception, and sexual health once again are important topics to discuss and include in the treatment plan.

Risk reduction—including medical, sexual, and substance use—should be addressed and included in the treatment plan. Adults are at higher risk of cardiovascular and thrombotic disorders as well as cancers that can be increased with the start of hormonal treatment. These risks can be further increased by smoking, obesity, and coexisting mental health disorders and treatment with some psychiatric medications.

Adults with intellectual disability, developmental disorders, autism spectrum disorders, and cognitive changes, based on their severity, may need more in-depth evaluation and working/consult with someone particularly experienced in that field [22].

Late onset mental health issues, cognitive decline, or geriatric problems need to be further managed accordingly in older TGNC adult populations.

Post-transitioned adults and older TGNC adults are a growing population and may have different mental health needs than young TGNC patients. Intimacy, social isolation, rejection, mental health disorders due to the trauma, and stress of being a gender minority, as well as substance use, are important issues in this age group. Although desistance and detransitioning are rare, they may happen, and because this can impose more stress on an individual, the psychiatrist or mental health practitioner should be aware of this possibility. For example, some older adults find less need or desire to remain on their exogenous testosterone or estrogen—the possible changes that may result can be discussed and planned for in therapy.

Working with Families and Conflict Resolution

As mentioned in earlier sections, working with families is often an essential step in working with TGNC patients. Supportive families may reduce risk of mental health issues in this population.

In a child or adolescent, parents or legal guardians, siblings, and extended family such as grandparents need to be included in the treatment. Family therapy may be added to individual therapy whether in separate sessions or divided time in one appointment. When the issues are complicated, a family therapist may be needed to address the family dynamics and work closely with the primary therapist.

The TGNC person almost always knows about their gender identity before their family does. This may mean that their family needs more time than the TGNC patient wishes. The family's emotional responses are at times similar to grief stages, such as denial, anger, and loss, and can be worked on through that lens to reach acceptance and advocacy. In working with families, a therapist may note identification, guilt, shame, or a number of other reactions in the family. In younger and more vulnerable patients, exploring colluding factors and agendas is necessary, such as a family or social group that is invested in or against transitioning more than the patient is. Anger and frustration are common feelings in this process, and a family therapist can help identify and work on these. Aggression can be disguised in a loving language but still carry hurtful passive-aggressive comments. Although not always necessary, there are interview techniques and questionnaires for families that can help them to identify their microaggressive actions. Psychiatrists and other therapists familiar with these issues can help the family work on them.

In adults who have formed their own families and may have their own children or spouses, it is necessary to discuss who to include in the treatment planning. The goal of this treatment needs to be clear to all parties, but often needs to be focused on repairing or maintaining support and relationships in the course of transitioning. At times, post-transitioned adults may wish to work on their family relations if it was not possible in the course of transitioning. All these can be discussed and planned accordingly with all relevant parties. Not all marriages and relationships fall apart as the person transitions: some do, while most continue but change substantially in many ways. This can be anticipated, addressed, and helped with closure and grief processes in therapy.

Referral Letters

Medical transitioning including hormonal and surgical interventions are almost always performed after obtaining referral and clearance letters or recommendation from psychiatrists or mental health practitioners. With the growing need of caring for transgender patients, there is a growing demand for evaluation and referrals as well. Insurance companies often mandate letters of "clearance" for people who are seeking medical transitioning treatments. These letters are important and a sensitive part of evaluation in assisting safe and thoughtfully processed medical transitioning.

A referral letter should be provided by a mental health practitioner who is trained in diagnosing mental health as well as gender-related issues. In working with youth, the person must be trained in child and adolescent mental health. The letter is to confirm the diagnosis of gender dysphoria, any co-occurring mental health diagnoses, document their impact on the patient's mental health, the stability or risks of destabilizing the patient's mental health, address the patient's capacity for consent and/or the parents' or legal guardians' ability to make appropriate decisions, and discuss potential risks and benefits of treatment, as well as reversibility or irreversibility of each step. The letter also must state the psychiatrist's recommendation for or against the proposed medical treatment. Based on these factors, a psychiatrist needs to comment if it is a medical necessity for the patient to receive this treatment.

We recommend that the referral letter at least has:

1. Opening paragraph of your credentials and in what capacity you have evaluated the patient and for how long you have seen the patient.
2. Who the patient is (use their preferred name and gender and also document their legal name and birth-assigned gender).
3. Documentation of the DSM-5 diagnosis of gender dysphoria (required for proper procedure coding by the endocrinologist or surgeon).
4. A description of how long the person has identified as the other sex and how the patient has transitioned so far.
5. A brief report of mental health stability, social history, and current status.
6. The patient's capacity for consent.
7. A brief but related report of symptoms of gender-related issues and developmental history.
8. Summary of the case and discussion of risks and benefits, including fertility issues/desires, and the medical necessity for this treatment referral.
9. Any risk to mental health and who will handle complications in that case.
10. Your recommendation.

Some legal letters, such as referral for gender marker change, need to have very specific language and can only be written if you have a doctor–patient relationship to attest that you certify the diagnosis and the patient is in the process of transitioning to the new gender. Such language can be found on websites like those of the U.S. Department of State (for U.S. passports) or the state that a person was born in (for birth certificate changes in the U.S.).

Advocating for Care and Parity

Disparities and Barriers to Care of TGNC People

The health care of TGNC people is greatly disparate from people who are not sexual or gender minorities. TGNC people often face obstacles in terms of unequal protection by nondiscrimination laws, problems of access to general and gender-related health care, and societal discrimination and rejection [29]. They face societal stigma and discrimination, which negatively affects their health and marginalizes their health care. Anti-transgender bias creates stigma, which maintains inequalities in health care and reinforces excessive medical authority during patient encounters [30]. TGNC people continue to suffer unjust health disparities in multiple areas [31–33]. These disparities in the U.S. and in many countries include a lack of civil rights and increased risks for rejection, bullying, homelessness, sexually transmitted infections (including HIV), suicide, and murder [34]. In a major national survey [31], TGNC people revealed increased rates of catastrophic discrimination (23%), suicidality (41%, compared to 1.6% in the general population), denial of medical service due to bias (19%), harassment in medical settings (28%), postponing or avoiding medical treatment when they were sick or injured (28%), and delaying or not trying to get preventive health care (33%). TGNC patients may not disclose their gender identity and their transition status to their healthcare providers, which could result in inappropriate care and harm. Even with attempts to include diverse gender identity descriptors (not just male or female) in healthcare records and/or documentation of organs that people have or had removed (organ inventories), TGNC people may choose not to disclose this information due to a rational fear of discrimination.

An error in the opposite direction occurs if advocates for optimal health care for TGNC people become so zealous in attempts to achieve that goal that they may go overboard and extend care and recommendations far past evidence-based medicine. This may be seen in going substantially beyond generally accepted guidelines such as those from WPATH [27] and the Endocrine Society [28]. Such beyond-the-guidelines care may be unintentionally harmful, and is best considered in the context of and consultation with a multidisciplinary team.

Responsible, Affirming, and Appropriate Care of TGNC People

Responsible, affirming, and appropriate health care of TGNC people in Western cultures began in the modern era, primarily in Germany with Magnus Hirschfeld's Institute of Sexual Research in Berlin from 1919 until 1933, when it was closed down by the Nazis. Harry Benjamin was the first major figure in the United States to openly help and care for TGNC people, from 1948 to 1975 at his age of 90. Other prominent U.S. clinicians and researchers advocating early on for TGNC people (starting in the 1960s) included psychologists such as John Money, Anke Ehrhardt, and Heino Meyer-Bahlburg, and psychiatrists such as Richard Green and Jack Drescher. Even with these pioneer health advocates, care for TGNC people in the U.S. and in most countries was isolated and sparse, and remains inadequate now. Many other providers have become involved in TGNC care since the 1980s, especially since 2011. In 2011, the Institute of Medicine issued a highly influential report on the health of LGBT people, charging that the U.S. is far behind in knowledge, research, and health provisions for LGBT people [35]. In the same year, the Joint Commission issued a clarion call for equal care of LGBT people, requiring that U.S. healthcare organizations develop or adopt a nondiscrimination policy that protects patients from discrimination based on personal characteristics, including sexual orientation and gender identity or expression [36]. These two 2011 reports heralded a major change in addressing the healthcare needs of LGBT people.

Around the same time, there was a growing recognition and protection of the rights of LGBT people, which continues to expand and/or contract, depending on political and cultural changes locally and nationally.

Clinicians can be most helpful and work toward the goals of being responsible, affirming, and appropriate healthcare providers in part by referencing and following evidence-based guidelines, particularly the WPATH Standards of Care [27] and the Endocrine Society Clinical Practice Guideline [28], both of which strongly recommend mental health assessment and treatment, and require mental stability of the patient before proceeding with nonreversible biological transitioning. Mental health evidence reviews and guidelines have also been recently developed, such as the LGBT youth practice parameter by the American Academy of Child & Adolescent Psychiatry [37], the report of the American Psychiatric Association on GID [38], and the American Psychological Association's 2015 Guidelines [39]. Mental health providers who are working with TGNC people should be familiar with and use these references, along with scholarly texts such as those by Levonis et al. [40], Pleak [19], and Yarbrough [41], and more general books such as those by Nealy [25] and Erickson-Schroth [42]. It can be very valuable and therapeutically affirming to review these books, articles, and websites together with patients, family, and significant others in sessions and to suggest and/or assign readings from them between sessions. Other resources to review in sessions include websites of support organizations (e.g., the Trevor Project, www.trevorproject.org, which provides a 24-hour national suicide hotline), parent and family organizations (e.g., Parents, Families, Friends, and Allies of LGBT people, www.pflag.org), and local TGNC youth and adult groups.

It is ideal for mental health providers working with TGNC people to belong to organizations such as WPATH, and, when possible, to attend conferences to learn about advances in transgender care. Transgender-affirming policy statements of major professional organizations (e.g., www.aacap.org, www.psychiatry.org) are of great help to refer to and quote when needing to appeal insurance denials or confront those who refuse a transgender person's desire to transition, or those who propose "conversion" or "reparative" approaches to change transgender identification. Understanding and actively addressing the healthcare disparities that TGNC patients encounter is a key component in helping them.

Therapists should consult with colleagues including endocrinologists, surgeons, pediatricians, family physicians, voice therapists, and other providers of care for TGNC people, even if they are based far away, in order to provide the best information and referrals for patients, for both general care and specialized care. Working with teams of providers, whether in person or by online or phone conferences, decreases the isolation that many therapists (and their patients) experience, and increases awareness and the knowledge base of all involved. In these ways, we can do our best in providing the most responsible, affirming, and appropriate mental health care for our TGNC patients. Advancing transgender identity affirmation for ultimate emotional well-being should be the primary overall goal for the therapist and patient [43]. Working together to achieve this goal is a journey that encompasses persevering over disparities and barriers to care, overcoming discrimination and fostering safety, expansion of knowledge and expectations, and joint learning and discovery [29].

References

1. Bockting WO, Miner MH, Swinburne Romine RH, Hamilton A, Coleman E. Stigma, mental health, and resilience in an online sample of the US transgender population. Am J Public Health. 2013;103(5):943–51.
2. Pleak RR. Gender identity issues in youth: opportunities, terminologies, histories, and advancements. In: Pleak RR, editor. Gender variant children and transgender adolescents. Child Adolesc Psychiatr Clin N Am. 2011;20(4):601–25.
3. Turban J, Shadianloo, S. Transgender and gender nonconforming youth. In: IACAPAP textbook of child and adolescent mental health, chapter H.3. 2018.
4. American Psychiatric Association. Diagnostic and statistical manual of mental disorders, second edition, DSM-II. Washington, DC: American Psychiatric Association; 1968.
5. American Psychiatric Association. Diagnostic and statistical manual of mental disorders, third edition, DSM-III. Washington, DC: American Psychiatric Association; 1980.
6. American Psychiatric Association. Diagnostic and statistical manual of mental disorders, third edition, revised, DSM-III-R. Washington, DC: American Psychiatric Association; 1987.
7. American Psychiatric Association. Diagnostic and statistical manual of mental disorders, fourth edition, DSM-IV. Washington, DC: American Psychiatric Association; 1994.
8. American Psychiatric Association. Diagnostic and statistical manual of mental disorders, fifth edition, DSM-5. Washington, DC: American Psychiatric Publishing; 2013.
9. American Psychiatric Association. Diagnostic and statistical manual of mental disorders, with special supplement on plans for revision. Washington, DC: American Psychiatric Association; 1965.
10. World Health Organization. International classification of diseases, 10th revision, ICD-10. Geneva: World Health Organization; 1990. Available at: http://www.who.int/classifications/icd/en/. Accessed 30 Apr 2018.
11. World Health Organization. International classification of diseases, 11th revision, ICD-11. Geneva: World Health Organization; 2018. Available at: https://icd.who.int/dev11. Accessed 30 Apr 2018.
12. Reed M, Drescher J, Krueger RB, Atalla E, Cochran SD, First MB, Cohen-Kettenis PT, Arango-de Montis I, Parish SJ, Cottler S, Briken P, Saxena S. Disorders related to sexuality and gender identity in the ICD-11: revising the ICD-10 classification based on current scientific evidence, best clinical practices, and human rights considerations. World Psychiatry. 2016;15(3):205–21. https://doi.org/10.1002/wps.20354.
13. Takács J. Social exclusion of young lesbian, gay, bisexual and transgender (LGBT) people in Europe. Brussels: ILGA-Europe; 2006.
14. European Union lesbian, gay, bisexual and transgender survey. European Union for Fundamental Rights, survey results 2013.
15. Connolly MD, Zervos MJ, Barone CJ 2nd, Johnson CC, Joseph CL. The mental health of transgender youth: advances in understanding. J Adolesc Health. 2016;59(5):489–95.
16. Simons L, Schrager SM, Clark LF, Belzer M, Olson J. Parental support and mental health among transgender adolescents. J Adolesc Health. 2013;53(6):791–3.
17. Ristori J, Steensma TD. Gender dysphoria in childhood. Int Rev Psychiatry. 2016;28:13–20.
18. Cohen-Kettenis PT, Pfäfflin F. Transgenderism and intersexuality in childhood and adolescence: making choices. London: Sage; 2003.

19. Pleak RR, editor. Gender variant children and transgender adolescents. Child Adolesc Psychiatr Clin N Am. 2011;20(4).
20. Janssen A, Huang H, Duncan C. Gender variance among youth with autism spectrum disorders: a retrospective chart review. Transgender Health. 2016;1(1):63–8. https://doi.org/10.1089/trgh.2015.0007.
21. Turban J, van Schwalkwyk GI. "Gender dysphoria" and autism spectrum disorder: is the link real? J Am Acad Child Adolesc Psychiatry. 2018;57(1):8–9.e2.
22. Strang JF, Meagher H, Kenworthy L, de Vries ALC, Menvielle E, Leibowitz S, Janssen A, Cohen-Kettenis P, Shumer DE, Edwards-Leeper L, Pleak RR, Spack N, Karasic DH, Schreier H, Balleur A, Tishelman A, Ehrensaft D, Rodnan L, Kuschner ES, Mandel F, Caretto A, Lewis HC, Anthony LG. Initial clinical guidelines for co-occurring autism spectrum disorder and gender dysphoria or incongruence in adolescents. J Clin Child Adolesc Psychol. 2016;47(1):105–15. https://doi.org/10.1080/15374416.2016.1228462.
23. Bockting W, Coleman E, Deutsch MB, Guillamon A, Meyer I, Meyer W 3rd, Reisner S, Sevelius S, Ettner R. Adult development and quality of life of transgender and gender nonconforming people. Curr Opin Endocrinol Diabetes Obes. 2016;23(2):188–97.
24. Ehrenhaft D. Listening and learning from gender non-conforming children. Psychoanal Study Child. 2014;68:28–56.
25. Nealy EC. Transgender children and youth: cultivating pride and joy with families in transition. New York: W. W. Norton & Company; 2017.
26. Wallien MS, Cohen-Kettenis PT. Psychosexual outcome of gender-dysphoric children. J Am Acad Child Adolesc Psychiatry. 2008;47:1413–23.
27. Coleman E, Bockting W, Botzer M, Cohen-Kettenis P, DeCuypere G, Feldman J, Fraser L, Green J, Knudson G, Meyer WJ, Monstrey S, Adler RK, Brown GR, Devor AH, Ehrbar R, Ettner R, Eyler E, Garofalo R, Karasic DH, Lev AI, Mayer G, Meyer-Bahlburg H, Hall BP, Pfaefflin F, Rachlin K, Robinson B, Schechter LS, Tangpricha V, van Trotsenburg M, Vitale A, Winter S, Whittle S, Wylie KR, Zucker K. Standards of care for the health of transsexual, transgender, and gender-nonconforming people, version 7. Int J Transgenderism. 2012;13(4):165–232. https://doi.org/10.1080/15532739.2011.700873.
28. Hembree WC, Cohen-Kettenis PT, Gooren L, Hannema SE, Meyer WJ, Murad MH, Rosenthal SM, Safer JD, Tangpricha V, T'Sjoen GG. Endocrine treatment of gender-dysphoric/gender-incongruent persons: an endocrine society clinical practice guideline. J Clin Endocrinol Metab. 2017;102(11):3869–903. https://doi.org/10.1210/jc.2017-01658.
29. Pleak RR. Transgender people. In: Ruiz P, Primm A, editors. Disparities in psychiatric care: clinical & cross-cultural perspectives. Philadelphia: Lippincott Williams & Wilkins; 2010. p. 107–15.
30. Poteat T, German D, Kerrigan D. Managing uncertainty: a grounded theory of stigma in transgender health care encounters. Soc Sci Med. 2013;84:22–9.
31. Grant JM, Mottet LA, Tanis J, Harrison J, Herman JL, Keisling M. Injustice at every turn: a report of the national transgender discrimination survey. Washington, DC: National Center for Transgender Equality and National Gay and Lesbian Task Force; 2011 Feb 03.
32. Safer JD, Coleman E, Feldman J, Garofalo R, Hembree W, Radix A, Sevelius J. Barriers to health care for transgender individuals. Curr Opin Endocrinol Diabetes Obes. 2016;23(2):168–71. https://doi.org/10.1097/MED.0000000000000227.
33. Daniel H, Butkus R, For the Health and Public Policy Committee of the American College of Physicians. Lesbian, gay, bisexual, and transgender health disparities: executive summary of a policy position paper from the American College of Physicians. Ann Intern Med. 2015;163:135–7. https://doi.org/10.7326/m14-2482.
34. Healthy people 2020 [Internet]. Washington, DC: U.S. Department of Health and Human Services, Office of Disease Prevention and Health Promotion [cited 6/10/2018]. Available from: https://www.healthypeople.gov/2020.
35. Institute of Medicine. The health of lesbian, gay, bisexual, and transgender people: building a foundation for better understanding. Washington, DC: The National Academies Press; 2011. https://doi.org/10.17226/13128.

36. The Joint Commission. Advancing effective communication, cultural competence, and patient- and family-centered care for the lesbian, gay, bisexual, and transgender (LGBT) community: a field guide. Oak Brook, IL: 2011 Oct.
37. Adelson SL. Practice parameter on gay, lesbian, or bisexual sexual orientation, gender nonconformity, and gender discordance in children and adolescents. J Am Acad Child Adolesc Psychiatry. 2012;51(9):957–74.
38. Byne W, Bradley SJ, Coleman AE, Green R, Menvielle EJ, Meyer-Bahlburg HFL, Pleak RR, Tompkins DA. Report of the American Psychiatric Association task force on treatment of gender identity disorder. Arch Sex Behav. 2012;41(4):759–96.
39. American Psychological Association. Guidelines for psychological practice with transgender and gender nonconforming people. Am Psychol. 2015;70(9):832–64.
40. Levonis P, Drescher J, Barber ME, editors. The LGBT casebook. Washington, DC: American Psychiatric Publishing; 2012.
41. Yarbrough E. Transgender mental health. Washington, DC: American Psychiatric Publishing; 2018.
42. Erikson-Schroth L, editor. Trans bodies, trans selves: a resource for the transgender community. New York: Oxford University Press; 2014.
43. Nuttbrock L, Rosenblum A, Blumenstein R. Transgender identity affirmation and mental health. Int J Transgenderism. 2002;6(4):1–11.

Chapter 8
Endocrine Care of Transgender Adults

Sarah L. Fishman, Maria Paliou, Leonid Poretsky and Wylie C. Hembree

Endocrine Care of the Transgender Patient

Introduction

Since the mid-twentieth century, transgender individuals have become increasingly visible. Strong advocacy group efforts and increasing government support have improved access to medical care for people with gender dysphoria. Physicians should be aware of the unique conditions and challenges affecting this population. Healthcare professional organizations such as the American Medical Association (AMA), the Endocrine Society, and the World Professional Association for Transgender Health have concluded that hormonal and surgical treatment of gender dysphoria is medically necessary to prevent long-term morbidity. Furthermore, physicians caring for transgender persons must have sufficient experience to recognize gender dysphoria as a spectrum of conditions, and should be adept in tailoring therapy to the individual patient. Many, but not all, gender dysphoric individuals presenting for care will ultimately seek endocrine therapy for the modulation of endogenous hormone production and exogenous hormone supplementation, to improve their quality of life.

S. L. Fishman · M. Paliou · L. Poretsky (✉)
Division of Endocrinology, Lenox Hill Hospital, Northwell Health,
New York, NY, USA
e-mail: lporetsky@northwell.edu

W. C. Hembree
Division of Endocrinology, Columbia University College of Physicians
and Surgeons, New York, NY, USA

L. Poretsky and W. C. Hembree (eds.), *Transgender Medicine*, Contemporary
Endocrinology, https://doi.org/10.1007/978-3-030-05683-4_8

General Considerations

The goals of hormone therapy in individuals suffering from gender dysphoria are determined by many factors including age, capacity to consent to treatment, pre-existing health conditions, risk factors for future disease, access to care, and the patient's desired outcomes with regards to gender transition. While some individuals with gender dysphoria desire to live as the opposite gender, others prefer to live as neither gender and seek suppression of all evidence of a sexual or gender representation.

Hormonal therapy for individuals with gender dysphoria is but one of many treatments available, and must be considered in the context of contemporaneous psychological care and possible surgical interventions. In addition, the developmental stage at which the patient presents for evaluation and treatment (i.e., prepubertal, during puberty, or in adulthood having completed puberty) will necessarily affect the goals and possible outcomes of hormone treatment. A discussion of the care of transgender children and adolescents is presented elsewhere in this volume.

Hormonal treatment for patients with gender dysphoria must begin with an assessment of the individual's expectations and goals of care. Prior to initiating hormonal therapy, patients should be counseled regarding realistic expectations of masculinization/feminization, and the time course over which potential changes may occur. The initial discussion should include a thorough medical history that may elucidate potential risks to hormonal treatment. A family history of gynecologic and breast cancers, cardiovascular disease, diabetes, hypertension, and hyperlipidemia should be noted if present. Patients who previously have not been in the care of a mental health provider should be assessed for psychological stability, as psychiatric disease has been reported in over 56% of patients seeking gender-affirming hormone treatment [1]. Providers should inform individuals of the particular benefits, limitations, and risks of treatment, specific to the individual's age, previous experience with hormones, and concurrent physical or mental health concerns. Additionally, a detailed psychiatric, social, and sexual history are warranted as certain behaviors such as cigarette smoking, excessive alcohol consumption, and high-risk sexual activity may increase the inherent risks of hormone treatment. A physical exam should be performed including measurements of height, weight, and blood pressure. Breast, rectal, and genital exams may provoke anxiety and severe discomfort in patients with gender dysphoria, and should be approached delicately and with explicit consent. Laboratory evaluation should include a complete blood count, electrolytes, kidney, liver, and thyroid function tests, lipid profile measurements, fasting glucose and HbA1C, β-HCG (for native females), and baseline levels of testosterone, estradiol, FSH, LH, and prolactin. Where appropriate, screening for cervical cancer, breast cancer, and prostate cancer may be warranted. Additionally, a careful risk assessment for the development of estrogen- and androgen-sensitive cancers should be conducted prior to initiating therapy. For patients interested in testosterone therapy, an evaluation for sleep apnea may be indicated [2].

Obtaining informed consent for hormone therapy is important to ensure that patients understand the psychological and physical risks and benefits of hormone therapy. Adverse effects of hormonal treatment, such as infertility, may be irreversible with prolonged treatment, and these should be discussed openly and frankly when developing a treatment plan. It has been suggested that patients should have demonstrated an understanding of the psychosocial implications of gender transition by completing a social transition to their affirmed gender, however more recent guidelines recognize the difficulty of making a social transition in the absence of a biochemical and physical transition.

Developing a Treatment Plan

The overall framework of endocrine care for gender dysphoria consists of treatments aimed at suppressing the natal gender characteristics and treatments aimed at affirming the desired gender. Feminization and masculinization refer to the physical changes that allow transgender individuals to feel comfortable in society in their affirmed gender. Hormonal regimens will vary based on the age, treatment status, and desired outcomes of the individual. Access to care and availability of treatment modalities varies greatly geographically.

Puberty

The onset of puberty is of particular significance in the lives of children with gender dysphoria. For many children who have not socially transitioned away from their natal gender, the physical transitions occurring in puberty serve to reverse much of their initial discomfort. By contrast, a marked increase in gender dysphoria at the onset of puberty is highly suggestive that the condition will not remit [3–5]. It is because of this dichotomous reaction to pubertal changes that hormonal therapy is not recommended in children who have not yet achieved Tanner stage 2 of puberty. At this stage, current guidelines [5] recommend initiating hormonal treatment to halt the progression of puberty rather than the initiation of cross-sex hormones. Suppression of puberty increases the interval during which gender dysphoria may resolve, while allowing the individual to remain less identified with the bothersome gender as peers develop secondary sexual characteristics. Furthermore, suppression of puberty prevents development of potentially irreversible secondary sexual characteristics such as changes in voice and bone structure, allowing the body some capacity to develop physical characteristics of either sex once this suppression is lifted. A discussion of pubertal suppression can be found in the chapter on pediatric management of transgender individuals elsewhere in this volume.

For transgendered patients managed with puberty suppression, adult care begins with puberty induction. Induction of female puberty in this scenario requires administration of increasing doses of estrogen to mimic the gradual rise in levels seen in the progression of puberty in natal females. In the setting of delayed onset of male puberty followed by induction of female puberty, endogenous androgen production is typically minimal due to continuous suppression of LH and FSH and rarely requires additional suppression or antiandrogen treatment. GnRH analogs used for puberty suppression should be continued until adult premenopausal estrogen levels have been achieved, at which time attempts to wean GnRH can be made. Antiandrogen medications can be used to mitigate the effects of endogenous hormone production [3, 4, 6, 7].

Induction of male puberty is achieved with increasing doses of subcutaneous or intramuscular injections of testosterone esters beginning at 12.5 mg/m^2/week and increasing every 6 months until a serum testosterone level in the normal adult range has been reached. Suppression of endogenous hormones is no longer required once adult testosterone levels have been achieved, sufficient virilization has occurred, or the patient undergoes gonadectomy. However, continued use of GnRH analogs along with testosterone may allow for a reduction in the testosterone dose required to maintain adult levels [3, 6].

In patients who began puberty suppression at a later developmental stage, induction of cross-gender puberty should be allowed to progress more rapidly, with higher starting doses of gender-affirming hormones. Throughout the period of puberty induction, patients should be monitored with quarterly measurements of height, weight, blood pressure, and Tanner stage. Hemoglobin/hematocrit, serum levels of lipids and testosterone for transgender males, and levels of prolactin and estradiol for transgender females should be assessed every 6 months prior to dose adjustments of hormonal therapy. In addition, all patients undergoing puberty induction should undergo bone age monitoring along with vitamin D level measurements annually as well as yearly bone mineral density testing with DEXA until early adulthood.

Hormone Therapy for the Transgender Female

The treatment of individuals with gender dysphoria presenting in postpubertal adulthood relies more heavily on the suppression of natal characteristics and often requires intensified hormonal treatment compared with that of persons presenting before or during puberty. Gender-affirming hormonal treatments have been developed and influenced by the regimens used for hypogonadism.

The treatment of transgender females relies on suppressing native androgen production as well as supplementation of female hormones [8, 9]. There is significant global variability in the treatment regimens due to cost and availability of medication. Both natural estrogens including estrone, estradiol, and 17β-estradiol, and synthetic estrogens (estradiol valerate, estradiol benzoate, and ethinylestradiol) are available in a variety of forms and combinations (Table 8.1). The oral estrogens most commonly used include micronized estradiol (2–4 mg/day), estradiol valerate (2–4 mg/day), ethinylestradiol (20 μg/day), and conjugated estrogens

Table 8.1 Feminizing hormones

Name	Route	Dose	Comments
Micronized estradiol	Oral	2–4 mg/day	Inexpensive
Estradiol valerate	Oral	2–4 mg/day	
Ethinylestradiol	Oral	20 μg/day	Not recommended, high DVT risk
Conjugated estrogens	Oral	1.25–2.5 mg/day	Not detectable in serum assays
17β-estradiol	Transdermal	100–200 μg/day	Lowest DVT risk, higher cost
Estradiol cypionate	IM	3 mg/month	Long latency period
Estradiol valerate	IM	5–20 mg/2 weeks	
Estradiol undecylate	IM	100 mg/month	

(1.25–2.5 mg/day). A transdermal patch of 17β estradiol (100–200 μg/day) is the estrogen of choice to reduce the risk of thromboembolic disease [8, 10] and may be preferred due to the lack of associated changes in lipid profile or markers of coagulation (discussed in more detail below). However, the use of transdermal delivery is limited by a higher cost relative to oral preparations. Intramuscular depots [estradiol cypionate (3 mg/month), estradiol valerate (5–20 mg/2 weeks), estradiol undecylate (Progynon, 100 mg/month)] have been used, but these agents have a longer latency period before the development of noticeable physical changes, often leading to self-discontinuation or dose escalation by patients [11, 12]. In addition, a number of estradiol/progestin combination tablets are available, typically used as oral contraceptives.

The initial dose of estrogen should be increased gradually until achieving sufficient feminization without exceeding the normal native female premenopausal range (typically 100–200 pg/mL). This is usually achieved with an oral preparation of 2.0–6.0 mg/day; a transdermal patch of 0.025–0.2 mg/day or parenteral injections of 2–10 mg/week. It should be noted that conjugated and synthetic estrogens such as ethinylestradiol are not detectable in the serum by conventional assays [13] and are no longer recommended [2, 14–24]. Serum target levels may change as the patient ages to account for reduced drug clearance as well as the natural decline in endogenous estrogen production that occurs in natal females at menopause. Older transgender females may continue to require high-dose estrogen supplementation to maintain a female body habitus and continued suppression of androgen production after the typical age of menopause.

Estrogen supplementation into the normal premenopausal female range can suppress testosterone production into the low-normal range, but is usually insufficient to achieve a reduction of levels into the normal female range [9, 13, 24–31] (ideally <50 ng/dL). Treatments aimed at further reducing testosterone levels include progesterone supplementation (more common in Europe), androgen receptor antagonists (more common in the US), GnRH agonists (primarily in the UK) and 5α-reductase inhibitors (Table 8.2) [2, 8, 10, 13, 32, 33]. Orchiectomy may be necessary to achieve optimal reductions in testosterone levels and male pattern secondary sex characteristics.

Table 8.2 Antiandrogens

Type	Route	Dose	Comments
GnRH analogs			
Goserelin	SubQ	3.8 mg/ 4 weeks	Most commonly used in the UK High cost Tolerated well Variations in geographic availability of agents
Leuprolide	IM	3.75 mg/ 4 weeks	
Buserelin	SubQ/ intranasal	200–1200 μg/ day	
Triptorelin	IM	3.75 mg/ 4 weeks	
Histrelin	SubQ depot	50 μg/day	
Progesterone			
Cyproterone acetate	Oral	25–100 mg/ day	Preferred agent in Europe. Cyproterone acetate not available in the USA
Medroxyprogesterone	Oral	10 mg/day	
Androgen receptor blocker			
Spironolactone	Oral	100–400 mg/day	Preferred in the US, low cost Risk of hepatotoxicity
Flutamide	Oral	250–500 mg/day	
Bicalutamide	Oral	25–50 mg/ day	
Enzalutamide	Oral	160 mg/day	
5α-reductase inhibitors			
Finasteride	Oral	5 mg/day	May be beneficial following gonadectomy
Dutasteride	Oral	0.5 mg/day	

GnRH agonists create continuous stimulation of the GnRH receptor, thus interrupting the normal pulsatile rhythm responsible for the secretion of LH and FSH. Lack of pituitary stimulation leads to downstream inhibition of testosterone and dihydrotestosterone secretion from the testes and estradiol and estrone from ovaries. Small studies have reported successful gonadotropin suppression using goserelin acetate (3.8 mg subcutaneous injection every 4 weeks) [34] and leuprolide [35] (3.75 mg intramuscular injection every month), in combination with estrogen. There are few published reports [36] describing the use of additional GnRH analogs in the treatment of transgender adults, however many studies have shown a dramatic suppression of gonadotropins with buserelin [37, 38]. Triptorelin has been successfully used in the treatment of transgender adolescents [12]. Long-term androgen suppression for up to 2 years can be achieved with histrelin (50 μg/day) subcutaneous implants, and is a suggested option for patients who desire but are unable to undergo gonadectomy [15].

Supplementation with progesterone or its derivatives can reduce serum testosterone levels by 70–80% in native males [39]. Certain progestins such as cyproterone acetate (25–100 mg/day) and medroxyprogesterone (10 mg/day) possess additional testosterone receptor antagonist activity [40] making them attractive drugs for androgen suppression in transgender females. Studies suggest that cyproterone acetate is more effective than medroxyprogesterone in reducing testosterone levels into the female range [10, 25, 35, 41] which may be attributed to additional antigonadotropic effects [10]. The use of additional progesterone to promote breast growth is controversial [42–44]. There is some evidence that breast development, mood, and sexual desire are increased with progesterone supplementation [43]. Adverse effects including liver toxicity and severe depression have been reported in association with cyproterone acetate [10, 45]. In addition, long-term use of cyproterone acetate may increase the risk of meningiomas [10, 46–48].

Additional treatment modalities aimed at reducing the effects of testosterone include androgen receptor blockers and 5α-reductase inhibitors (due to the reduced conversion of testosterone to the more potent dihydrotestosterone). Spironolactone, a potassium-sparing diuretic used in the treatment of hypertension and congestive heart failure, is a steroid compound with androgen receptor blocking activity when administered at higher doses (100–400 mg/day). Additional antiandrogenic effects are mediated via inhibition of the 17α-hydroxylase enzyme leading to decreased testosterone synthesis and secretion, as well as by modest estrogen receptor agonist activity [49, 50]. Some studies suggest spironolactone may inhibit breast development via activation of the estrogen receptor leading to early breast bud fusion, though this remains controversial [44] as gynecomastia is a well-described adverse effect of spironolactone [51].

Non-steroidal selective androgen receptor antagonists, developed as a treatment for androgen-sensitive prostate cancer, are occasionally used in transgender females who do not achieve their desired results or do not tolerate alternative drugs [52]. There are isolated reports of successful outcomes with flutamide (Eulexin), though reportedly not as effective as cyproterone acetate in reducing testosterone levels [12]. Both flutamide and bicalutamide (Casodex), in conjunction with oral contraceptive pills, have shown significant improvements in hirsutism in natal females with polycystic ovarian syndrome (PCOS) [53–57]. The use of these agents as antiandrogens in transgender patients has been limited by concerns of hepatotoxicity. However, at low doses, these agents have shown to be both well tolerated and effective when used for the treatment of hirsutism [57].

The putative mechanism of 5α-reductase inhibitors (finasteride 5 mg/day PO, dutasteride 0.5 mg/day PO) should lead to a reduction and regression of male secondary sex characteristics through inhibition of conversion of testosterone to dihydrotestosterone. Evidence exists for the role of these agents in improving scalp hair loss, reducing body hair growth and sebaceous gland secretions, and improving skin consistency in transgender females [6]. However, blocking of dihydrotestosterone synthesis leads to an increased concentration of testosterone availability to specific receptors, limiting the efficacy of this class of medications in reducing testosterone levels [2, 14, 15]. In addition, this class of drugs has been linked to worsening depression [10, 58], and liver toxicity [14]. Dutasteride (0.5 mg) is more effective than finasteride in blocking the type 1 isozyme, which is present in the pilosebaceous gland and may lead to larger reductions in scalp hair loss and body hair growth. Unlike other antiandrogen medications, 5α-reductase inhibitors may continue to be useful after gonadectomy for management of hair loss [59]. For older transgender females, antiandrogens may become the primary component of treatment as estrogen requirements are reduced in parallel to the decline in estrogen levels in natal females that occurs with menopause [60].

The effects of estrogen along with antiandrogen medications are typically observed beginning 3 months into treatment. The most desired effects of gender-affirming hormones for transgender females are the development of female secondary sex characteristics including: enlarged breasts, decreased facial and body hair, development of female pattern weight distribution and body habitus, and softening of the skin. Clinically significant estrogen levels will also lead to a reduction in spontaneous and sexually stimulated erections, reduced ejaculatory volume and sperm concentrations, and changes in sweat and odor patterns. Longer hormone exposure is necessary for significant decreases in testicular and prostate size. The maximal effect of hormone therapy on secondary sex characteristics typically occurs 2 years after starting treatment [61]. The degree and rate of these changes are hard to predict and are dependent on the type of medication, the dose, and route of administration. Many transgender females are dissatisfied with breast growth achieved through hormonal therapy, and opt for surgical augmentation [10, 19]. One multicenter study reported modest breast development, occurring primarily within the first 6 months of treatment. No clinical or laboratory parameters were found to predict breast development [62].

Failure to achieve testosterone suppression with standard antiandrogen regimens despite maximal therapy and medication adherence should prompt evaluation for endogenous testosterone production from a tumor, or undisclosed exogenous testosterone use to maintain sexual function during the transition. In transgender females wishing to retain erectile function, sildenafil or tadalafil can be used as supportive measures.

Transgender females should be informed of the risks of estrogen treatment and evaluated for preexisting conditions that may pose an increased risk. The most well-known adverse effect of estrogen therapy is the development of thromboembolic disease. There is an increasing risk of this complication with advancing age, active cigarette smoking, and concurrent use of progestins. Providers should encourage all patients on estrogen therapy to stop smoking. Transdermal and parental administration of estrogen is associated with a decreased risk of thromboembolic disease as compared to oral administration, attributed to reduced first-pass hepatic metabolism [10, 63]. In addition, synthetic estrogens appear to confer an increased risk of thromboembolism as compared to natural estrogens [10, 64]. The mechanism for this effect remains unknown.

Additional adverse effects of estrogen use in transgender females include liver dysfunction, gallstones, hypertriglyceridemia, and weight gain. The role of estrogen in the development of cardiovascular disease remains controversial. One study of 161 transgender females showed no increased incidence of cardiovascular mortality [65]. Alterations in lipid metabolism include decreased LDL and increased triglycerides [10, 66–70]. The effects of estrogen on HDL levels are unclear, with studies reporting both increases [50, 71] decreases [24, 72], and no change [70]. The effect of estrogen on HDL may be partially related to route of administration, with transdermal estradiol more likely to increase HDL [67, 69]. Increased insulin resistance and the development of type 2 diabetes has also been reported during estrogen treatment [42]. Elevated prolactin levels are nearly universal, though mild, in transgender females. There are reported cases of prolactinomas in this population that may result from enhanced growth of pituitary lactotrophs under the influence of increased estrogen levels [11, 24, 73–75]. In these cases, prolactinomas may resolve when the dose of estrogen or progesterone is reduced. The evaluation of elevated prolactin with MRI of the pituitary is controversial in the absence of visual or other symptoms as asymptomatic prolactinomas do not require treatment in this population [76]. Furthermore, the prolactin raising effects of psychotropic medications may be enhanced by estrogen administration.

Gender-affirming hormone treatment in transgender females has been reported to reduce blood pressure [42], however, this effect is likely due to a reduction in testosterone levels leading to reduced hematocrit rather than increased estrogen concentrations. This finding is supported by reports that administration of ethinylestradiol in combination with cyproterone acetate lead to increased blood pressure and arterial stiffness [24, 42, 71, 77] and that use of oral contraceptives in cis-gender females can lead to hypertension that resolves on discontinuation [78].

Sexual function is greatly affected by exogenous hormones. High estrogen levels can lead to reduced libido, as well as reduced spontaneous and sexually stimulated erections. High levels of hypoactive sexual desire disorder are reported in transgender females, with one study reporting that over 75% of individuals never or rarely experience spontaneous or responsive sexual desire [79].

Hormone Therapy for the Transgender Male

Gender-affirming treatment for the transgender male consists primarily of exogenous testosterone administration. While testosterone is available in oral (outside of the USA), buccal, topical, transdermal preparations and as subcutaneous implants, intramuscular injections are most often prescribed as they are available at relatively low cost (Table 8.3). There are no standardized protocols for the initiation of testosterone therapy, but expert opinions recommend a low initial dose with gradual increases, as is typically done in treating patients with hypogonadism. Intramuscular injections of short-acting testosterone esters such as testosterone cypionate (Depo-testosterone) (200 mg), decanoate (Sustanon) (250 mg) or enanthate (Delatestryl) (250 mg) administered every 2–4 weeks are among the most commonly prescribed. However, these agents do not mimic circadian release of the

Table 8.3 Masculinizing hormones

Name	Route	Dose	Comments
Testosterone cypionate	IM	200 mg/ 4 weeks	Short-acting preparations do not mimic circadian release
Testosterone decanoate	IM	250 mg/ 4 weeks	
Testosterone enanthate	IM	250 mg/ 4 weeks	
Testosterone undecenoate	IM	1000 mg/ 12 weeks	Must be administered in physician's office in the US. High cost
Androderm, Testoderm	Transdermal patch	5 mg/day	Skin irritation at patch site may occur
Androgel, Testim	Transdermal gel	5 g/day	Risk of transfer to intimate partner
Striant	Lozenge	30 mg/12 h	
Crystalline testosterone (Testopel)	SubQ depot	600 mg/4–6 months	
Testosterone undecanoate (Andriol)	Oral	80–160 mg/day	Multiple daily doses required

hormone. Supraphysiologic levels of testosterone (with associated adverse effects) occur at the time of injection, with hypogonadal symptoms occurring in the days leading up to the next injection. Some centers include two doses of intramuscular progesterone (500 mg) 3–4 days after each testosterone injection [11]. A newer preparation, testosterone undecanoate (Nebido), is now available for injection every 12 weeks to achieve more consistent levels, although at considerably higher cost. Transdermal patches (Androderm, Testoderm) and gels (AndroGel, Testim) can be used daily (5 mg/patch or 5 g of gel) for more consistent testosterone levels, however these delivery methods can be complicated by skin irritation at the patch site and transfer of hormone from the gel to an intimate partner. Bioidentical testosterone lozenges (Striant) (30 mg every 12 h) can provide consistent levels, but have been associated with gum irritation, changes in taste, and headaches [80]. Subcutaneous implants of crystalline testosterone (Testopel) (600 mg/4–6 months) can maintain stable and physiologic testosterone levels without the need for daily dosing. Finally, oral testosterone undecanoate (Andriol) is now available in doses of 80–160 mg/day, but requires multiple daily doses and has a short history of clinical use. It should be noted that non-injectable forms of testosterone are inferior to injectable forms in suppressing menstruation for reasons that remain unknown.

Testosterone is essential for the development of male secondary sex characteristics. Androgen receptors are located throughout the body, leading to a multitude of physical and psychiatric changes in association with testosterone therapy. Gender-affirming treatment in transgender males aims to promote a deepened voice, clitoral enlargement, increased facial and body hair, cessation of menses, atrophy of breast tissue, decreased body fat, and an increase in muscle mass and strength. The expected onset of these changes ranges from 1 to 12 months after starting therapy, with maximal effects achieved as late as 5 years after initiation. The first manifestations of virilization include changes in body hair and skin, and cessation of menses. Clitoromegaly and voice deepening typically occur within 6 months of starting therapy. Clitoral growth may be associated with pain prior to significant elongation, and is reported to peak 6 months following initiation of testosterone [13, 72, 81]. Alopecia may occur in those genetically predisposed after prolonged testosterone use. Providers should avoid increasing the dose of testosterone to hasten masculinization, as this may lead to increased conversion to estrogen. Reduced doses of testosterone should be considered following oophorectomy [80].

In some patients, the side effects of testosterone treatment limit the dose, leading to incomplete menstrual suppression. As in transgender females, GnRH agonists are highly effective in suppressing endogenous ovarian hormone production, leading to amenorrhea [2, 82]. Menstruation can also be suppressed by continuous progesterone therapy administered systemically or locally (for example, with an intrauterine device in individuals with an intact uterus). Ovarian production of estrogen is decreased in the presence of continuous progesterone due to negative feedback at the level of the pituitary inhibiting secretion of FSH and LH. In transgender males, androgenic progesterones have the added advantage of reducing sex hormone binding globulin concentrations leading to a relative increase in available testosterone [82, 83].

Available preparations include oral norethindrone (Micronor, Camila, Deblitane, Heather, Jencycla, Jolivette, Sharobel) as a 0.35 mg tablet which should be taken at the same time daily. Norethindrone acetate (Aygestin), medroxyprogesterone acetate (Provera), Lynestrenol (Orgametril) and micronized progesterone (Prometrium) are alternative daily oral preparations. Medroxyprogesterone acetate depots are available as intramuscular gluteal or deltoid injection (Depo-Provera) or subcutaneous (Depo-SubQ) injections administered every 12–14 weeks obviate the need for daily dosing. Long-term progesterone therapy is available for up to 3 years as intradermal etonogestrel (Implanon) or up to 5 years as an intrauterine device with levonorgestrel (Mirena, Liletta). Breakthrough bleeding may occur for 3 months following placement [8]. If menses are not suppressed with hormone treatment, endometrial ablation may be required. Contraception should be continued in all transgender females, who have not undergone gonadectomy as testosterone monotherapy may be insufficient to prevent ovulation and is contraindicated in pregnancy.

Very little is known regarding the utility of antiestrogen medications in transgender males. Aromatase inhibitors such as anastrozole or letrozole have been used off-label as adjunctive therapies to suppress menstruation in transgender men by preventing the conversion of testosterone to estrogen. Aromatase inhibitors have been shown to safely and effectively increase testosterone levels in hypogonadal natal males [84, 85], however, there are no published reports of their use in transgender males. Reduced estrogen concentrations in transgender males is theorized to reduce vaginal bleeding and pelvic pain. Menopausal side effects attributed to aromatase inhibitors in natal women are attenuated or absent in transgender men with concurrent use of testosterone. These agents may be of particular benefit in obese patients as aromatase is naturally expressed in adipose tissue. Anecdotal evidence supports a role for selective estrogen receptor blockers such as raloxifene to reduce uterine bleeding in transgender men on testosterone treatment with unsuppressed menses [59].

While testosterone treatment is generally well tolerated, adverse effects can occur and may lead to significantly increased risk of life-threatening disease. A rise in hemoglobin and hematocrit concentrations is nearly universal with testosterone administration. While the development of overt polycythemia (hematocrit >50) is a common finding in natal men using exogenous testosterone, the rise in hematocrit in transgender females is typically less pronounced. The degree to which polycythemia increases the risk of deep venous thrombosis (DVT) in transgender males is unclear because of the lack of evidence to suggest that testosterone treatment increases the incidence of DVT [20, 86, 87]. Untreated severe obstructive sleep apnea is a relative contraindication to testosterone treatment as this may further increase the risk of polycythemia and deep venous thrombosis [88]. In addition, testosterone may exacerbate underlying sleep apnea by increasing weight and muscle mass. The mechanism by which testosterone increases erythropoiesis remains unknown and appears to be unrelated to increased erythropoietin [89, 90]. Polycythemia occurs most often with intramuscular preparations of testosterone [91].

A causal relationship between testosterone use and cardiovascular disease remains controversial [20, 80, 92–94]. Testosterone use is associated with worsening of numerous cardiac risk factors including: hypertension, weight gain, salt retention, increased LDL and triglyceride levels, reduced HDL levels [42, 93, 95], and reduced homocysteine levels [14, 96, 97]. A controlled study of transgender males reported an increased incidence of cardiovascular mortality [98], however, this finding was not confirmed in small studies of transgender males compared to the general population [94]. Two studies examined the effects of hormone therapy in patients with preexisting risk factors such as hyperlipidemia and hypertension. In one study, no patients experienced cardiovascular events over an average of 10 years of treatment [20]. A second study of 138 subjects reported no significant increase in cardiovascular events over an average of 7.4 years of therapy compared to the general population [99]. However, the use of testosterone in patients with a history of unstable coronary artery disease is not recommended [80, 100].

Studies are equivocal with respect to the effects of testosterone on increasing insulin resistance in transgender males [94, 99]. Multiple studies have reported a lowering of fasting glucose in transgender males [24, 42, 71, 101]. Others have reported no change in fasting glucose or insulin activity as measured by the homeostatic model assessment-insulin resistance [71, 72, 102–104]. A case-control study [105] found an increased incidence in type 2 diabetes in transgender men using testosterone, despite maintenance of a stable body weight.

The increase in muscle mass associated with testosterone use can lead to an increase in measured creatinine levels and glomerular filtration rate [42, 72, 106, 107]. The significance of these changes with respect to renal function is unclear: In murine models, testosterone has both protective and damaging effects [108, 109]. No long-term studies have reported significant effects on kidney function in transgender patients.

An increased risk of uterine and ovarian cancer in association with testosterone use in transgender males remains controversial [80, 82, 93, 110–113]. This may be related to the development of polycystic ovaries in patients on testosterone therapy [112–114] as testosterone may increase ovarian volumes and induce stromal hyperplasia [13]. However, more recent studies suggest that the de novo development of polycystic ovaries in transgender males is different from the a priori presence of polycystic ovaries in natal females with PCOS [6, 110]. A baseline higher incidence of PCOS in transgender males as compared with cis-gender females has been reported warranting closer follow-up in this group. PCOS is an independent risk factor for cardiac disease, type 2 diabetes mellitus, as well as ovarian and endometrial malignancies, which may confound the observed association between these outcomes and testosterone use. Endometrial atrophy occurs in a subset of patients in response to testosterone [112]. An increased risk of endometrial cancer may be due to the effects of testosterone conversion to estrogen without opposing progesterone.

The risk of breast cancer remains present in transgender males. Although testosterone leads to a reduction in breast glandular tissue accompanied by an increase in fibrous connective tissue [115, 116], as with endometrial cancer, aromatization to estradiol may promote malignancy. Multiple cases of breast cancer have been reported in transgender males, including following mastectomy [117–121], however testosterone therapy has been shown to reduce the risk of breast cancer [117]. The risk of breast cancer in transgender males is higher in post-oophorectomy and menopausal patients [111].

Additional less severe adverse effects of testosterone therapy include the development of cystic acne, baldness (male pattern), and unwanted body hair. Cystic acne will often improve with topical or oral retinoic acid treatment. Finasteride and topical minoxidil can be considered to improve male pattern baldness. Insufficient evidence exists regarding the effects of testosterone on exacerbating underlying psychiatric conditions. Some individuals may experience a bothersome increase in libido, which can be managed with low-dose SSRIs [122, 123]. This effect is exacerbated by painful intercourse resulting from thinning of the vaginal epithelia [13, 124].

Screenings and Follow-Up

Transgender females and transgender males should be closely followed by a multidisciplinary team of physicians during and following their transition.

Following the initiation of hormone treatments, patients should undergo quarterly physical exams including measurements of weight and blood pressure, to document any physical changes related to gender transition. Additionally, smoking cessation counseling and screening for depression should be provided at each visit. Serum levels of testosterone, estradiol, progesterone, LH, FSH, prolactin, lipids, fasting glucose, liver enzymes, and creatinine should also be monitored at these visits until appropriate stable levels have been achieved. In patients using periodic intramuscular testosterone injections, a trough level should be collected. Testosterone levels in transgender males should be maintained in the normal male range of 300–1000 ng/dL [80] and in transgender females should be suppressed into the normal female range of <50 ng/dL. Ideal estrogen levels in transgender females are in the normal premenopausal range for native females (100–200 pg/mL), taking into account that this goal may change as the patient ages. Sex hormone binding globulin (SHBG) levels are expected to increase in transgender females, and decrease in transgender males [72]. It should be noted that normal values for metabolic and hormonal parameters have not been established for transgender individuals, and care should be taken in interpreting parameters with sex-specific reference ranges [125].

Establishing objective targets to evaluate a dosing regimen can be challenging given that appropriate hormone levels are unknown for transgendered individuals, and that clinical/phenotypic response is related to genetics as well as the age at which treatment was started. Titration should be guided by patients' goals, in the setting of measured hormone levels and safety considerations. For transgender females, one approach is to begin both estrogen and antiandrogen medications at low doses, escalate in parallel until appropriate estrogen serum levels have been achieved, and then increase the dose of antiandrogen to achieve improved feminization and further androgen suppression if needed.

Once a consistent dosing regimen has been established, the frequency of monitoring can be decreased to 6 months for 1 year, and annually thereafter. Annual visits should also include a thorough assessment of ongoing cardiovascular risk and sexual health. Recommendations for breast cancer screenings are the same for both transgender and cis-gender females, as well as transgender males who have undergone a mastectomy. In patients with an intact uterus, cervical cancer screenings should continue as per recommended guidelines for natal females. Endometrial ultrasound is recommended every 2 years or if unexpected bleeding occurs following cessation of menses. Periodic hepatic ultrasound can be considered in patients taking oral testosterones to screen for hepatic tumors [80]. An individualized approach to prostate cancer screening is recommended for transgender females.

The need for osteoporosis screening is equivocal in transgender patients as both estrogen and testosterone have profound effects on bone metabolism. While some centers recommend annual bone densitometry [11], there is little evidence to support this. Estradiol will stimulate endosteal bone apposition. Testosterone stimulates radial bone expansion and has anabolic effects on the periosteum, as well as downstream effects related to its conversion to estradiol [126]. Increased cortical bone size, cortical thickness, and bone mineral density have been reported in transgender males [127–130]. It has been reported that transgender females have high rates of osteoporosis which may pre-date the initiation of hormone therapy [131, 132] possibly due to poor nutritional status and low levels of physical activity [65]. Despite this, the incidence of fragility fractures in transgender females is low [133]. Serum levels of estradiol are better predictors of bone mineral density than testosterone levels [134, 135]. In evaluating transgender patients who underwent transition following puberty, birth gender should be used when estimating osteoporosis risk. In patients who have not undergone gonadectomy, osteoporosis screening may not be necessary. Bone mineral density should be assessed every 2 years in patients without ovaries [80]. Testosterone therapy may benefit transgender females by a direct stimulatory effect of testosterone on bone in addition to the effects of estrogen [130].

Special attention to deep venous thrombosis prophylaxis is necessary for patients undergoing surgical procedures while on hormone therapy. While no clear evidence exists for discontinuation of treatment, some experts recommend cessation of hormone therapy for up to 4 weeks prior to elective procedures [27] and reintroduction of estrogen therapy when the patient is fully ambulatory [32]. A recent retrospective study of over 900 patients [136] on testosterone treatment demonstrated no increased risk of postoperative in-hospital mortality, myocardial infarction, stroke, or major thromboembolism.

Conclusions

The use of cross-sex hormones in the treatment of gender dysphoria is an evolving field. More studies are needed to better elucidate the optimal regimens for feminization and masculinization while reducing the rate of adverse effects. Increasing global awareness and acceptance of transgender medicine should help this field to make significant strides in the coming years.

References

1. Leinung MC, et al. Endocrine treatment of transsexual persons: extensive personal experience. Endocr Pract. 2013;19(4):644–50.
2. Hembree WC, et al. Endocrine treatment of transsexual persons: an endocrine society clinical practice guideline. J Clin Endocrinol Metab. 2009;94(9):3132–54.
3. Spack NP, et al. Children and adolescents with gender identity disorder referred to a pediatric medical center. Pediatrics. 2012;129(3):418–25.
4. de Vries AL, Cohen-Kettenis PT. Clinical management of gender dysphoria in children and adolescents: the Dutch approach. J Homosex. 2012;59(3):301–20.
5. Steensma TD, et al. Desisting and persisting gender dysphoria after childhood: a qualitative follow-up study. Clin Child Psychol Psychiatry. 2011;16(4):499–516.

6. Smith KP, Madison CM, Milne NM. Gonadal suppressive and cross-sex hormone therapy for gender dysphoria in adolescents and adults. Pharmacotherapy. 2014;34(12):1282–97.
7. Schagen SE, et al. Efficacy and safety of gonadotropin-releasing hormone agonist treatment to suppress puberty in gender dysphoric adolescents. J Sex Med. 2016;13(7):1125–32.
8. Carswell JM, Roberts SA. Induction and maintenance of amenorrhea in transmasculine and nonbinary adolescents. Transgender Health. 2017;2(1):195–201.
9. Hembree WC, et al. Endocrine treatment of gender-dysphoric/gender-incongruent persons: an endocrine society clinical practice guideline. J Clin Endocrinol Metab. 2017;102 (11):3869–903.
10. Tangpricha V, den Heijer M. Oestrogen and anti-androgen therapy for transgender women. Lancet Diabetes Endocrinol. 2017;5(4):291–300.
11. Costa EM, Mendonca BB. Clinical management of transsexual subjects. Arq Bras Endocrinol Metabol. 2014;58(2):188–96.
12. Israel GE, Tarver DE. Transgender care: recommended guidelines, practical information, and personal accounts. Philadelphia: Temple University Press; 1997. xviii, 282 p.
13. Irwig MS. Testosterone therapy for transgender men. Lancet Diabetes Endocrinol. 2017;5 (4):301–11.
14. Meriggiola MC, Berra M. Safety of hormonal treatment in transgenders. Curr Opin Endocrinol Diabetes Obes. 2013;20(6):565–9.
15. Spack NP. Management of transgenderism. JAMA. 2013;309(5):478–84.
16. Meriggiola MC, et al. Endocrine treatment of transsexual persons: an endocrine society clinical practice guideline: commentary from a European perspective. Eur J Endocrinol. 2010;162(5):831–3.
17. Murad MH, et al. Hormonal therapy and sex reassignment: a systematic review and meta-analysis of quality of life and psychosocial outcomes. Clin Endocrinol (Oxf). 2010;72 (2):214–31.
18. Unger CA. Care of the transgender patient: the role of the gynecologist. Am J Obstet Gynecol. 2014;210(1):16–26.
19. Seal LJ, et al. Predictive markers for mammoplasty and a comparison of side effect profiles in transwomen taking various hormonal regimens. J Clin Endocrinol Metab. 2012;97 (12):4422–8.
20. Wierckx K, et al. Long-term evaluation of cross-sex hormone treatment in transsexual persons. J Sex Med. 2012;9(10):2641–51.
21. Knezevich EL, Viereck LK, Drincic AT. Medical management of adult transsexual persons. Pharmacotherapy. 2012;32(1):54–66.
22. Godano A, et al. SIAMS-ONIG consensus on hormonal treatment in gender identity disorders. J Endocrinol Invest. 2009;32(10):857–64.
23. Meriggiola MC, Berra M. Long-term cross-sex hormone treatment is safe in transsexual subjects. Asian J Androl. 2012;14(6):813–4.
24. Gooren LJ, Giltay EJ, Bunck MC. Long-term treatment of transsexuals with cross-sex hormones: extensive personal experience. J Clin Endocrinol Metab. 2008;93(1):19–25.
25. Prior JC, Vigna YM, Watson D. Spironolactone with physiological female steroids for presurgical therapy of male-to-female transsexualism. Arch Sex Behav. 1989;18(1):49–57.
26. Rosenthal SM. Approach to the patient: transgender youth: endocrine considerations. J Clin Endocrinol Metab. 2014;99(12):4379–89.
27. Gooren L. Hormone treatment of the adult transsexual patient. Horm Res. 2005; 64(Suppl 2):31–6.
28. Levy A, Crown A, Reid R. Endocrine intervention for transsexuals. Clin Endocrinol (Oxf). 2003;59(4):409–18.
29. Tangpricha V, et al. Endocrinologic treatment of gender identity disorders. Endocr Pract. 2003;9(1):12–21.
30. Meriggiola MC, Gava G. Endocrine care of transpeople part I. A review of cross-sex hormonal treatments, outcomes and adverse effects in transmen. Clin Endocrinol (Oxf). 2015;83(5):597–606.

31. Meriggiola MC, Gava G. Endocrine care of transpeople part II. A review of cross-sex hormonal treatments, outcomes and adverse effects in transwomen. Clin Endocrinol (Oxf). 2015;83(5):607–15.
32. Wylie K, et al. Serving transgender people: clinical care considerations and service delivery models in transgender health. Lancet. 2016;388(10042):401–11.
33. Feldman J, et al. Priorities for transgender medical and healthcare research. Curr Opin Endocrinol Diabetes Obes. 2016;23(2):180–7.
34. Dittrich R, et al. Endocrine treatment of male-to-female transsexuals using gonadotropin-releasing hormone agonist. Exp Clin Endocrinol Diabetes. 2005;113(10): 586–92.
35. Gava G, et al. Cyproterone acetate vs leuprolide acetate in combination with transdermal oestradiol in transwomen: a comparison of safety and effectiveness. Clin Endocrinol (Oxf). 2016;85(2):239–46.
36. Wilczynski C, Emanuele MA. Treating a transgender patient: overview of the guidelines. Postgrad Med. 2014;126(7):121–8.
37. Bourguignon JP, et al. Treatment of central precocious puberty with an intranasal analogue of GnRH (Buserelin). Eur J Pediatr. 1987;146(6):555–60.
38. Rappaport R, Fontoura M, Brauner R. Treatment of central precocious puberty with an LHRH agonist (Buserelin): effect on growth and bone maturation after three years of treatment. Horm Res. 1987;28(2–4):149–54.
39. Kjeld JM, et al. Effects of norgestrel and ethinyloestradiol ingestion on serum levels of sex hormones and gonadotrophins in men. Clin Endocrinol (Oxf). 1979;11(5):497–504.
40. Raudrant D, Rabe T. Progestogens with antiandrogenic properties. Drugs. 2003;63(5): 463–92.
41. Toorians AW, et al. Venous thrombosis and changes of hemostatic variables during cross-sex hormone treatment in transsexual people. J Clin Endocrinol Metab. 2003;88 (12):5723–9.
42. Vita R, et al. Changes in hormonal and metabolic parameters in transgender subjects on cross-sex hormone therapy: a cohort study. Maturitas. 2018;107:92–6.
43. Wierckx K, Gooren L, T'Sjoen G. Clinical review: breast development in trans women receiving cross-sex hormones. J Sex Med. 2014;11(5):1240–7.
44. Orentreich N, Durr NP. Proceedings: mammogenesis in transsexuals. J Invest Dermatol. 1974;63(1):142–6.
45. Moore E, Wisniewski A, Dobs A. Endocrine treatment of transsexual people: a review of treatment regimens, outcomes, and adverse effects. J Clin Endocrinol Metab. 2003;88 (8):3467–73.
46. Gil M, et al. Risk of meningioma among users of high doses of cyproterone acetate as compared with the general population: evidence from a population-based cohort study. Br J Clin Pharmacol. 2011;72(6):965–8.
47. Ter Wengel PV, et al. Meningiomas in three male-to-female transgender subjects using oestrogens/progestogens and review of the literature. Andrologia. 2016;48(10):1130–7.
48. Gazzeri R, Galarza M, Gazzeri G. Growth of a meningioma in a transsexual patient after estrogen-progestin therapy. N Engl J Med. 2007;357(23):2411–2.
49. Levy J, et al. Interaction of spironolactone with oestradiol receptors in cytosol. J Endocrinol. 1980;84(3):371–9.
50. Deutsch MB, Bhakri V, Kubicek K. Effects of cross-sex hormone treatment on transgender women and men. Obstet Gynecol. 2015;125(3):605–10.
51. Mosenkis A, Townsend RR. Gynecomastia and antihypertensive therapy. J Clin Hypertens (Greenwich). 2004;6(8):469–70.
52. Kreukels BPC, Steensma TD, de Vries ALC. Gender dysphoria and disorders of sex development: progress in care and knowledge. In: Focus on sexuality research. New York; Heidelberg: Springer; 2014. xxxii, 357 p.

53. Moretti C, et al. Combined oral contraception and bicalutamide in polycystic ovary syndrome and severe hirsutism: a double-blind randomized controlled trial. Moretti C1, Guccione L1, Di Giacinto P1, Simonelli I2, Exacoustos C3, Toscano V4, Motta C4, De Leo V5, Petraglia F5, Lenzi A6. J Clin Endocrinol Metab. 2018;103(3):824–38.
54. Muderris II, et al. New alternative treatment in hirsutism: bicalutamide 25 mg/day. Gynecol Endocrinol. 2002;16(1):63–6.
55. Calaf J, et al. Long-term efficacy and tolerability of flutamide combined with oral contraception in moderate to severe hirsutism: a 12-month, double-blind, parallel clinical trial. J Clin Endocrinol Metab. 2007;92(9):3446–52.
56. Castelo-Branco C, et al. Long-term safety and tolerability of flutamide for the treatment of hirsutism. Fertil Steril. 2009;91(4):1183–8.
57. Dikensoy E, et al. The risk of hepatotoxicity during long-term and low-dose flutamide treatment in hirsutism. Arch Gynecol Obstet. 2009;279(3):321–7.
58. Irwig MS. Safety concerns regarding 5alpha reductase inhibitors for the treatment of androgenetic alopecia. Curr Opin Endocrinol Diabetes Obes. 2015;22(3):248–53.
59. Available from: http://transhealth.ucsf.edu/trans?page=guidelines-feminizing-therapy (2/15/2018).
60. Ettner R. Care of the elderly transgender patient. Curr Opin Endocrinol Diabetes Obes. 2013;20(6):580–4.
61. Mepham N, et al. People with gender dysphoria who self-prescribe cross-sex hormones: prevalence, sources, and side effects knowledge. J Sex Med. 2014;11(12):2995–3001.
62. de Blok CJM, et al. Breast development in transwomen after 1 year of cross-sex hormone therapy: results of a prospective multicenter study. J Clin Endocrinol Metab. 2018;103 (2):532–8.
63. Canonico M, et al. Hormone replacement therapy and risk of venous thromboembolism in postmenopausal women: systematic review and meta-analysis. BMJ. 2008;336(7655): 1227–31.
64. Asscheman H, et al. Venous thrombo-embolism as a complication of cross-sex hormone treatment of male-to-female transsexual subjects: a review. Andrologia. 2014;46(7):791–5.
65. van Kesteren PJ, et al. Mortality and morbidity in transsexual subjects treated with cross-sex hormones. Clin Endocrinol (Oxf). 1997;47(3):337–42.
66. Costa R, Colizzi M. The effect of cross-sex hormonal treatment on gender dysphoria individuals' mental health: a systematic review. Neuropsychiatr Dis Treat. 2016;12: 1953–66.
67. Rossouw JE, et al. Inflammatory, lipid, thrombotic, and genetic markers of coronary heart disease risk in the women's health initiative trials of hormone therapy. Arch Intern Med. 2008;168(20):2245–53.
68. Miller VT, et al. Effects of estrogen or estrogen/progestin regimens on heart disease risk factors in postmenopausal women. The postmenopausal estrogen/progestin interventions (PEPI) trial. The writing group for the PEPI trial. JAMA. 1995;273(3):199–208. https://doi.org/10.1001/jama.1995.03520270033028.
69. Ott J, et al. Cross-sex hormone therapy alters the serum lipid profile: a retrospective cohort study in 169 transsexuals. J Sex Med. 2011;8(8):2361–9.
70. Singh-Ospina N, et al. Effect of sex steroids on the bone health of transgender individuals: a systematic review and meta-analysis. J Clin Endocrinol Metab. 2017;102(11):3904–13.
71. Elbers JM, et al. Effects of sex steroids on components of the insulin resistance syndrome in transsexual subjects. Clin Endocrinol (Oxf). 2003;58(5):562–71.
72. Wierckx K, et al. Cross-sex hormone therapy in trans persons is safe and effective at short-time follow-up: results from the European network for the investigation of gender incongruence. J Sex Med. 2014;11(8):1999–2011.
73. Kovacs K, et al. Prolactin-producing pituitary adenoma in a male-to-female transsexual patient with protracted estrogen administration. A morphologic study. Arch Pathol Lab Med. 1994;118(5):562–5.

74. Serri O, et al. Lactotroph hyperplasia in an estrogen treated male-to-female transsexual patient. J Clin Endocrinol Metab. 1996;81(9):3177–9.
75. Cunha FS, et al. Diagnosis of prolactinoma in two male-to-female transsexual subjects following high-dose cross-sex hormone therapy. Andrologia. 2015;47(6):680–4.
76. Freda PU, et al. Pituitary incidentaloma: an endocrine society clinical practice guideline. J Clin Endocrinol Metab. 2011;96(4):894–904.
77. Giltay EJ, et al. Sex steroids, insulin, and arterial stiffness in women and men. Hypertension. 1999;34(4 Pt 1):590–7.
78. Boldo A, White WB. Blood pressure effects of the oral contraceptive and postmenopausal hormone therapies. Endocrinol Metab Clin North Am. 2011;40(2):419–32, ix.
79. Wierckx K, et al. Sexual desire in trans persons: associations with sex reassignment treatment. J Sex Med. 2014;11(1):107–18.
80. Steinle K. Hormonal management of the female-to-male transgender patient. J Midwifery Womens Health. 2011;56(3):293–302.
81. Meyer WJ 3rd, Webb A, Stuart CA, Finkelstein JW, Lawrence B, Walker PA. Physical and hormonal evaluation of transsexual patients: a longitudinal study. Send to Arch Sex Behav. 1986;15(2):121–38.
82. Tack LJ, et al. Consecutive lynestrenol and cross-sex hormone treatment in biological female adolescents with gender dysphoria: a retrospective analysis. Biol Sex Differ. 2016;7:14.
83. Darney PD. The androgenicity of progestins. Am J Med. 1995;98(1A):104S–10S.
84. Leder BZ, et al. Effects of aromatase inhibition in elderly men with low or borderline-low serum testosterone levels. J Clin Endocrinol Metab. 2004;89(3):1174–80.
85. T'Sjoen GG, et al. Comparative assessment in young and elderly men of the gonadotropin response to aromatase inhibition. J Clin Endocrinol Metab. 2005;90(10):5717–22.
86. Ott J, et al. Incidence of thrombophilia and venous thrombosis in transsexuals under cross-sex hormone therapy. Fertil Steril. 2010;93(4):1267–72.
87. Buckler HM, et al. The effects of low-dose testosterone treatment on lipid metabolism, clotting factors and ultrasonographic ovarian morphology in women. Clin Endocrinol (Oxf). 1998;49(2):173–8.
88. Gorton RN, Buth J, Spade D. Medical therapy and health maintenance for transgender men: a guide for health care providers. San Francisco, CA: Lyon-Martin Women's Health Services; 2005. http://www.lyon-martin.org
89. Coviello AD, et al. Effects of graded doses of testosterone on erythropoiesis in healthy young and older men. J Clin Endocrinol Metab. 2008;93(3):914–9.
90. Dickerman RD, et al. Androgen-induced erythrocytosis: is it erythropoietin? Am J Hematol. 1999;61(2):154–5.
91. Dobs AS, et al. Pharmacokinetics, efficacy, and safety of a permeation-enhanced testosterone transdermal system in comparison with bi-weekly injections of testosterone enanthate for the treatment of hypogonadal men. J Clin Endocrinol Metab. 1999;84(10):3469–78.
92. Mueller A, et al. Long-term administration of testosterone undecanoate every 3 months for testosterone supplementation in female-to-male transsexuals. J Clin Endocrinol Metab. 2007;92(9):3470–5.
93. Gooren LJ. Management of female-to-male transgender persons: medical and surgical management, life expectancy. Curr Opin Endocrinol Diabetes Obes. 2014;21(3):233–8.
94. Asscheman H, et al. A long-term follow-up study of mortality in transsexuals receiving treatment with cross-sex hormones. Eur J Endocrinol. 2011;164(4):635–42.
95. Gooren LJ, Giltay EJ. Men and women, so different, so similar: observations from cross-sex hormone treatment of transsexual subjects. Andrologia. 2014;46(5):570–5.
96. Costantino A, et al. A prospective study on sexual function and mood in female-to-male transsexuals during testosterone administration and after sex reassignment surgery. J Sex Marital Ther. 2013;39(4):321–35.
97. Mueller A, et al. Effects of intramuscular testosterone undecanoate on body composition and bone mineral density in female-to-male transsexuals. J Sex Med. 2010;7(9):3190–8.

98. Dhejne C, et al. Long-term follow-up of transsexual persons undergoing sex reassignment surgery: cohort study in Sweden. PLoS ONE. 2011;6(2):e16885.
99. Wierckx K, et al. Prevalence of cardiovascular disease and cancer during cross-sex hormone therapy in a large cohort of trans persons: a case-control study. Eur J Endocrinol. 2013;169 (4):471–8.
100. Deutsch MB, Feldman JL. Updated recommendations from the world professional association for transgender health standards of care. Am Fam Physician. 2013;87(2):89–93.
101. Polderman KH, et al. Induction of insulin resistance by androgens and estrogens. J Clin Endocrinol Metab. 1994;79(1):265–71.
102. Berra M, et al. Testosterone decreases adiponectin levels in female to male transsexuals. Asian J Androl. 2006;8(6):725–9.
103. Colizzi M, et al. Concomitant psychiatric problems and hormonal treatment induced metabolic syndrome in gender dysphoria individuals: a 2 year follow-up study. J Psychosom Res. 2015;78(4):399–406.
104. Pelusi C, et al. Effects of three different testosterone formulations in female-to-male transsexual persons. J Sex Med. 2014;11(12):3002–11.
105. Dunaif A, et al. Profound peripheral insulin resistance, independent of obesity, in polycystic ovary syndrome. Diabetes. 1989;38(9):1165–74.
106. Fernandez JD, Tannock LR. Metabolic effects of hormone therapy in transgender patients. Endocr Pract. 2016;22(4):383–8.
107. Emmelot-Vonk MH, et al. Effect of testosterone supplementation on functional mobility, cognition, and other parameters in older men: a randomized controlled trial. JAMA. 2008;299(1):39–52.
108. Doublier S, et al. Testosterone and 17beta-estradiol have opposite effects on podocyte apoptosis that precedes glomerulosclerosis in female estrogen receptor knockout mice. Kidney Int. 2011;79(4):404–13.
109. Soljancic A, et al. Protective role of testosterone in ischemia-reperfusion-induced acute kidney injury. Am J Physiol Regul Integr Comp Physiol. 2013;304(11):R951–8.
110. Ikeda K, et al. Excessive androgen exposure in female-to-male transsexual persons of reproductive age induces hyperplasia of the ovarian cortex and stroma but not polycystic ovary morphology. Hum Reprod. 2013;28(2):453–61.
111. Galazis N, et al. Proteomic biomarkers for ovarian cancer risk in women with polycystic ovary syndrome: a systematic review and biomarker database integration. Fertil Steril. 2012;98(6):1590–601 e1.
112. Grynberg M, et al. Histology of genital tract and breast tissue after long-term testosterone administration in a female-to-male transsexual population. Reprod Biomed Online. 2010;20 (4):553–8.
113. Baba T, et al. Association between polycystic ovary syndrome and female-to-male transsexuality. Hum Reprod. 2007;22(4):1011–6.
114. Pache TD, Fauser BC. Polycystic ovaries in female-to-male transsexuals. Clin Endocrinol (Oxf). 1993;39(6):702–3.
115. Coleman E, et al. Standards of care for the health of transsexual, transgender, and gender-nonconforming people, version 7. Int J Transgenderism. 2012;13(4):165–232.
116. Slagter MH, et al. Effects of long-term androgen administration on breast tissue of female-to-male transsexuals. J Histochem Cytochem. 2006;54(8):905–10.
117. Gooren LJ, et al. Breast cancer development in transsexual subjects receiving cross-sex hormone treatment. J Sex Med. 2013;10(12):3129–34.
118. Gooren L, et al. Five new cases of breast cancer in transsexual persons. Andrologia. 2015;47 (10):1202–5.
119. Shao T, Grossbard ML, Klein P. Breast cancer in female-to-male transsexuals: two cases with a review of physiology and management. Clin Breast Cancer. 2011;11(6):417–9.
120. Burcombe RJ, et al. Breast cancer after bilateral subcutaneous mastectomy in a female-to-male trans-sexual. Breast. 2003;12(4):290–3.

121. Nikolic DV, et al. Importance of revealing a rare case of breast cancer in a female to male transsexual after bilateral mastectomy. World J Surg Oncol. 2012;10:280.
122. Mahan RJ, et al. Drug therapy for gender transitions and health screenings in transgender older adults. J Am Geriatr Soc. 2016;64(12):2554–9.
123. Primary care protocol for transgender patient care. Center of Excellence for Transgender Health, University of California, San Francisco, Department of Family and Community Medicine. [online] available at http://transhealth.ucsf.edu/protocols (2011). Accessed 5 Feb 2018.
124. Baldassarre M, et al. Effects of long-term high dose testosterone administration on vaginal epithelium structure and estrogen receptor-alpha and -beta expression of young women. Int J Impot Res. 2013;25(5):172–7.
125. Roberts TK, et al. Interpreting laboratory results in transgender patients on hormone therapy. Am J Med. 2014;127(2):159–62.
126. Callewaert F, et al. Skeletal sexual dimorphism: relative contribution of sex steroids, GH-IGF1, and mechanical loading. J Endocrinol. 2010;207(2):127–34.
127. Lips P, et al. The effect of androgen treatment on bone metabolism in female-to-male transsexuals. J Bone Miner Res. 1996;11(11):1769–73.
128. Van Caenegem E, et al. Bone mass, bone geometry, and body composition in female-to-male transsexual persons after long-term cross-sex hormonal therapy. J Clin Endocrinol Metab. 2012;97(7):2503–11.
129. Ruetsche AG, et al. Cortical and trabecular bone mineral density in transsexuals after long-term cross-sex hormonal treatment: a cross-sectional study. Osteoporos Int. 2005;16 (7):791–8.
130. Turner A, et al. Testosterone increases bone mineral density in female-to-male transsexuals: a case series of 15 subjects. Clin Endocrinol (Oxf). 2004;61(5):560–6.
131. Van Caenegem E, et al. Low bone mass is prevalent in male-to-female transsexual persons before the start of cross-sex hormonal therapy and gonadectomy. Bone. 2013;54(1):92–7.
132. Van Caenegem E, et al. Preservation of volumetric bone density and geometry in trans women during cross-sex hormonal therapy: a prospective observational study. Osteoporos Int. 2015;26(1):35–47.
133. Fischer EM, et al. Severe osteoporosis with multiple vertebral fractures after gender reassignment therapy—is it male or female osteoporosis? Gynecol Endocrinol. 2011;27 (5):341–4.
134. Amin S, et al. Association of hypogonadism and estradiol levels with bone mineral density in elderly men from the Framingham study. Ann Intern Med. 2000;133(12):951–63.
135. Khosla S, et al. Relationship of serum sex steroid levels to longitudinal changes in bone density in young versus elderly men. J Clin Endocrinol Metab. 2001;86(8):3555–61.
136. Argalious MY, et al. Association of testosterone replacement therapy and the incidence of a composite of postoperative in-hospital mortality and cardiovascular events in men undergoing noncardiac surgery. Anesthesiology. 2017;127(3):457–65.

Chapter 9
Endocrine Care of Transgender Children and Adolescents

Daniel Evan Shumer and Adrian Araya

Introduction

An estimated 0.7% of youth ages 13–17 in the United States identify as transgender according to a 2017 report, the largest percentage of any measured age group [1]. Dozens of US comprehensive clinical care programs [2] and likely, hundreds of individual providers across the country and around the world are now providing hormonal care for transgender youth. Current treatment approaches have their roots in the so-called "Dutch Protocol", consisting of confirmation of a diagnosis of gender dysphoria by a mental health professional, pubertal suppression at Tanner stage 2, and treatment with gender-affirming hormones in later adolescence [3]. This treatment strategy has subsequently been codified by the World Professional Association for Transgender Health (WPATH) Standards of Care for the Health of Transsexual, Transgender and Gender-Nonconforming People (version 7, 2012) [4] and the Endocrine Society Clinical Practice Guideline for Endocrine Treatment of Gender-Dysphoric/Gender-Incongruent Persons (2017) [5]. Other seminal resources outlining current best practices include the UCSF Guidelines for Primary and Gender-Affirming Care of Transgender and Gender Nonbinary People, section titled "Health considerations for gender nonconforming children and transgender adolescents" [6] and Rosenthal's *Approach to the patient: transgender youth: endocrine considerations* [7]. In this chapter, we aim to review the current standards and provide practical guidance for the clinical care of transgender youth.

D. E. Shumer (✉) · A. Araya
Department of Pediatrics, Mott Children's Hospital, Michigan Medicine, Ann Arbor, MI, USA
e-mail: dshumer@med.umich.edu

L. Poretsky and W. C. Hembree (eds.), *Transgender Medicine*, Contemporary Endocrinology, https://doi.org/10.1007/978-3-030-05683-4_9

Terminology

A brief review of terminology related to transgender youth serves as an introduction to subsequent sections. Note that this lexicon influx, and some terms which were previously in common use have been replaced and may be considered offensive by some. Below are some currently used terms and their definitions [5, 7–9].

Gender identity: an internal sense of oneself as a boy or girl, man or woman, somewhere along a gender spectrum, or as having no gender (agender). This is not the same as *sexual orientation*, defined below.
Assigned sex (sex assigned at birth or natal sex): the sex assignment made upon birth, typically male or female, based on the appearance of the external genitalia and/or based on information on the infant's chromosomal or hormonal sex. Persons born with a disorder of sex development, in which the classification as male or female may be less clear, may identify with the term *intersex*.
Transgender: an umbrella term describing individuals who identify with a gender that is different from gender assigned at birth; may or may not connote gender dysphoria or desire to seek an intervention.
Transgender girl/woman: a transgender person who identifies as a girl or a woman.
Transgender boy/man: a transgender person who identifies as a boy or man.
Cisgender: a person whose assigned sex is congruent with gender identity; a person who is not transgender.
Agender: a person whose gender identity is not aligned with any gender.
Gender expression: ways in which a person may express gender identity through appearance, clothing, and behavior.
Gender attribution: process by which others make an assessment of an individual's gender based on the person's expression.
Sexual orientation: a person's feelings of romantic interest or sexual attraction directed toward members of one or more sex or gender (*gay, lesbian, bisexual, straight*) or no such attractions (*asexual*).
Gender dysphoria: conflict between one's gender identity and assigned sex which results in distress. Gender dysphoria is further defined by the American Psychiatric Association's Diagnostic and Statistical Manual (DSM-5), and in previous versions was referred to as *gender identity disorder*. The DSM separates gender dysphoria in children from gender dysphoria in adolescents and adults. Furthermore, in children, two of the following six criteria must be present to meet the DSM clinical criteria [10]:

1. A strong desire to be of the other gender or an insistence that one is the other gender.
2. A strong preference for wearing clothes typical of the opposite gender.
3. A strong preference for cross-gender roles in make-believe play or fantasy play.
4. A strong preference for the toys, games, or activities stereotypically used or engaged in by the other gender.

5. A strong preference for playmates of the other gender.
6. A strong rejection of toys, games, and activities typical of one's assigned gender.
7. A strong dislike of one's sexual anatomy.
8. A strong desire for the physical sex characteristics that match one's experienced gender.

Likewise, in adolescents and adults, two of the following six criteria must be present to meet criteria:

1. A marked incongruence between one's experienced/expressed gender and primary and/or secondary sex characteristics.
2. A strong desire to be rid of one's primary and/or secondary sex characteristics.
3. A strong desire for the primary and/or secondary sex characteristics of the other gender.
4. A strong desire to be of the other gender.
5. A strong desire to be treated as the other gender.
6. A strong conviction that one has the typical feelings and reactions of the other gender.

Transition: the hormonal, surgical, or social interventions taken to live as one's affirmed gender; specific terms *hormonal transition*, *surgical transition*, and *social transition* refer to those individual processes within one's transition.

Hormone blockers, or "*blockers*": term commonly used by patients and families referring to medications that delay the progression of puberty such as gonadotropin-releasing hormone (GnRH) agonists.

Gender-affirming hormone treatment: use of medications that will provide secondary sexual characteristics consistent with gender identity, specifically testosterone, or estrogen treatments.

Gender-affirming surgeries: surgical interventions providing physical characteristics congruent with gender identity. Patients and families may refer to chest surgeries "top surgery" and genital surgeries as "bottom surgery." Gender-affirmation surgery is preferred over the term *gender-reassignment surgery*.

Sex Differentiation and Puberty

Prior to discussion of the treatment of gender dysphoria in youth, a foundation in normal growth and development is required, beginning with sex differentiation. In fetal life, the undifferentiated gonad, under direction from the sex chromosomes, becomes differentiated as a testis or an ovary. During the first trimester, the testis or ovary is stimulated by human chorionic gonadotropin from the placenta. Later in fetal life, the hypothalamic–pituitary–gonadal axis develops with gonads receiving stimulation from, and providing feedback to, the central nervous system. The differential production of testosterone, anti-Mullerian hormone, and estrogen in the fetus accounts for the development of male and female internal and external reproductive organs, known as the primary sex characteristics. After birth, gonads continue to produce differential levels of these hormones during a so-called "mini-puberty of infancy", but quickly thereafter become quiescent. Therefore, prepubertal male and female children share a similar hormonal milieu [11]. This fact has significant application for prepubertal transgender youth. Transgender youth who desire to make a social transition is not encumbered by incongruent secondary sex characteristics, the changes that occur during puberty. For example, young transgender girls do not have a low voice, an Adam's apple, facial hair, or masculine facial features; young transgender boys do not have breasts or a feminine body habitus; and therefore gender expression alone (their dress, hairstyle, and behavior) can allow for successful attribution from others as their desired gender. Transgender youth, therefore, require no medical intervention.

Secondary sex characteristics are the group of sex-specific changes that occur during puberty. These changes begin as the GnRH pulse generator matures within the hypothalamus. When secreted in a pulsatile fashion, GnRH acts upon the anterior pituitary causing the pulsatile release of luteinizing hormone (LH) and follicle stimulating hormone (FSH) which, in turn, provides stimulation to the gonads. This process occurs in parallel with adrenarche, during which adrenal androgen production increases, manifested by the development of pubic hair and apocrine body odor [12, 13].

In males, LH stimulates testicular Leydig cells to produce testosterone and FSH stimulates maturation of germ cells and testicular enlargement. Development of male secondary sex characteristics is driven by the production of testosterone and conversion to dihydrotestosterone at end organs. Pubertal development in boys typically occurs as early as 9 years of age to as late as 15 years of age with mean age of 11–12 years. Physical manifestation of central puberty presents first with testicular enlargement and scrotal reddening and thinning. These changes are the hallmark of Tanner stage 2. Peak height velocity is achieved, on average, by age 14 [14]. Importantly, while an adolescent male may have fully developed genitalia (Tanner stage 5), continued production of testosterone in young adulthood further acts to contour the facial skeleton. This has relevance when considering whether to use GnRH agonists in transgender girls or young women presenting later to care in order to limit further facial and skeletal masculinization.

In females, puberty is driven by estrogen production. LH stimulates ovarian theca cells to produce androgens which are aromatized to estrogen in granulosa cells. FSH is responsible for follicular recruitment [13]. Pubertal development typically occurs as early as 8 years of age to as late as 14 years of age with mean age of 10–11 years. Physical manifestation of central puberty presents first with the development of glandular breast tissue characterized by elevation of breast and papilla, the hallmark of Tanner stage 2 [15]. Peak height velocity is achieved in Tanner stage 2–3 prior to menses, with menses occurring 2–2.5 years after Tanner stage 2 begins [16].

Historical Perspectives

The current hormonal management of transgender youth evolved from strategies first described by Delemarre-van de Waaal and Cohen-Kettenis at the Amsterdam Gender Clinic in 2006, and was subsequently referred to as the "Dutch Protocol" [3]. This protocol was derived from several important observations: (i) prior to the onset of puberty, no hormonal intervention is necessary; (ii) after the onset of puberty, the development of secondary sex characteristics can exacerbate a young person's gender dysphoria and also cause permanent changes to the young person's body, incongruent with their gender identity; (iii) the onset of puberty occurs at an age when providers were not comfortable starting medications which would cause irreversible effects; (iv) older adolescents and young adults can make appropriately informed decisions about gender-affirming hormone treatments and gender-affirming surgeries. The specific timeline outlined by Delemarre-van de Waal and Cohen-Kettenis dictated that youth with consistent cross-gender identity could begin GnRH agonist at Tanner stage 2 or 3 *and* at an age older than 12 [3]. The supposition was made that prepubertal youth may or may not have persisting gender dysphoria and that persistent dysphoria could not be predicted. By waiting until Tanner stage 2 or 3, the young person would experience some pubertal development, and the exacerbation of dysphoria would be diagnostic of persisting dysphoria into later adolescence and adulthood [17, 18]. Age 12 was chosen as an age when adolescents were able to make medical decisions with their caretakers [19]. Pubertal suppression could also be applied to adolescents presenting after age 12 and in later stages of pubertal development with a goal to halt further progression of puberty. Gender-affirming hormone treatments could be introduced at age 16, an age chosen because at this age Dutch adolescents were considered adults in the context of medical decision making. Pubertal development aligned with gender identity was achieved by gradually increasing doses of testosterone or estrogen every 6 months until adult hormonal levels were achieved. GnRH agonist treatment was continued at least until adult hormonal levels were reached and preferably until gonadectomy. Gender-affirming surgeries were deferred until age 18 in the initial descriptions of the protocol.

The Dutch Protocol provided the framework for subsequent guidelines [4–7] and current clinical practices. The authors noted that hormonal treatment for transgender youth is a controversial topic, but argued that nonintervention is not a neutral option; postponing medical intervention until adulthood may portend negative mental health outcomes for transgender youth [20]. Long-term outcomes data related to the first cohort of patients treated under the Dutch Protocol demonstrated positive mental health outcomes in young adulthood, in contrast to the large mental health disparities faced by untreated transgender persons [21]. That said, the evolving landscape of gender identity has led to the evolution of contemporary care. For example, the Dutch Protocol relied heavily on age cutoffs for medical decision making, largely based on Dutch law at the time. These cutoffs are being reconsidered by many clinicians in favor of other factors including appropriate pubertal timing, stability of gender identity, patient maturity, ability to understand risks and benefits, and family readiness. Second, gonadectomy was an assumed goal of the initial patients described by the Dutch Protocol. Clinicians today acknowledge that not all transgender youth who are appropriate candidates for hormonal intervention will desire or will be able to afford gonadectomy or other gender-affirming surgeries [22].

Contemporary Management

The WPATH Standards of Care (SOC) [4] and the Endocrine Society's guidelines [5] currently serve as the basis for clinical care of transgender youth. As mentioned before, guidance published by UCSF [6] and also independently by Rosenthal [7] compliment these guidelines and provide logistical detail. These resources and our clinical experience guide future sections of the chapter.

The Clinical Care Team

The WPATH SOC and Endocrine Society both strongly recommend that medical providers work with mental health professionals with expertise in the diagnosis of gender dysphoria prior to medical intervention. This recommendation highlights the importance of confirming the diagnosis of gender dysphoria prior to embarking on a medical intervention. In addition, because transgender children and adolescents have increased the risk of suicidal ideation, suicide attempt, depression, and anxiety, evaluation by a mental health professional can be helpful in the diagnosis of comorbid conditions and can help coordinate complimentary mental health treatment as appropriate [23, 24].

The logistics of how mental health professionals work with medical providers is variable and often influenced by local resources. Large hospital-based gender clinics may employ social workers or psychologists to perform independent gender and psychosocial assessments for patients presenting for care [25]. Other providers may form informal networks with community based mental health providers, and ask for letters of support from these providers prior to initiation of hormonal interventions. Additionally, psychiatrists may work within gender teams or as consultants to evaluate and treat patients with unmet psychiatric needs such as depression and anxiety.

Hormone prescribers may have received initial medical training in any number of specialties including, but not limited to, general pediatrics, pediatric endocrinology, adolescent medicine, family medicine, or gynecology. The most important requirement of the hormone provider is that they have an interest in working with this vulnerable patient population—the medical aspects of care can be learned.

Other team members may include: legal consultants (to assist with gender marker changes on legal documents, or to advocate for insurance coverage); nursing (to provide education related to medication administration, for example to teach self-administration of testosterone); plastic surgery; and speech and language pathologists (to evaluate and treat voice dysphoria). Individual providers not working as part of a formal gender team may familiarize themselves with local transgender-friendly resources in these fields. In addition, all staff members working with hormone providers should be trained on topics of gender identity, including the use of preferred names and pronouns. This includes, but is not limited to, scheduling staff, receptionists, medical assistants, phlebotomists, and radiology technicians. Leaders of gender teams may need to think critically about the cultural competency of the health system in which they work and advocate at administrative levels in order to improve care for patients.

Hormonal Interventions

Hormonal interventions used in the treatment of adolescents with gender dysphoria include medications that suppress natal hormone production or action (pubertal suppression), and medications which promote the development of secondary sex characteristics of the affirmed gender (gender-affirming hormone treatment). Factors involved in deciding which interventions are appropriate for the individual patient include the current pubertal stage of the patient, the patient's stated goals of treatment, the maturity level of the patient and their ability to understand risks and benefits of intervention, and the consent and support of parents or guardians (Fig. 9.1). Unfortunately, insurance coverage and affordability of interventions may also dictate what interventions are available to individual patients.

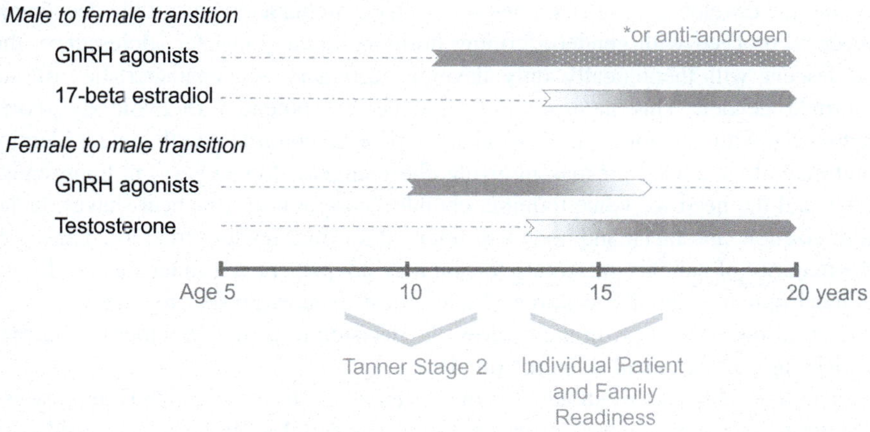

Fig. 9.1 General timeline for medical interventions in transgender youth/adolescents

Pubertal Hormone Suppression/Inhibition

GnRH agonists

Both the WPATH SOC and Endocrine Society suggest children with gender dysphoria are eligible for treatment with GnRH agonist medications starting at Tanner stage 2, regardless of age [4, 5]. The goals of suppression include (i) prevention of development of unwanted secondary sex characteristics, (ii) mitigation of the accompanying dysphoria associated with puberty, and (iii) the ability to delay decisions around gender-affirming hormone treatment.

GnRH agonist medications, initially used in pediatrics for the treatment of central precocious puberty, provide continual stimulation of the GnRH receptor. When stimulated continuously, as opposed to in pulsatile fashion, gonadotrophs in the anterior pituitary are inhibited from releasing LH and FSH. Treatments with GnRH agonists, therefore, inhibit pituitary stimulation of the gonads with a goal of suppressing production of the sex hormones, testosterone, and estrogen [26].

GnRH agonists are formulated as intramuscular injections (such as leuprolide acetate 1-month or 3-month preparations) and subcutaneous implants (histrelin, implanted annually). Factors such as preference for more frequent injections versus less frequent surgical implantation procedures and cost/insurance coverage may influence the choice of formulation [7, 23, 27]. In situations where GnRH agonist treatment is desired but not available or affordable, treatment with medroxyprogesterone acetate, which works both to inhibit the hypothalamic–pituitary–gonadal axis and to inhibit gonadal steroidogenesis, has been described. This treatment has been shown to reduce but not completely inhibit sex hormone production in transgender adolescents [28, 29].

The classic scenario when GnRH agonist treatment is prescribed is the young adolescent patient, male or female, presenting at Tanner stage 2. The efficacy of GnRH agonist in this situation is well documented—the young person will be spared the development of unwanted secondary sex characteristics; if the decision is made to proceed with gender-affirming hormone therapy in later adolescence, the adolescent will theoretically only develop secondary sex characteristics of the affirmed gender. This treatment strategy has the potential to avoid dysphoria associated with development of sex characteristics incongruent with gender identity and may obviate need for masculinizing chest surgery (top surgery) in transgender boys and the need for voice training, chondrolaryngoplasty (tracheal shave), facial feminization, and facial and body hair removal for transgender girls [30]. That said, the majority of patients presenting to care may not present at Tanner stage 2. In our clinical practice, about two-thirds of adolescent patients present to care at a more advanced pubertal stage. In these cases, the decision regarding whether to consider GnRH agonist treatment is more complex.

The following factors should be considered when discussing GnRH agonist use for the transgender adolescent presenting at a pubertal stage more advanced than Tanner stage 2: (i) Is more pubertal development expected? (ii) What are the goals of treatment? (iii) Is the patient currently a candidate for gender-affirming hormone treatment? (iv) Is the patient male or female? Brief case examples will highlight how answers to these questions can assist in medical decision making.

A transgender girl presents at Tanner stage 4. Despite the fact that she started male puberty 2 years prior, she has very little facial or body hair, her facial bone structure appears still quite gender neutral. She is a candidate for estrogen therapy and she and her family are considering starting estrogen in 1 year. In this case, there is more masculinization of the facial structure expected, as is often true of adolescent transgender girls in mid-puberty. A significant goal of treatment, in this case, would be to limit masculine facial structure and facial hair development. Regardless of whether this patient decides to start estrogen now or in the future, GnRH agonist treatment could be considered. Concurrent use of GnRH agonist plus estrogen in transgender young women can also be beneficial. This "block-and-replace" strategy can be advantageous—the estrogen dose required to both suppress testosterone production and promote feminization when given as monotherapy may be significantly higher than when used concurrently with GnRH agonist [6].

A transgender girl presents at Tanner stage 5 to discuss initiation of gender-affirming hormonal treatment. On clinical exam, the patient has developed adult facial and body hair and is already engaged in the removal of this hair using electrolysis. She has a masculine appearing facial bone structure and is planning to request facial feminization surgery in the future. She is also contemplating vaginoplasty with gonadectomy in the future. This patient does not have expected further masculinizing pubertal development—she is fully masculinized. Treatment with GnRH agonist will not prevent further pubertal development. She may still benefit from concurrent use of GnRH agonist with estrogen in order to limit the required estrogen dose. However, the cost–benefit analysis in this situation is different than the previously described scenario, especially if there is a financial burden to the patient for initiation of GnRH agonist.

A transgender boy presents at Tanner stage 3 breast development. He is not yet a candidate for testosterone but is concerned about the prospect of further breast development. In this situation, GnRH agonist could be useful in limiting further breast development and the associated dysphoria accompanying this development. While breast development may not entirely regress on treatment, future mastectomy (top surgery) may require a less invasive incision if breasts do not develop past their current stage (i.e., a periareolar incision may be used rather than an inframammary incision).

A transgender boy presents at Tanner stage 5 breast development. He is not currently interested in starting testosterone; however, he is experiencing significant distress associated with his menses. In this scenario, GnRH agonist would inhibit the menstrual cycle, however, other interventions, such as progesterone-only contraceptive medications may have the same effect, and is further described below. The cost–benefit analysis may favor this approach over GnRH agonist treatment. GnRH agonist treatment could be reconsidered if other strategies are not successful [6].

A transgender boy presents at Tanner stage 3–4 breast development for discussion of gender-affirming hormone treatment. In this scenario, testosterone therapy is initiated prior to the completion of female puberty. Unlike estrogen monotherapy, testosterone monotherapy is more effective at suppressing further development of female secondary sex characteristics and the additional benefit of concurrent use of GnRH agonist is likely minimal.

In addition to GnRH agonist medications, several other medications should be included in the discussion of pubertal hormone suppression in transgender adolescents.

As previously mentioned, medroxyprogesterone acetate has been described for suppression of puberty when GnRH agonist treatment is not available. Medroxyprogesterone acetate can be given as a daily oral preparation (up to 40 mg/day) or as an intramuscular preparation (150 mg every 3 months) for males or females [7]. Commercially available progesterone-only contraceptive pills, when taken daily, can promote amenorrhea in transgender boys with menses-based dysphoria (for example, norethindrone 5–15 mg daily).

Spironolactone, initially developed as a potassium-sparing diuretic, additionally works to inhibit the synthesis and action of testosterone. Spironolactone (100–300 mg daily) is commonly prescribed to transgender girls and women who have already developed secondary hair (facial hair, body hair) as a means to slow hair growth and limit further hair development.

Prior to initiation of pubertal suppression, a baseline medical evaluation is recommended including height, weight, and blood pressure measurements and Tanner staging. Baseline laboratory evaluation of LH, FSH, estradiol, and testosterone can be used in confirming central puberty and for comparing to posttreatment assessments [5]. Rosenthal suggests assessment of LH, FSH, estradiol (in females), testosterone (in males) at baseline and every 3 months, assessments of calcium, phosphorus, alkaline phosphatase, and 25-hydroxyvitamin D at baseline and annually, and bone age and bone densitometry at baseline and annually in transgender youth treated with pubertal suppression [7]. Assessment of bone metabolism markers has been suggested due to the concerns regarding delaying bone density accrual, further described later in the chapter. Bone age evaluation can help the prescriber understand the individual patient's timing and tempo of growth and development, specifically with regards to height accrual.

Gender-Affirming Hormonal Interventions

Gender-affirming hormones, specifically testosterone and estradiol, are used to promote development of secondary sex characteristics of the affirmed gender. Specifically, testosterone is used in transgender boys to promote the development of facial and body hair, voice deepening, masculinization of facial structures and of fat and muscle distribution. Testosterone monotherapy, as mentioned above, also typically causes amenorrhea during use. Estradiol is used in transgender girls to promote breast development and development of a feminine body habitus. Unlike GnRH agonists, which have been described as *reversible* interventions, many of the changes which occur from use of gender-affirming hormones are more permanent. Therefore, careful assessment and thorough discussion of risks, benefits, and expectations of treatment are critical.

The timing of initiation of gender-affirming hormone therapy is a complex decision based on individual, family, social, and societal factors. As discussed, in the initial "Dutch Protocol" the age 16 was used. Many transgender adolescents, however, are deemed to have clear gender dysphoria and are requesting these interventions with parental support at much younger ages. From a social perspective, it may be challenging for a transgender child living in all contexts as their affirmed gender to wait until age 16 to start puberty—an age significantly older than what is typical for their peers. Furthermore, for a child who started GnRH agonist treatment at Tanner stage 2, perhaps as young as 8 or 9 years old, restricting the use of gender-affirming hormone therapy until age 16 would artificially delay their pubertal development, including growth spurt and bone density accrual, by over a half-decade. Given these concerns, many providers treat transgender youth with testosterone or estrogen at ages younger than 16 years. Rosenthal notes the use of age 14 in his review [7]. The Endocrine Society, in its 2017 revised Clinical Practice Guideline, comments: "we recognize that there may be compelling reasons to initiate sex hormone treatment prior to age 16 years, although there is minimal published experience treating prior to age 13.5–14 years of age [5]." As the evolution on age continues, providers seem to be acknowledging that individual readiness factors, rather than age cutoffs, are important when considering the use of gender-affirming hormones.

Testosterone is most commonly prescribed as testosterone cypionate or enanthate and given as an intramuscular (IM) or subcutaneous (SC) injection. For treatment of youth receiving GnRH agonist treatment concurrently, the goal of treatment is to mimic normal male puberty. This can be achieved by prescribing gradually escalating doses over time, such as starting with 12.5 mg/week (or 25 mg/2 weeks) and gradually increasing to 50–100 mg/week (or 100–200 mg/2 weeks) SC based on clinical progress [7]. For older adolescents, especially when not prescribed GnRH agonist concurrently, prescribers can more rapidly increase dosing or start at the lower end of the final dose range. The adult maintenance dose should provide enough testosterone for masculinization, should suppress menses, should limit excessive androgen effects such as acne vulgaris, and should provide for a measured testosterone level in the normal adult male range. In our clinical practice, most commonly prescribed adult dose of testosterone used to achieve these goals is 50 mg SC weekly. Testosterone has classically been prescribed as an intramuscular injection, however, subcutaneous administration has become a popular alternative delivery method as it is easier for self-administration and has been shown to be effective [31]. When prescribing testosterone for home administration, it should e noted that injectable testosterone is suspended in oil and is too thick to draw up through small caliber needles. In our practice, we prescribe a 1 cc or 3 cc syringe, a 21 gage removable needle for drawing up the testosterone, and a 25 gage

5/8 inch removable needle for injecting into the subcutaneous tissue. A demonstration injection is performed in our office using saline.

Other preparations of testosterone include transdermal gel and patch products. Transdermal gels and patches can be prescribed with a similar graduated dosing strategy to the adult dose of 50–100 mg daily for gel, 4 mg for the patch. Disadvantages of the gel, especially in the pediatric population, is the care needed to ensure that the gel does not come in contact with family members, and the need for daily administration. Testosterone patches provide for less flexibility with dosing increments and may irritate the skin. Both gels and patches are more expensive than injectable products. We suggest reserving use of gels and patches for cases of needle phobia or per patient preference after the full adult dose of injectable testosterone has been achieved.

Feminizing hormonal treatment for transgender girls is achieved with 17-beta-estradiol. Pharmaceutical products containing other conjugated or synthetic estrogens are not preferred due to unfavorable risk profiles [32]. 17-beta-estradiol can be prescribed as oral tablets, transdermal patches, or injectable products, with oral or transdermal administration most common in pediatric practice. Similarly to testosterone dosing, estrogen dosing varies with the clinical situation. For transgender girls concurrently treated with GnRH agonist, estrogen dosing can start low and proceed gradually to mimic normal female puberty. For example, oral 17-beta-estradiol can be initiated at 0.25 mg PO daily and advance to 2 mg oral daily based on clinical progress. Transdermal dosing could start with a portion of a 25 mcg patch (for example, 12.5 mcg by cutting the patch in half), and progressing to 100 mcg patch over time based on clinical progress. When treating an adolescent not concurrently prescribed GnRH, estrogen the dose required to suppress testosterone production and promote feminization is higher. For example, starting doses could be 2 mg oral or 100 mcg transdermal with increases to 6 mg or 300 mg, respectively. Goals of treatment, in this case, are to promote desired feminine development while suppressing testosterone; a concrete goal may be to keep measured testosterone level under 100 ng/dL.

Ongoing monitoring is required for patients prescribed gender-affirming hormone therapy. Assessments should focus on the clinical effects of the intervention, and how these effects align with the patient's goals of treatment. Ongoing review of mental health concerns, other medical concerns, general well-being, and social impacts of transition should also be discussed. For patients treated with 17-beta-estradiol, signs and symptoms of insulin resistance and hyperprolactinemia should be reviewed. Patients treated with testosterone may be at risk for hyperlipidemia, insulin resistance, and polycythemia, which guides recommendations for interval laboratory evaluation. In our experience, cystic acne is the most commonly encountered unwanted side effect of testosterone treatment, which can respond to reductions in testosterone dosing or standard acne interventions. Given these concerns, Rosenthal suggests baseline and quarterly assessments of height, weight, blood pressure, Tanner staging, LH, FSH, testosterone and/or estrogen, complete blood counts, renal function, liver function, fasting lipids, glucose, and hemoglobin A1c for at least the first year of treatment. Potassium should be included if a patient is treated with spironolactone. If a patient had been previously treated with GnRH agonists, assessments of calcium, phosphorus, alkaline phosphatase, 25-hydroxyvitamin D, bone densitometry, and bone age may also be helpful [7]. When appropriate adult dosing is determined and remains unchanged, monitoring frequency can be reduced, eventually to annual assessments as clinically appropriate.

Special Considerations for Youth

Bone density

Puberty is a time of relatively rapid skeletal maturation and accrual of bone mass. When puberty is suppressed at Tanner stage 2, there is a concern for a relative decrease in bone mineral density compared to untreated peers. There are data to suggest that current protocols do result in a decrease in apparent bone mineral density *z*-score, but with improvement toward normal after initiation of gender-affirming hormone therapy [33]. However, another study demonstrated a decline in bone mineral density *z*-score during GnRH agonist treatment without full catchup by age 22 [34]. Ultimately, clinicians are advised to discuss the risk of lower bone density at the onset of treatment, screen calcium, and vitamin D intake and treat deficiencies in an attempt to mitigate this potential risk.

Stature

There are a few little data regarding the final impact of pubertal suppression and gender-affirming hormone therapy on stature. While stature may not be a concern for all patients, it is not uncommon in our experience that transgender boys may desire a taller stature than their expected female height and transgender girls may be concerned about excessive height. Bone age assessments can be helpful in determining growth potential. Height growth can be expected until growth plates fuse. Hormonal interventions including use of GnRH agonists, estrogen, and testosterone have the potential to affect the duration of growth plate patency. The action of growth hormone, adrenal androgens, and sex hormones on the growth plate likely all contribute to height growth; estrogens are also known to promote growth plate closure. Broadly speaking, we recommend that decisions regarding timing of hormonal interventions be based primarily on patient readiness, however, significant concerns around stature could be influenced by the timing of therapy and dosing. For example, a longer course of pubertal delay followed by slower escalation in testosterone dosing may allow for more time for growth in a transgender boy. A more rapid escalation in estrogen dosing may marginally reduce unwanted height growth in a transgender girl. Trials examining these strategies are lacking.

Fertility

One of the most challenging aspects of providing patient-centered care to transgender youth and their families is engaging in discussions regarding fertility. Transgender youth, especially those presenting prior to or around the onset of puberty, are seldom concerned about the impact of medical interventions on fertility, and often even less interested in discussing this topic. This ambivalence is likely age appropriate, shared by their cisgender peers, and may not predict their future feelings. For example, a study of transmen indicates the majority desire to have children [35].

Development of mature sperm and oocytes occurs during puberty. Therefore, progressing through natural puberty is a requirement for fertility. When discussing fertility with a patient and family presenting at Tanner stage 2, it should be noted that patients with central precocious puberty treated with GnRH agonists have normal reproductive function after discontinuation of GnRH agonist and progression through natal puberty [36]. However, patients considering GnRH agonist therapy for gender dysphoria may not decide to allow their natal puberty to progress in later adolescence, choosing instead to bridge to gender-affirming hormone treatment. If that decision is made, there will never be maturation of sperm or eggs and no opportunity for gamete preservation.

It should be noted that trans men who maintain a uterus and ovaries have achieved pregnancy by cessation of testosterone and achieve pregnancy by ovarian stimulation [21].

Patients presenting after puberty should be advised that future fertility could be compromised by prolonged use of gender-affirming hormones. While there are examples of preserved fertility after hormonal transition, fertility options can be expanded by use of gamete cryopreservation [37]. In our practice, preservation of sperm is more likely to be desired than oocytes, likely due to cost and logistics.

Consent

Because adolescents are unable to independently consent for medical care, decisions on hormonal transition are shared among patients, parents, and medical providers. The best outcomes are achieved when all parties are in agreement with the medical plan [38]. Adolescents and their parents should be counseled on risks and benefits of treatment prior to proceeding [39]. In our experience, disagreements regarding the timing of transition can often be resolved by reviewing the goals of treatment, the potential risks of nontreatment, and encouraging professional family counseling when indicated.

In our experience, older adolescents who meet criteria for hormonal transition have often done independent research on transition, may be connected with other transitioning youth on social media, and are eager to start testosterone or estrogen, while their parents may not be ready to provide consent. In these situations, we recommend meeting the parents where they are: affirming the fact that this is an important family decision, celebrating the love and support they are demonstrating by bringing their child in for assessment, providing education around gender identity and the rationale for current standards of care, and reviewing risks and benefits of treatment and of nontreatment. While consent for hormonal transition may not occur at an initial visit, we have seen this approach successful in shifting parental attitudes in favor of consenting to hormonal transition over time when it is clinically indicated.

More challenging situations arise when there are disagreements between two parents or guardians of a child or adolescent, especially when parents are separated and perhaps engaged in joint custody or a custody dispute. In these situations we have found it helpful to engage with legal and/or ethical experts within our health system for guidance on how to proceed on an individual basis.

Summary

Several consensus guidelines outline best practices for the medical management of transgender youth. These guidelines describe the use of pubertal suppression and gender-affirming hormones to reduce gender dysphoria. As more transgender youth are now presenting to medical attention than in previous generations, medical providers caring for youth in any capacity should expect to see transgender youth in their practice and be knowledgeable about the basics of gender-affirming care. Providers interested in prescribing gender-affirming hormonal interventions should familiarize themselves with current standards and guidelines and develop a strategy for the provision of multidisciplinary care including mental health support and knowledge of community resources.

References

1. Herman JL, Flores AR, Brown TNT, Wilson B. DM, Conron K. Age of individuals who identify as transgender in the United States. The Williams Institute; 2017.
2. Hsieh S, Leininger J. Resource list: clinical care programs for gender-nonconforming children and adolescents. Pediatr Ann. 2014;43:238–44.
3. Delemarre-van de Wall HA, Cohen-Kettenis PT. Clinical management of gender identity disorder in adolescents: a protocol on psychological and paediatric endocrinology aspects. Eur J Endocrinol. 2006;155:S131–7.
4. Coleman E, et al. Standards of care for the health of transsexual, transgender, and gender-nonconforming people, version 7. Int J Transgenderism. 2012;13:165–232.
5. Hembree WC, et al. Endocrine treatment of gender-dysphoric/gender-incongruent persons: an endocrine society* clinical practice guideline. J Clin Endocrinol Metab. 2017;102:1–35.
6. Center of Excellence for Transgender Health. Guidelines for the primary and gender-affirming care of transgender and gender nonbinary people. University of California San Fransisco. http://transhealth.ucsf.edu/trans?page=guidelines-home. Accessed 3/19/2018.
7. Rosenthal SM. Approach to the patient: transgender youth: endocrine considerations. J Clin Endocrinol Metab. 2014;99:4379–89.
8. Simons L, Leibowitz SF, Hidalgo M. Understanding gender variance in children and adolescents. Pediatr Ann. 2014;43:e126–31.

9. Shumer DE, Nokoff NJ, Spack NP. Advances in the care of transgender children and adolescents. Adv Pediatr. 2016;63:79–102.
10. American Psychiatric Association. Diagnostic and statistical manual of mental disorders, 5th ed.; 2013.
11. Witchel SF, Lee PA. In: Sperling M, editor. A Pediatric endocrinology. Saunders Elsevier; 2008, p. 132.
12. Hughes, I. A. In: Sperling MA, editor. Pediatric endocrinology. Saunders Elsevier; 2008, p. 676–679.
13. Rosenfield RL, Cooke DW, Radovick S. In: Sperling MA, editor. Pediatric endocrinology. Saunders Elsevier; 2008, p. 532–559.
14. Marshal WA, Tanner JM. Variations in the pattern of pubertal changes in boys. Arch Dis Child. 1970;45:13–23.
15. Marshall W, Tanner JM. Variations in pattern of pubertal changes in girls. Arch Dis Child. 1969;44:291–303.
16. Marcell, A. V. In: Kligman RM, Behrman RE, Jenson HB, Stanton BF, editors. Nelson textbook of pediatrics. Saunders Elsevier; 2007, p. 60–65.
17. Steensma TD, Biemond R, de Boer F, Cohen-Kettenis PT. Desisting and persisting gender dysphoria after childhood: a qualitative follow-up study. Clin Child Psychol Psychiatry. 2011.
18. Steensma T, Kreukels B, de Vries A, Cohen-Kettenis P. Gender identity development in adolescence. Horm Behav. 2013;64:288–97.
19. Cohen-Kettenis PT, Klink D. Adolescents with gender dysphoria. Best Pract Res Clin Endocrinol Metab. 2015;29:485–95.
20. Cohen-Kettenis PT, Delemarre-van de Wall HA, Gooren LJG. The treatment of adolescent transsexuals: changing insights. J Sex Med. 2008;5:1892–7.
21. De Vries ALC, et al. Young adult psychological outcome after puberty suppression and gender reassignment. Pediatrics. 2014;134:1–9.
22. De Vries ALC, Cohen-Kettenis PT. Clinical management of gender dysphoria in children and adolescents: the Dutch approach. J Homosex. 2012;59:301–20.
23. Nahata L, Quinn GP, Caltabellotta N, Tishelman A. Mental health concerns and insurance denials among transgender adolescents. LGBT Heal. 2017;4:188–193.
24. Veale J, Watson R, Peter T, Saewyc E. Mental health disparities among canadian transgender youth. J. Adolesc. Heal. 2017;60:44–9.
25. Spack NP, et al. Children and adolescents with gender identity disorder referred to a pediatric medical center. Pediatrics. 2012;129:418–25.
26. Boepple PA, et al. Use of a potent, long acting agonist of gonadotropin-releasing hormone in the treatment of precocious puberty. Endocr Rev. 1986;7:24–33.
27. Chen M, Fuqua J. Adolescent transgender health: Awareness does not equal resources. Curr Pediatr Rep. 2016;4:186–7.
28. Lynch MM, Khandheria MM, Meyer WJ. Retrospective study of the management of childhood and adolescent gender identity disorder using medroxyprogesterone acetate. Int. J. Transgenderism. 2015;16:201–8.
29. Warren M, Mathews J, Morishima A, Vande Wiele R. The effect of medroxyprogesterone acetate on gonadotropin secretion in girls with precocious puberty. Am J Med Sci. 1975;269:375–81.
30. Shumer DE, Spack NP. Current management of gender identity disorder in childhood and adolescence: guidelines, barriers and areas of controversy. Curr Opin Endocrinol Diabetes Obes. 2013;20:69–73.
31. Spratt D, et al. Subcutaneous injection of testosterone is an effective and preferred alternative to intramuscular injection: demonstration in female-to-male transgender patients. J Clin Endocrinol Metab2. 2017;102:2349–55.
32. Asscheman H, et al. A long-term follow-up study of mortality in transsexuals receiving treatment with cross-sex hormones. Eur J Endocrinol. 2011;164:635–42.

33. Vlot M, et al. Effect of pubertal suppression and cross-sex hormone therapy on bone turnover markers and bone mineral apparent density (BMAD) in transgender adolescents. Bone. 2017;95:11–9.
34. Klink D, Caris M, Heijboer A, van Trotsenburg M, Rotteveel J. Bone mass in young adulthood following gonadotropin-releasing hormone analog treatment and cross-sex hormone treatment in adolescents with gender dysphoria. J Clin Endocrinol Metab. 2015;100:E270–5.
35. Wierckx K, et al. Reproductive wish in transsexual men. Hum Reprod2. 2012;27:483–7.
36. Pasquino A, et al. Long-term observation of 87 girls with idiopathic central precocious puberty treated with gonadotropin-releasing hormone analogs: impact on adult height, body mass index, bone mineral content, and reproductive function. J Clin Endocrinol Metab. 2008;93:190–5.
37. Nahata L, Curci M, Quinn G. Exploring fertility preservation intentions among transgender youth. J Adolesc Heal. 2018;62:123–5.
38. American Academy of Pediatrics Committee on Bioethics. Informed consent, parental permission, and assent in pediatric practice. Pediatrics. 1995:314–317.
39. Shumer D, Tishelman A. The role of assent in the treatment of transgender adolescents. Int J Transgenderism. https://doi.org/10.1080/15532739.2015.1075929.

Chapter 10
Gender Confirmation Surgery

Mark Fisher, Mark Smith and Adam D. Perry

History

The first reported gender confirmation surgery (GCS) was performed in Berlin in 1931 [1]. Prior to that only ablative procedures such as hysterectomy and gonadectomy were reported for gender dysphoria, notably the case of Alan L. Hart, an American physician born Alberta Lucille Hart who underwent hysterectomy and gonadectomy in 1917, at the age of 27 [2]. After a setback due to World War II, GCS in the United States resumed, notably with the creation of the Johns Hopkins Gender Identity Clinic in 1965. Led by plastic surgeon Milton Edgerton, this was the first multidisciplinary center for the care of transgendered patients and was composed of psychiatrists, psychologists, plastic surgeons, gynecologists, urologists, and endocrinologists. The center was closed in 1979 but reopened in 2017. Significant change occurred in 2014 when the United States Department of Health and Human Services review board ruled that Medicare would pay for GCS.

Surgical Goals

Adjusting the body to the mind is the overarching goal of gender confirmation surgery [3, 4]. For transwomen, this includes removal of the phallus and scrotum and creation of a natural-appearing vulva, sensate neo-clitoris, and vagina of adequate depth and width to enable penetrative intercourse. Adjunct procedures that achieve feminization include breast augmentation, thyroid chondrolaryngoplasty, as well as voice and facial feminization.

M. Fisher · M. Smith · A. D. Perry (✉)
Department of Plastic and Reconstructive Surgery, Zucker School of Medicine at Hofstra/Northwell, Hempstead, NY, USA
e-mail: aperry1@northwell.edu

L. Poretsky and W. C. Hembree (eds.), *Transgender Medicine*, Contemporary Endocrinology, https://doi.org/10.1007/978-3-030-05683-4_10

For transmen, the ability to achieve standing micturition and sexual penetration via phalloplasty or metoidioplasty is the mainstay of GCS. In addition, subcutaneous mastectomy and facial masculinization are common procedures.

Preoperative Evaluation

No patient should undergo gender confirmation surgery without proper screening and preoperative evaluation. Prior to proceeding to surgery, two referral letters from a qualified mental health professional are generally required. A diagnosis of persistent gender dysphoria should be well documented, and the patient must complete at least a year's trial of living in the gender role most congruent with their gender identity. Patients are required to have undergone at least 1 year of continuous hormone therapy as required for their gender goals. In addition, any medical or mental health concern must be reasonably well controlled, and patient must have the capacity to provide informed consent.

Hormone Therapy

It is critical for the surgeon to understand the effects of hormonal therapy. Though specific regimens may differ, the surgeons must be familiar with the possible side effects and how they may affect the surgery and recovery.

Feminization

Feminization is achieved by the suppression of androgen effects and induction of female secondary sex characteristics. Suppression of androgen effects may be achieved by medications that either suppress gonadotrophin-releasing hormone (GnRH) or are GnRH antagonists, suppress production of luteinizing hormone, interfere with testosterone production or interfere with androgen binding to its receptor at target tissues. Estrogens are used to induce female secondary sex characteristics through its action on tissue receptors.

After the initiation of feminizing hormone therapy, body fat redistributes into a female fat pattern, muscle mass decreases, skin softens, and libido decreases. Facial hair becomes finer, and breast growth commences.

Masculinization

Testosterone is the mainstay of masculinization hormone therapy. Testosterone therapy via either parenteral or transdermal routes increases muscle mass, decreases fat mass, increases facial hair, induces male-pattern baldness, causes clitoromegaly, deepens the voice, atrophies the vagina, increases libido, and causes cessation of menses. Testosterone levels should be monitored to avoid complication of excess testosterone—liver dysfunction, hypertension, lipid changes, erythrocytosis, excessive weight gain, salt retention, and cystic acne [5]. Estrogen levels may be decreased through the use of GnRH analogs or medroxyprogesterone.

Surgical Therapy

Feminization

A successful feminization of the genitalia achieves a natural-appearing vagina that can support penetrative intercourse, a feminine-appearing mons pubis, labia majora, and labia minora, and a sensate neo-clitoris with adequate clitoral hooding. This may be achieved through a number of surgical procedures, although the mainstay of genital feminization is vaginoplasty.

Currently, three major options exist for vaginoplasty—penile inversion, rectosigmoid colon intestinal transposition, and nongenital flaps. Of these, penile inversion [6, 7] and intestinal transposition [8] are most common. Intestinal transposition allows for the creation of a vascularized vagina of adequate length, with a moist lining, and that requires less postoperative vaginal dilation and lubrication. However, this technique subjects the patient to an intra-abdominal operation with bowel anastomosis and all its associated complications such as postoperative ileus, anastomotic leak, adhesions, and perforations. In addition, intestinal transposition GCS may be complicated by excess neo-vaginal secretions and malodorous discharge. Penile inversion, on the other hand, avoids the risks of intra-abdominal surgery, but requires postoperative neo-vaginal dilation to maintain length and manipulation of the urethra to provide moisture. Nongenital flaps are a tertiary option and are generally only used for reconstruction following oncologic resection, trauma, or failed primary reconstruction.

Colonic Interposition Vaginoplasty

In this technique, a neo-vagina is created from a portion of the bowel—most frequently from the sigmoid colon, although small or large intestine may be used. The sigmoid colon has the benefit of a large diameter lumen and decreased the rate of secretions compared to other parts of the bowel.

A bowel prep is required prior to surgery and colonoscopy is performed to rule out suspicious lesions or malignancy. Surgery is performed in conjunction with a general surgeon, who mobilizes 12–15 cm of sigmoid colon while the plastic surgeon begins the perineal dissection. The sigmoid segment remains attached to its vascular pedicle and is sutured to the neo-introitus. The distal end is stapled, and the mesentery is sewn to the pelvis to maintain length and prevent torsion. The ends of the native colon are then primarily anastomosed to restore continuity of the digestive tract. Of note, postoperatively the patient must continue surveillance for colonic malignancy.

Penile Inversion Vaginoplasty (Fig. 10.1a–g)

Penile inversion vaginoplasty is performed by deconstructing the penis and using the penile skin to create a neo-vagina. After placing a urinary catheter, the scrotum is incised along the median raphe and an orchiectomy performed. A circumcision incision is performed below the glans and the skin is dissected free from the underlying penile shaft. The dorsal neurovascular bundle is dissected from the underlying corpora cavernosa, which is separated from the corpora spongiosum.

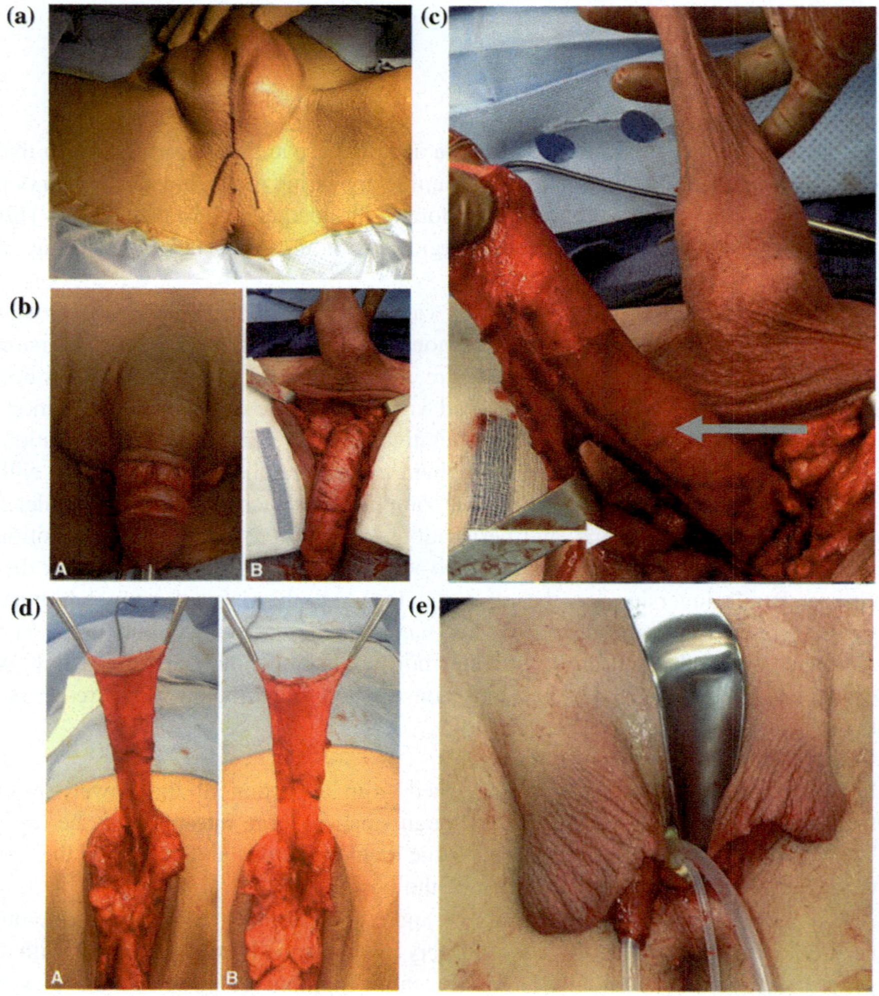

Fig. 10.1 **a**-**g** Vaginoplasty using penile inversion technique. **a** Preoperative vaginoplasty markings. **b** Penile skin inversion. **c** Separating the urethra from the corpora. **d** Formation of neo-vagina by inverting penile shaft skin tube. **e** Neo-vagina insertion. **f** Labia majora contouring and positioning of the urethra and neo-clitoris. **g** Final post-operative view—tie over bolster. Reprinted by permission from Springer Nature: Leclère et al. [24]

The corpora spongiosum is resected from the base of the penis to prevent it from constricting the neo-vagina when engorged during sexual arousal. The corpora cavernosa are resected at the pubis, but a short amount is left to provide a base for the neo-clitoris. The neo-clitoris is then formed from the dorsal glans. A neo-vaginal pocket is dissected between the rectum and penile shaft. The penile skin is inverted, closed to create a blind pouch, and inserted into this space. A urethral flap may be inset with the penile skin to provide lubrication to the

(f)

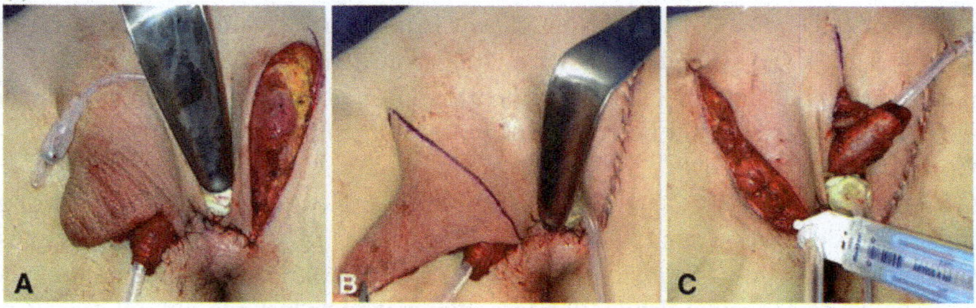

(g)

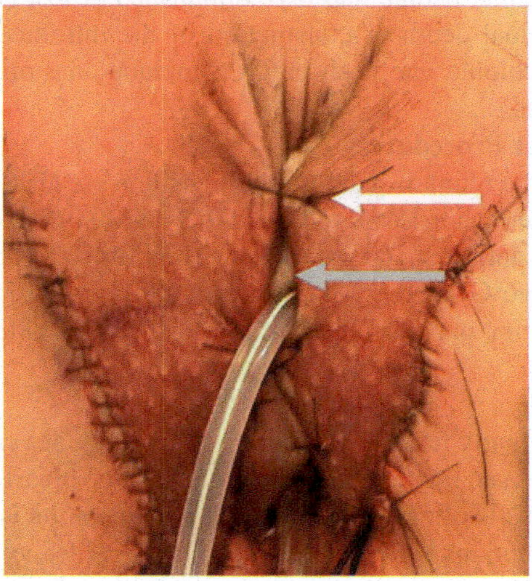

Fig. 10.1 (continued)

vaginal cavity. The urethra is shortened and incised ventrally. The glans penis is brought out through this opening thus creating a neo-clitoris surrounded by labia minora and a clitoral hood. The cut end of the urethra is spatulated to create a new urethral meatus. The scrotal skin is tailored to form the labia majora and a silastic stent is inserted into the neo-vagina to maintain patency of the vaginal cavity. This, along with the urinary catheter, is kept in place for 4–6 days. After removal of the vaginal stent, a vaginal dilation regimen is begun. The patient may initiate vaginal intercourse 6–8 weeks after surgery. Of note, continued prostate exams are recommended as per national guidelines.

Hair Removal

Hair removal prior to vaginoplasty is an important and required step. Hair should be removed from any area that will either be in contact with urine (i.e., skin used to construct a neourethra) or form a partially closed cavity (i.e., skin used to line the neo-vagina). This is important because hair within the neourethra will obstruct the flow of urine thus promoting urinary retention and may become encrusted with calculi and debris. In both cases, that patient would be at an increased risk of urinary infections. Likewise, hair within the neo-vagina may become a potential source of infection. Options for permanent hair removal include electrolysis and laser hair removal. Although neither is 100% effective, laser hair removal is generally considered superior to electrolysis [9]. Topical anesthetics are often used, and areas to be treated should be confirmed by the surgeon prior to hair removal.

Complications

Complications from GCS are similar to those of any surgery—bleeding, scarring, infection, delayed wound healing, and damage to surrounding structures. Complications specific to male-to-female GCS include strictures of the urethra and neo-vagina, rectovaginal fistula, flap loss, diminished or lost neo-clitoral sensation, and inadequate vaginal depth or constriction of the introitus. Additional complications specific to colonic interposition GCS include anastomotic leak, ileus, and abdominal adhesions.

Nongenital Adjunct Procedures

For many patients, the ultimate goal of their transition are GCS. However, there is a subset of patients who choose not to have GCS and only undergo procedures that affect features seen during social interaction when fully clothed. For patients who do choose to undergo GCS, these procedures are often performed prior to genital surgery. Generally, for male-to-female transition, this includes chest surgery and facial feminization.

Chest Surgery

Chest surgery, commonly referred to as top surgery, includes creation of an esthetic breast mound and female nipple. Although there is some breast growth as a result of hormone therapy, this is often inadequate, and augmentation is required to produce the desired result. Options for augmentation include silicone and saline implants, and more recently have evolved to include autologous tissue reconstruction. For implant-based reconstruction, implants may be placed in either subglandular, subfascial, or subpectoral pockets, with subpectoral being the most common. This may be done through either transaxillary, periareolar, or inframammary crease incisions, depending on a patient's anatomy and preferences.

Recently, autologous breast reconstruction, a procedure that is commonly performed for breast reconstruction after mastectomy, has been offered to transgender patients. This differs from implant-based reconstruction because the patients' own tissue is used to augment the breast, thus avoiding the need for a permanent foreign body. Most commonly, tissue from the abdomen (a deep inferior epigastric perforator flap) is transferred and attached to blood vessels in the chest (Fig. 10.2a, b). This produces a natural-appearing result that feels like a native breast. Although this technique avoids the complications associated with breast implants (implant infection, capsular contracture, rupture, rippling, etc.), it is associated with a small but real risk of flap loss.

Facial Surgery

The goal of facial surgery in a male-to-female patient is feminization of the facial features. This is achieved by reshaping or recontouring masculine facial features to achieve a feminine appearance. Areas of the face that readily define the sex include

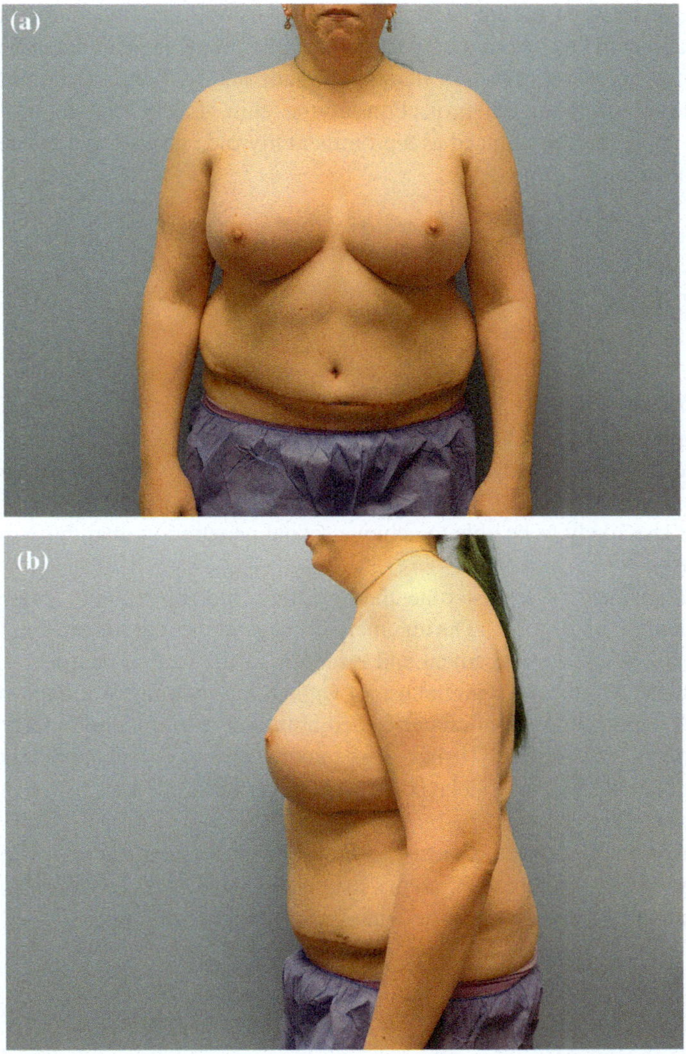

Fig. 10.2 a,b Deep inferior epigastric artery perforator flap (DIEP) technique used for male-to-female chest surgery. Figures courtesy of A. Perry MD, M. Smith MD)

the forehead, nose, lips, cheeks, chin, and jawline. The forehead shape can make a significant difference in facial appearance. Men generally have a more prominent supraorbital ridge, which can be shaved down to achieve a feminine forehead and brow. The hairline can be moved forward and the brows can be lifted. The shape of the eye sockets can also be altered to achieve a smaller, higher set orbit. The nose can be narrowed, the dorsal height decreased, and the tip rotated to produce a more feminine shape. Cheek implants may be used to add projection and produce fuller, more prominent cheeks. Subtle changes to lip shape can be enacted by decreasing the distance between the lips and nose, and by using fillers to produce fuller lips. The jaw and chin can be contoured to achieve a feminine appearance. The angles of the jaw can be burred down to narrow the face and a sliding genioplasty can be performed to decrease the projection of the chin. Lastly, the thyroid cartilage (Adam's apple) can be reduced as a prominent thyroid cartilage is a male secondary sex characteristic.

Masculinization

Metoidioplasty (Fig. 10.3a–c)
Of the options for female-to-male GCS, metoidioplasty is the simpler operation with lower complication rates. It relies entirely on local tissue and does not require specialized instruments or techniques. However, patients undergoing metoidioplasty are less likely to be able to achieve sexual penetration than those undergoing phalloplasty.

During the course of testosterone therapy, the clitoris gradually enlarges to an average length of 4–5 cm. During metoidioplasty, the clitoris is lengthened by releasing the suspensory ligament and resection of the ventral chordee. The female urethra is also lengthened with the use of vaginal musculomucosal flaps or the labia minora. A vaginectomy is often performed at the same time. Scrotoplasty may also be performed concomitantly using labia majora flaps. Testicular implants may be placed immediately or in a delayed fashion to decrease the risk of infection.

Phalloplasty (Fig. 10.4a–d)
Phalloplasty has become the most common choice for constructing a neo-phallus due to high patient satisfaction, ability to achieve standing micturition, and success in penetrative intercourse after the addition of a prosthetic implant.

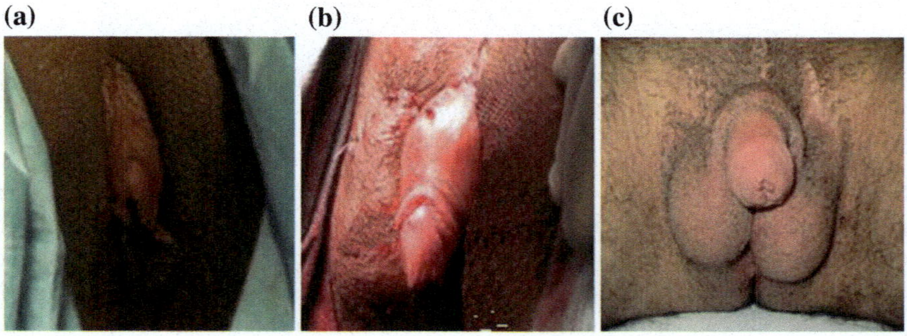

Fig. 10.3 **a–c** Metoidioplasty. **a** Pre-op, **b** post-op, **c** 1-year post-op. Reprinted by permission from Springer Nature: Cohanzad [25]

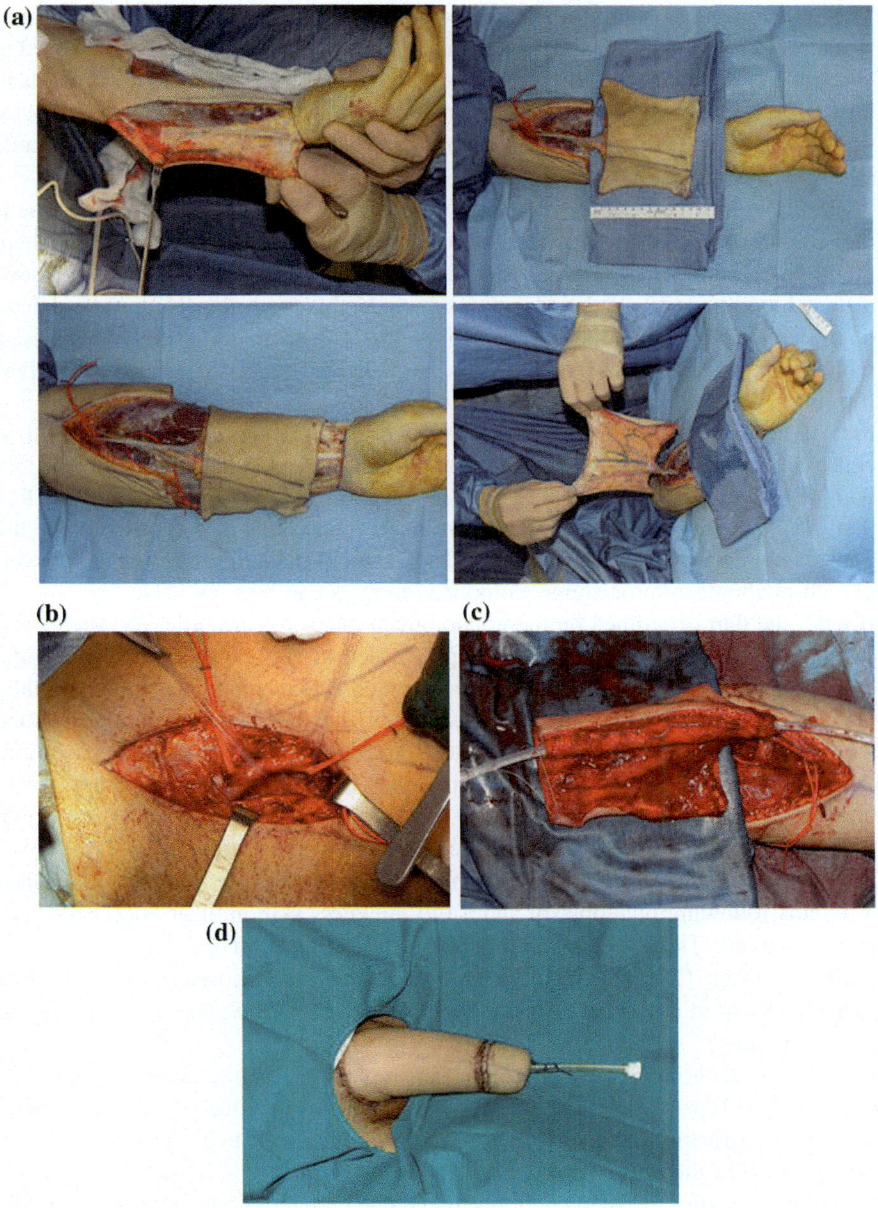

Fig. 10.4 a–d Forearm free-flap phalloplasty. **a** Radial forearm free-flap harvest. **b** Femoral artery recipient site exposure. **c** Radial forearm flap is tubularized around a 16 French Foley catheter. **d** Final result of radial forearm phalloplasty. Reprinted by permission from Springer Nature: Trombetta et al. [26]

The first reported phalloplasty was performed in Russia for total penile reconstruction in 1936. A tubed abdominal flap and autologous rib cartilage were used to create a neo-phallus [10]. The first phalloplasty performed for GCS was in England by Plastic Surgeon Sir Harold Gillies in 1946, and involved a series of 13 operations on another British physician, Laurence Michael Dillon (born Laura Maude Dillon) [11].

Phalloplasty may be performed either by use of a pedicled flap (one where tissue is moved, but blood vessels remain attached to their origin), or a free flap (one where blood vessels are completely detached from their origin, and reconnected to a new, distant blood supply). Pedicled options include the groin flap [12], anterolateral thigh flap [13], and island tensor fascia lata flap [14]. Although pedicled flaps are a reliable option, free flaps have become a preferred option in large centers performing GCS.

Free tissue transfer enables the surgeon to bring in tissue that is best suited to construct a phallus. Options for free tissue transfer include the radial forearm free flap [15], lateral arm flap [16], osteocutaneous free fibula [17], latissimus dorsi free flap [18], and free scapular flap [19]. Of these, the radial forearm has become the gold standard for phalloplasty [20] with high rates of patient satisfaction. However, like all phalloplasty procedures, complication rates can be high [21].

Briefly, the flap is outlined on the nondominant radial forearm after an Allen's test confirms a patent palmar arch. The flap is raised to include the radial artery, the cephalic and or basilic vein, and the medial antebrachial cutaneous nerve. It is then tubed to create a neo-phallus. Modification of the flap includes creating a tube within a tube for urethroplasty. The radial artery is clipped and cut at its origin. Then, an anastomosis is performed to either the femoral artery, femoral side branches, or inferior epigastric artery. The vein is anastomosed to the respective vein, and the nerve is coapted to the dorsal nerve of the clitoris.

If immediate urethroplasty is not performed, the ventral surface of the flap is opened 3 months following phalloplasty and a full-thickness skin graft or buccal mucosal graft is placed. Three to six months later, the healed graft is tabularized over a urinary catheter. Glansplasty (to create a neoglans) may also be performed either immediately or in a delayed fashion. The darker color of the glans can be achieved with tattooing.

Lastly, in order to achieve an erection, an implantable penile prosthesis must be inserted. This is usually performed after twelve months to reduce the risk of implant erosion or extrusion. Dilapidation may be performed prior to surgery or after surgery but before the return of sensation.

Complications after free-flap phalloplasty include partial or complete flap loss (<2% in large series), urethral fistula, urethral stricture, exposure or loss of the implant, and implant malfunction among others.

Nongenital Adjunct Procedures

Chest Surgery (Fig. 10.5a–d)
Chest surgery, commonly referred to as top surgery, includes the removal of the stigmatizing female breast in order to achieve a masculine chest contour and nipple appearance. Techniques vary depending on the amount of breast tissue and skin laxity. Small breasts may be amenable to a mastectomy performed through a circumareolar incision, although larger breasts with excess skin will require subcutaneous mastectomy through an incision above the inframammary fold, with free

(a) (b)

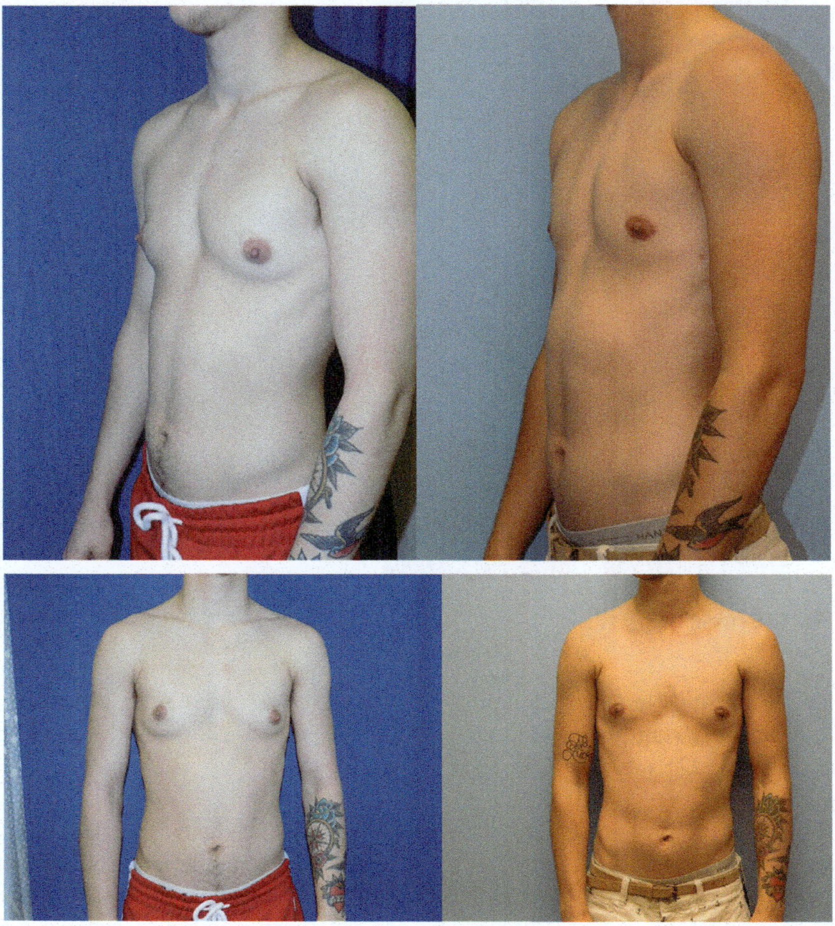

Fig. 10.5 a–d Female-to-male chest surgery using "keyhole" periareolar technique and suction-assisted liposuction. Left photos are pre-op and right photos are post-op. Figures courtesy of A. Perry MD

(c)

(d)

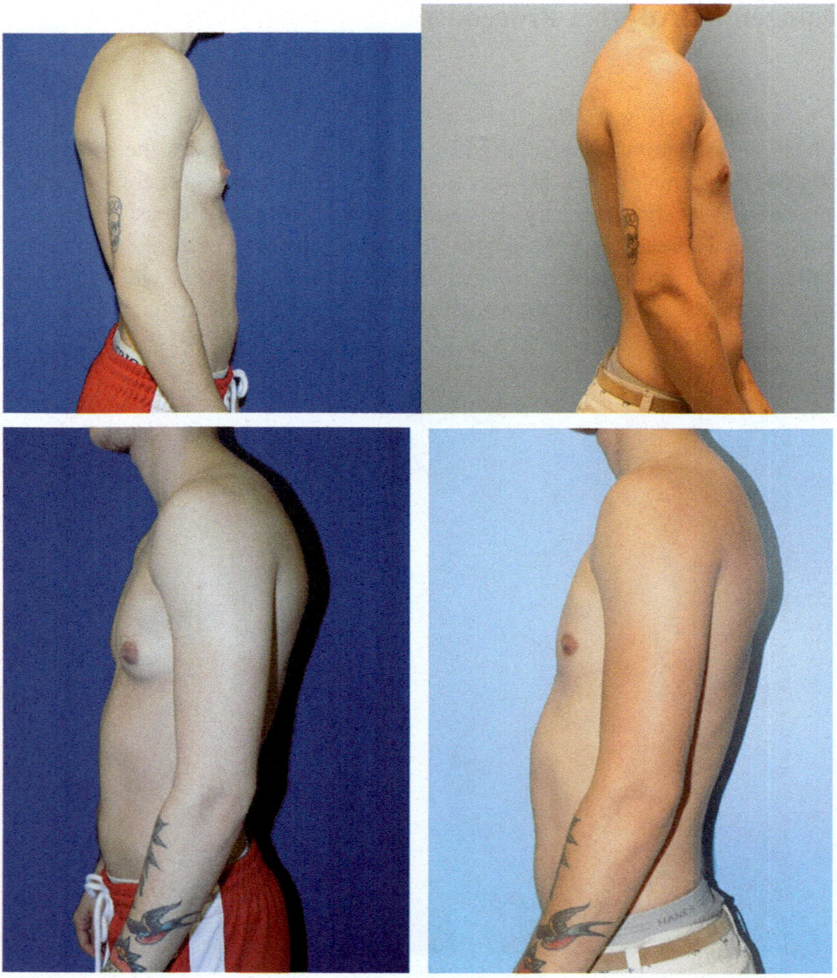

Fig. 10.5 (continued)

nipple grafting. In this technique, the nipple-areolar complex is harvested as a full-thickness skin grafts, reduced in size, and grafted at its new location on the chest wall. [22]

Facial Surgery

Facial masculinization surgery is a set of procedure that changes the female face to appear more masculine. The goals of these procedures are the opposite of those in facial feminization. Although some of the desired changes occur as a result of hormone therapy, surgical procedures can act as an adjunct to achieve a more masculine appearance.

As males tend to have a longer, more prominent forehead, forehead lengthening, and forehead augmentation with bone grafts or implants can be performed.

Similarly, the cheeks can be augmented with implants, fillers, or autologous fat. Rhinoplasty can be performed to create a larger nose, straighter dorsum, wider tip, and decrease nasolabial angle. Jaw and chin implants can be used to accentuate the jawline. Lastly, the thyroid cartilage can be masculinized using autologous rib cartilage [23].

Conclusion

Gender conformation surgery is the practice of aligning the body with the mind. Through these powerful techniques, patients are able to achieve a body that more closely resembles their perceived gender. Although every patient will have a different definition of what that means, these techniques enable the healthcare team to provide the necessary treatment and make their patients feel at home in their bodies.

References

1. Luther B. The activities of surgeon Erwin Gohrbandt (1890–1965) on behalf of the Berlin University, the city's municipal council and the Berlin Surgical Society. Z Arztl Fortbild (Jena). 1990;84(19):1005–8.
2. The life and career of Alberta Lucille/Dr. Alan L. Hart with collected early writings. Friends of the Aubrey Watzek Library, Lewis & Clark College, Po[r]tland, Or; 2003.
3. Meyer Iii W, Bockting WO, Cohen-Kettenis P. The standards of care for gender identity disorders—Sixth version, vol 5; 2001.
4. Cohen-Kettenis P, Kuiper A. Transseksualiteit en psychothérapie. Tijdschrift Voor Psychotherapie. 1984;10:153–66.
5. Hembree WC, Cohen-Kettenis P, Delemarre-van de Waal HA, Gooren LJ, Meyer WJ 3rd, Spack NP, Tangpricha V, Montori VM, Endocrine S. Endocrine treatment of transsexual persons: an Endocrine Society clinical practice guideline. J Clin Endocrinol Metab. 2009;94 (9):3132–54. https://doi.org/10.1210/jc.2009-0345.
6. Horbach SE, Bouman MB, Smit JM, Ozer M, Buncamper ME, Mullender MG. Outcome of vaginoplasty in male-to-female transgenders: a systematic review of surgical techniques. J Sex Med. 2015;12(6):1499–512. https://doi.org/10.1111/jsm.12868.
7. Colebunders B, Brondeel S, D'Arpa S, Hoebeke P, Monstrey S. An update on the surgical treatment for transgender patients. Sex Med Rev. 2017;5(1):103–9. https://doi.org/10.1016/j.sxmr.2016.08.001.
8. Manrique OJ, Sabbagh MD, Ciudad P, Martinez-Jorge J, Kiranantawat K, Sitpahul N, Nippoldt TB, Charafeddine A, Chen HC. Gender-confirmation surgery using the pedicle transverse colon flap for vaginal reconstruction: a clinical outcome and sexual function evaluation study. Plast Reconstr Surg. 2018;141(3):767–71. https://doi.org/10.1097/PRS.0000000000004122.
9. Park MW, Baek S-K, Jung K-Y. Laser epilation for unwanted hair in the Larynx. Med Lasers Eng. Basic Res Clin Appl 1. 2012;(1):31–33.
10. Bogoraz N. On complete plastic reconstruction of a penis sufficient for coitus. Sov Surg. 1936;8:303–9.

11. Nair R, Sriprasad S. 1129 Sir Harold Gillies: Pioneer of phalloplasty and the birth of uroplastic surgery. J Urol. 2010;183(4):e437. https://doi.org/10.1016/j.juro.2010.02.2326.
12. Zielinski T. Phalloplasty using a lateral groin flap in female-to-male transsexuals. Acta Chir Plast. 1999;41(1):15–9.
13. Rubino C, Figus A, Dessy LA, Alei G, Mazzocchi M, Trignano E, Scuderi N. Innervated island pedicled anterolateral thigh flap for neo-phallic reconstruction in female-to-male transsexuals. J Plast Reconstruct Aesthet Surg JPRAS. 2009;62(3):e45–9. https://doi.org/10.1016/j.bjps.2007.11.056.
14. Santanelli F, Scuderi N. Neophalloplasty in female-to-male transsexuals with the island tensor fasciae latae flap. Plastic Reconstr Surg. 2000;105(6):1990–6.
15. Chang TS, Hwang WY. Forearm flap in one-stage reconstruction of the penis. Plastic Reconstr Surg. 1984;74(2):251–8.
16. Upton J, Mutimer KL, Loughlin K, Ritchie J. Penile reconstruction using the lateral arm flap. J R Coll Surg Edinb. 1987;32(2):97–101.
17. Sadove RC, Sengezer M, McRoberts JW, Wells MD. One-stage total penile reconstruction with a free sensate osteocutaneous fibula flap. Plastic Reconstruct Surg. 1993;92(7):1314–1323; discussion 1324–1315.
18. Djordjevic ML, Bumbasirevic MZ, Vukovic PM, Sansalone S, Perovic SV. Musculocutaneous latissimus dorsi free transfer flap for total phalloplasty in children. J Pediatr Urol. 2006;2(4):333–9. https://doi.org/10.1016/j.jpurol.2006.05.003.
19. Yang MY, Li SK, Li YQ, Li Q, Huang WQ, Zhou CD, Tang Y. Penile reconstruction by using a scapular free flap. Zhonghua zheng xing wai ke za zhi = Zhonghua zhengxing waike zazhi = Chin J Plastic Surg. 2003;19(2):88–90.
20. Doornaert M, Hoebeke P, Ceulemans P, T'Sjoen G, Heylens G, Monstrey S. Penile reconstruction with the radial forearm flap: an update. Handchirurgie, Mikrochirurgie, plastische Chirurgie: Organ der Deutschsprachigen Arbeitsgemeinschaft fur Handchirurgie: Organ der Deutschsprachigen Arbeitsgemeinschaft fur Mikrochirurgie der Peripheren Nerven und Gefasse. 2011;43(4):208–14. https://doi.org/10.1055/s-0030-1267215.
21. Fang RH, Lin JT, Ma S. Phalloplasty for female transsexuals with sensate free forearm flap. Microsurgery. 1994;15(5):349–52.
22. Monstrey SJ, Ceulemans P, Hoebeke P. Sex reassignment surgery in the female-to-male transsexual. Semin Plastic Surg. 2011;25(3):229–44. https://doi.org/10.1055/s-0031-1281493.
23. Deschamps-Braly JC, Sacher CL, Fick J, Ousterhout DK. First female-to-male facial confirmation surgery with description of a new procedure for masculinization of the thyroid cartilage (Adam's Apple). Plast Reconstr Surg. 2017;139(4):883e–7e. https://doi.org/10.1097/PRS.0000000000003185.
24. Leclère FM, Casoli V, Baudet J et al. Aesth Plast Surg. 2015;39:927. https://doi.org/10.1007/s00266-015-0552-2
25. Cohanzad S. Aesth Plast Surg. 2016;40:130–138. https://link.springer.com/article/10.1007/s00266-015-0607-4
26. Trombetta C, et al. Surgical therapy: forearm free flap phalloplasty. In: Trombetta C, et al., editors. Management of gender dysphoria. Milan: Springer-Verlag Italia; 2015.

Chapter 11
Fertility Issues in Transgender Care

Leon Telis, Stephanie Baum, Tomer Singer and Boback M. Berookhim

Introduction

Treatment for gender dysphoria and the desire to live in the opposite gender requires hormonal, anatomical, and psychosocial changes [1]. Previously, undergoing gender affirming treatment meant the loss of reproductive potential for patients. Given the generally young age of patients seeking gender affirming treatment, it is important to discuss and offer fertility preservation options for patients that may want to have children in the future.

Concurrent with increased acceptance of fertility preservation is an increase in the acceptance and encouragement of transgender individuals. An emphasis is placed on the importance of their physical and emotional health. The medical community has a responsibility to meet the needs of transgender patients, which includes their reproductive health.

Although the mean age of presentation of patients seeking gender affirmative transition is 36.3 years in Sweden [2] and 32.6 years in Ireland [3], 61.9% of patients report that the age at which they self-diagnosed themselves as being gender dysphoric was prepubertal [4]. Currently, there are no definitive practice guidelines for fertility preservation for transgender patients. Fertility preservation options for male-to-female transgender patients are similar to those for patients undergoing treatment for malignant or nonmalignant diseases that may lead to infertility. Sperm cryopreservation prior to medical treatment for malignant disease in men who wish to retain future reproductive potential is common practice due to the acute azoospermia caused by alkylating and other chemotherapeutic agents [5]. The same

L. Telis · B. M. Berookhim
Department of Urology, Lenox Hill Hospital, Northwell Health, New York, NY, USA

S. Baum · T. Singer (✉)
Department of OBGYN and Reproductive Endocrinology and Infertility,
Lenox Hill Hospital, Northwell Health, New York, NY, USA
e-mail: Tsinger@northwell.edu

L. Poretsky and W. C. Hembree (eds.), *Transgender Medicine*, Contemporary Endocrinology, https://doi.org/10.1007/978-3-030-05683-4_11

management may be applied to male-to-female transgender patients who wish to retain fertility potential after undergoing hormonal and surgical gender affirming treatment. Similarly, oocyte cryopreservation is a method of fertility preservation in female-to-male transgender patients. Reproductive options in transgender persons should be discussed prior to initiation of gender reassignment. These options include sperm, oocyte, as well as embryo cryopreservation.

This chapter will explore the fertility preservation options for the transgender individual and couple. Importantly, the physician must be informed about these options in order to be in a position to educate and empower his or her patients.

Definitions

Gender identity is one's conceptualization, or one's intrinsic knowledge of oneself, as either male, female, or nonbinary individual. The term *trans* means "opposite"; therefore, a transgender individual commonly identifies oneself as the opposite gender of the gender assigned at birth. A transgender male is a person who was identified as female at birth. A transgender female is a person who was identified as male at birth. Presumably, the karyotype of a person born as a female would be 46XX, and as male, 46XY. However, the karyotype cannot be determined by external genitalia and phenotype prior to transition. For example, a person with androgen insensitivity syndrome is phenotypically female and likely identifies as such, with a 46XY karyotype. There is a broad spectrum of transitioning events and procedures from wearing clothes or a hairstyle typically displayed by the identified gender, to undergoing corrective surgery.

Gender identity is one of the most important characteristics of a patient seeking fertility treatment, whether independently or with a partner. The medical provider must learn what treatment is or is not acceptable to a transgender individual. A transgender male may still want to retain a uterus but may not desire to carry a pregnancy. Or a transgender male who is undergoing hormonal treatment as part of his transition may not find it acceptable to stop his treatment in order to undergo oocyte stimulation.

Sexual orientation refers to the gender to which an individual feels an attraction. A transgender male or female could be attracted to either a trans- or cisgender male or female.

Fertility Treatment Definitions

IUI—*Intrauterine insemination* is the process of placing sperm directly into the uterus to enhance the chances of achieving pregnancy. The patient undergoing the insemination arrives for a scheduled office visit and is briefly positioned with her legs in stirrups for the procedure. The partner or sperm donor may provide a fresh sample to be used that day; a frozen specimen may be used. Using sterile technique, a thin catheter is inserted directly into the uterus and the seminal fluid is pushed through the catheter. The procedure is performed under ultrasound guidance. The patient is able to return to normal activity shortly after the procedure. Some patients may take oral or injectable medication prior to the IUI to increase the chance of pregnancy during the IUI cycle (Fig. 11.1).

IVF—In vitro *fertilization* is the process of fertilizing an egg (oocyte) in the embryology laboratory using washed and prepared sperm. Traditional in vitro fertilization involves placing a single oocyte in a culture dish with multiple sperms, allowing for fertilization. This process usually takes place after a patient has undergone ovarian stimulation with injectable medication, an oocyte retrieval (an outpatient procedure performed under light anesthesia), and a partner or donor has provided a sperm sample. The fertilized egg, now an embryo, is usually observed in vitro for 2–6 days until it is either transferred into the uterus, frozen for future use, or discarded due to abnormal growth (Fig. 11.2).

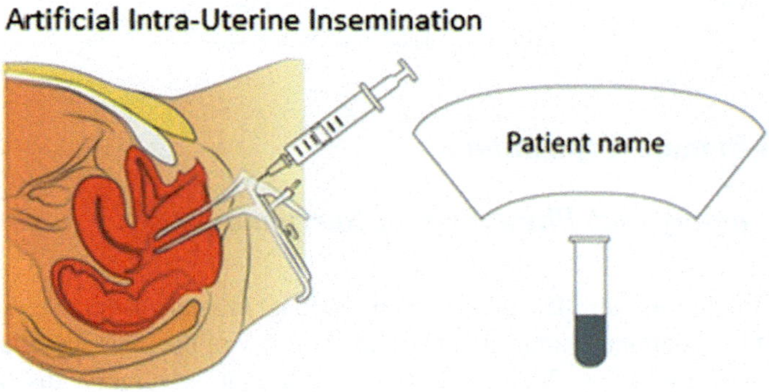

Fig. 11.1 Artificial intrauterine insemination

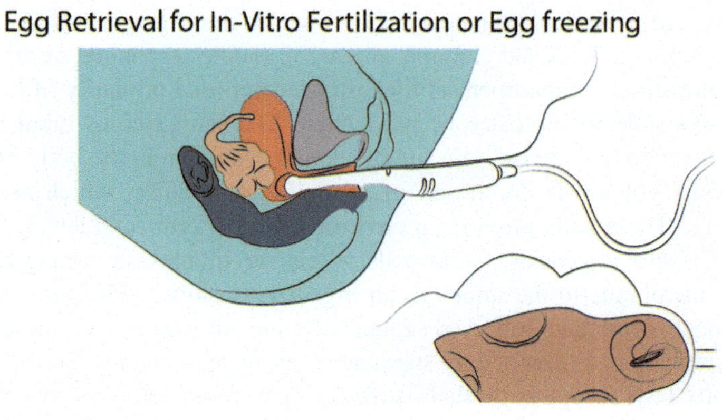

Fig. 11.2 Egg retrieval for IVF or egg freezing

ICSI—*Intracytoplasmic sperm injection* is a procedure where a single sperm is injected directly into the cytoplasm of an oocyte. This is performed in an embryology laboratory after oocyte retrieval has been performed and a sperm sample has been provided. The mature eggs undergo fertilization by a morphologically normal appearing sperm. If the fertilization is successful, the embryo is observed for 2–6 days after which it is transferred into the uterus, frozen, or discarded due to abnormal growth.

PGS/PGD—*Preimplantation genetic screening* is a procedure in which a biopsy is taken from an embryo, usually 5–6 days following fertilization, to determine if the embryo is euploid (chromosomally normal) or aneuploid. This is not part of routine fertility treatment but can be offered to a patient or couple. The benefit of this procedure is selecting the appropriate embryos for transfer. *Preimplantation genetic diagnosis* is a more specialized procedure where, after the biopsy is taken, the genetic material is analyzed for a specific gene or genetic mutation. This involves obtaining genetic material from multiple family members to design a specific probe. This procedure is not performed routinely and can be costly. However, this is an option for couples who seek to ensure that their child will not inherit a certain genetic disease.

Male-to-Female Transition

Male Anatomy and Physiology of Spermatogenesis

In order to discuss fertility preservation options in male-to-female transgender patients, it is important to understand a brief overview of the male reproductive tract anatomy and physiology. Male-to-female sex affirmation surgery, discussed elsewhere in this book, involves the removal of the testicles, penis, their associated structures, and preservation of portions of the skin of the penis as well as the glans in order to preserve the innervation of the glans.

With regard to testicular anatomy and function, the average testicle is approximately $4 \times 3 \times 2.5$ cm and contains about 250 lobules separated by fibrous septa [6]. The interstitial compartment of the testis is composed primarily of Leydig cells and is responsible for testosterone production. The seminiferous tubules serve an exocrine function and are the sole site of sperm production in the body. 90% of the overall testis volume is composed of seminiferous tubules, which are lined by Sertoli cells. These cells provide an environment for germ cells developing in the process of spermatogenesis. Germ cells within the tubules are arranged from the basement membrane to the lumen in an organized fashion with spermatogonia on the basement membrane, followed sequentially inward toward the tubule lumen by primary spermatocytes, secondary spermatocytes, and spermatids. Sertoli cells have high-affinity FSH receptors on their surface which, when activated by FSH, induce the production of androgen-binding protein that is then secreted into the luminal fluid of the tubule. The androgen-binding protein provides high levels of androgen within the seminiferous tubules as compared to serum by binding testosterone [7].

The epididymis lies posterolateral to the testis and is made up of a markedly coiled duct that is continuous with the vas deferens [6]. Functionally, the epididymis is the site for spermatozoa to become mature and functional. While moving through the epididymis, newly formed sperm undergoes numerous changes, including change in membrane protein composition, surface charge, immunoreactivity, phospholipid, and fatty acid content, as well as adenylate cyclase activity, all of which lead to increased fertilization ability [6]. The penis is made up of two corpora cavernosa and the corpus spongiosum in which the urethra is contained. Each corpus is contained within a fascial sheath and distally end in the glans penis [6].

The hypothalamic–pituitary–gonadal axis (Fig. 11.3) has a critical responsibility in the endocrine function of the testis (testosterone) as well as the exocrine function of the testis (sperm). Of the numerous hypothalamic hormones that act on the pituitary gland, the most important for reproduction is gonadotropin-releasing hormone (GnRH) also known as luteinizing hormone-releasing hormone (LHRH). The function of GnRH is to stimulate the anterior pituitary gland to secrete LH and FSH—the two primary pituitary hormones that regulate testis function. In the testis, LH acts upon Leydig cells to induce the mitochondrial conversion of cholesterol to pregnenolone and testosterone. FSH binds to Sertoli cells in the testis and stimulates seminiferous tubule growth during development. FSH is essential for initiation of spermatogenesis at puberty and stimulates normal spermatogenesis in adults. Men normally produce 5 g of testosterone daily [7]. Secretion occurs in an irregular, pulsatile manner and regulates its own production via negative feedback on the hypothalamic–pituitary–gonadal axis. Approximately 2% of testosterone is unbound or "free"—the biologically active fraction, while the rest is bound to either albumin or sex hormone-binding globulin (SHBG) in the blood (Fig. 11.3).

Cross-Sex Hormone Therapy

The regimen for hormone therapy for transgender patients is not fully standardized to date. For male-to-female transgender patients, cyproterone acetate can be utilized for "devirilization" followed by a combination of estrogens and antiandrogens for "feminization" [8]. Cyproterone acetate is a testosterone antagonist, acting as an antiandrogen and progestin, high levels of which will lead to a downregulation of GnRH and its downstream effects on gonadotropin release in the pituitary gland and testosterone release from Leydig cells in the testicles [8]. Another drug, spironolactone, produces antiandrogen effects by the direct inhibition of testosterone secretion and the inhibition of androgen binding to the androgen receptor [9]. Elevated testosterone levels within the seminiferous tubules, provided by the binding of testosterone to androgen-binding protein, are essential for the maturation of spermatogonia. Inhibition of testosterone release leads to the prevention of the maturation of spermatogonia as well as of numerous other secondary effects of testosterone on characteristic male development.

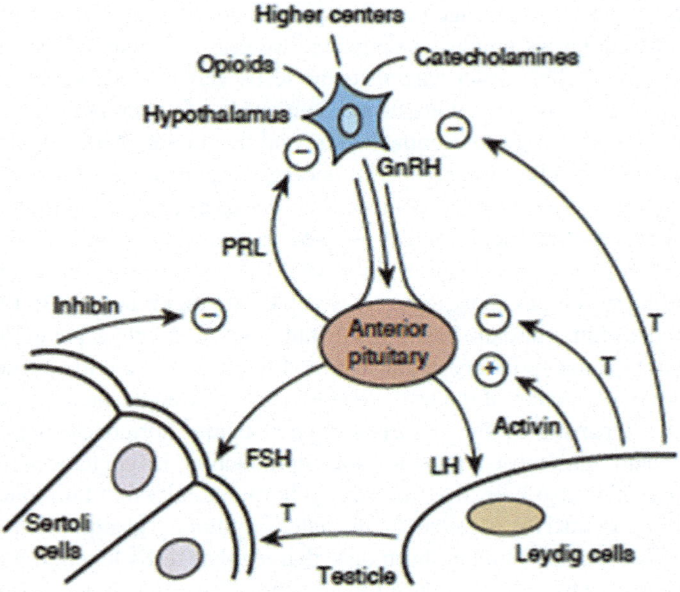

Fig. 11.3 Diagram of hypothalamic–pituitary–testis hormonal axis (In: Wein et al. [34])

Semen Analysis

The World Health Organization (WHO) established semen analysis values that are considered minimum criteria for "normal" semen quality by which it becomes statistically more difficult to achieve pregnancy with any semen parameters below "normal" (Table 11.1). The most recent publication of the "WHO Manual for the Examination of Human Semen and Sperm-Cervical Mucus Interaction" was released in 2010 and included lower reference values than the 1999 edition based on a population study of fertile men across 14 different countries [10]. The 2010 edition studied 4500 fertile men across these countries and established the lower limit for fertility based on the 5th percentile seen in this cohort [11].

The quality of semen is highly variable from day to day [7]. A minimum of two semen samples is needed in order to establish baseline semen quality and should be collected by masturbation, coitus interruptus, or with a nonspermicidal condom into a clean glass or plastic container [7]. Multiple factors influence semen quality from one individual from sample to sample. A large source of variability is length of

Table 11.1 Semen analysis—minimal standards of adequacy (WHO 2010)

Ejaculate volume	1.5 mL
Sperm concentration	$>15 \times 10^6$ sperm/mL
Motility	>40%
Morphology	>4% (Kruger criteria)

abstinence from sexual activity prior to collection. Semen volume may increase and sperm concentration can increase by 10–15 million/mL with each day of abstinence for up to 1 week [7]. Conversely, sperm motility decreases with an abstinence period greater than 5 days [7]. It is thus recommended that semen be collected after a period of 48–72 h of sexual abstinence.

Sperm Banking and Longevity of Sperm Viability

The most effective and the simplest method of fertility preservation in postpubertal males is sperm banking. Sperm cryopreservation has been the established method to maintain fertility in males with genitourinary cancers prior to initiating gonadotoxic treatments and can also be used in patients undergoing gender affirming surgery [12]. A semen sample is obtained, analyzed, placed in vials, and cryopreserved for use at a later date. Through intracytoplasmic sperm injection of oocytes, sperm cryopreservation has allowed for successful oocyte fertilization even with a low number of sperms available [13].

Cryopreservation has been shown to cause some damaging effects on semen quality. The most widely reported detrimental effect of cryopreservation is a significant decrease in sperm motility with some studies reporting a 45% decrease in average sperm velocity [5]. These effects notwithstanding, improvements in assisted reproduction techniques have resulted in live birth rates up to 49% in patients who underwent multiple IVF and/or ICSI cycles [13]. While it has been shown that freezing–thawing of sperm results in a decrease in motility and viability, cryopreservation of sperm does not negatively affect fertilization and pregnancy rates after intracytoplasmic sperm injection (ICSI) [14]. One study demonstrated no difference in pregnancy rates after ICSI between frozen–thawed and freshly ejaculated groups [2]. Although the duration of storage of cryopreserved semen samples has no influence on sperm quality, the process of freeze–thawing has been shown to have a negative impact on sperm motility [15, 16]. Studies have shown that cryopreserved semen in liquid nitrogen retains good post-thaw motility and binding to human zona pellucida after more than 28 years of storage [15].

Sperm Retrieval

Sperm banking is accomplished by patients producing a semen sample that can be obtained by multiple potential methods. Most commonly, men masturbate to ejaculation at a sperm bank or andrology laboratory.

Electroejaculation is an option for those men that are unable to provide a specimen by manual masturbation. Masturbation may be a limiting option for some patients with emotional distress, pain, various cultural factors or varying neurological abnormalities. To obtain a specimen by electroejaculation, a rectal probe is positioned over the prostate while the patient is under anesthesia and a mild electrical current is emitted to stimulate ejaculation. Electroejaculation has been used successfully in patients to obtain semen samples; however, the concentration and motility of sperm have been found to be decreased as compared to samples obtained through masturbation [17].

There exist several surgical techniques for sperm retrieval either from the epididymis or the testis. Although these retrieval techniques are most commonly used for men with congenital absence of the vas deferens or those with failed or entirely unreconstructable obstructions of the vas deferens, they can also be used as a solution for transgender women for whom masturbation is either emotionally or physically limiting. Common methods for sperm retrieval include epididymal aspiration, testicular fine-needle aspiration, known as testicular sperm aspiration, and testicular sperm extraction (TESE) [12]. Epididymal sperm aspiration can be performed either via an open tubule technique or via percutaneous puncture of the epididymis with a fine needle. The percutaneous approach is less reliable than open retrieval and the smaller quantities of sperm obtained can be inadequate for cryopreservation [18]. Open retrieval utilizes an incision in the scrotum with delivery of the testis and isolation of an epididymal tubule in order to obtain sperm [18]. With the use of ICSI, pregnancy and delivery rates have been reported to exceed 60% using open epididymal sperm retrieval techniques utilizing either fresh or cryopreserved sperm [19].

Testicular sperm aspiration (Fig. 11.4) utilizes an 18–23-gauge needle with negative pressure in order to retrieve sperm via multiple testicular punctures [12]. TESE technique uses an incision of the tunica albuginea to retrieve seminiferous tubules and has been shown to have sperm retrieval rates as high as 82.3% in patients with azoospermia [20]. Retrieval rates with TESE in the non-azoospermic patient population, as would be the case with most healthy patients seeking gender affirming surgery, would likely approach 100% (Fig. 11.4).

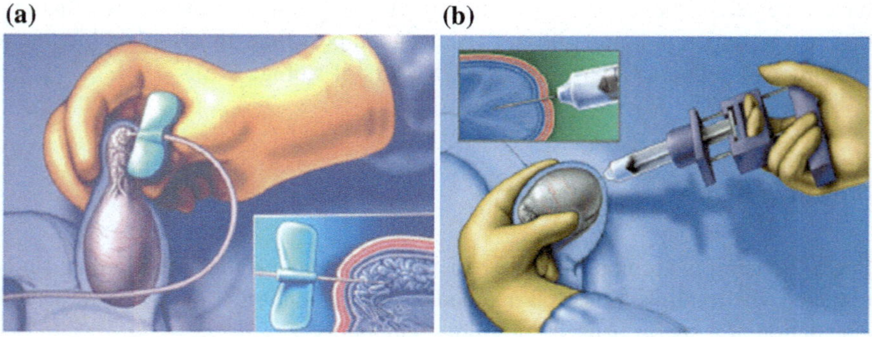

Fig. 11.4 **a** Percutaneous puncture of the epididymis with a fine needle. **b** Percutaneous aspiration (testicular sperm aspiration) with a high-suction glass syringe and a 23-gauge needle (In: Wein et al. [34])

Future Directions

The current avenue for fertility preservation in those undergoing male-to-female gender transformation is sperm cryopreservation prior to any hormonal therapy. While this is an excellent technique for sperm preservation and the maintenance of fertility, this option requires advance planning for fertility preservation prior to initiation of hormonal and surgical reassignment therapy. For those who have already undergone gender affirming surgery without prior fertility preservation planning, there are no current viable options to a male-to-female transgender person to achieve paternity. There are several exciting current avenues of research that can potentially offer fertility for this subset of patients.

There have been several groups studying the potential role of stem cell therapy as well as gene therapy in restoring fertility potential in patients undergoing cancer treatment [21]. Studies have looked at animal models for azoospermia, induced by either irradiation to destroy spermatogenesis or the use of alkylating chemotherapy [22, 23]. Hermann et al. [23] reported on autologous and allogeneic transplantation of spermatogonial stem cells (SSCs) into adult and prepubertal Rhesus macaques treated with chemotherapy and reported the presence of SSCs in the ejaculated sperm of 71% of monkeys with autologous grafts and 33% with allogeneic grafts. While there have been a number of advances in research in the area of stem cell therapy, it is primarily targeted at treatment of induced spermatogenic failure and is limited in its applications for patients that have undergone surgical intervention for gender conversion. Gene therapy can aid in delivering missing or impaired genetic factors in the testes to aid in sperm production due to underlying defects responsible for impaired spermatogenesis [21]. Although not currently allowed in the United States [24], gene transfer offers the promising potential to treat men with spermatogenic failure with underlying genetic defects. Both stem cell therapy and gene therapy offer exciting avenues of research for the future treatment of men with spermatogenic failure, though any potential treatment would require intervention prior to surgical management of the transgender patient.

Female-to-Male Transition

Female-to-Male Presentation for Fertility Evaluation

Fertility preservation for a transgender male depends on where the individual is in the transition process. Specifically, it is important to know whether the individual has undergone any hormonal or surgical treatment. Individuals are now starting to express gender identity at an earlier age as transitioning becomes more mainstream and accepted. The role of the primary care physician or general OBGYN is to discuss the options for fertility prior to the transition to become male. While many patients may not be thinking of childbearing at the time of transition, educating patients on their reproductive future and providing options is the responsibility of the medical provider. This is also an opportunity to educate the parent, should the individual be presenting with a parent or at an age less than 18.

Prior to Transition

The American Society for Reproductive Medicine (ASRM) Committee Opinion on access to fertility services by transgender persons encourages providers to offer fertility preservation to individuals prior to gender transition (ASRM). Prior to transitioning to male, the patient has the option of undergoing ovarian stimulation and freezing oocytes to be stored for future use. This secures an opportunity for the individual to use gametes in the future should this become the choice for family building selected by the patient. This is an option mainly available to the pubertal or postpubertal individual. The American Society for Reproductive Medicine lifted the experimental label of oocyte freezing in October 2012, and vitrification techniques in the embryology laboratory have significantly improved the process of oocyte freezing. The individual would meet with a reproductive endocrinologist, undergo one or more controlled ovarian stimulation cycles, and bank oocytes for potential use in the future. Ovarian stimulation and the collection of multiple oocytes does not advance the individual's reproductive age or "use up" oocytes that could have been destined for ovulation in a future cycle. The number of oocytes at puberty is approximately 400,000, with natural attrition occurring every month. Should the transgender male choose to express his gender through external means, and avoid hormonal or surgical treatment, the option for oocyte collection is available for this individual throughout the reproductive years, with a decline in fertility starting in the fourth decade of life and reproductive potential almost completely ceasing by the early 40s.

After Transition

After transition to a transgender male, the options to obtain gametes depend on two factors: surgery and hormone treatment. If the transgender male has undergone surgery to remove the ovaries and oocyte preservation has not been undertaken, then obtaining oocytes is no longer an option. Whether or not the uterus is retained has no bearing on the ability to retrieve eggs from the ovaries. If definitive gonadectomy has not taken place, then, theoretically, oocytes can be obtained. If the person is on hormone therapy, most commonly testosterone, this therapy would need to be temporarily stopped and ovarian stimulation would be administered, usually with injectable gonadotropins. There are limited studies regarding oocyte retrieval following the use and cessation of testosterone therapy. There is also limited information regarding the ability to stay on testosterone therapy while undergoing oocyte stimulation. Even if feasible, this is a practice most reproductive endocrinologists would be reluctant to recommend given the unknown potential outcomes. The main barrier is usually the willingness of the transgender person to stop testosterone therapy, and thus temporarily stop or reverse the transition process. This causes extreme emotional distress for many transgender males and becomes an additional barrier to obtaining oocytes. Psychological assessment and support are important in making treatment decisions for an elective process.

Being the carrier of a pregnancy is an option for transgender males who retain a uterus and who are willing to stop testosterone hormone therapy preconception and for the duration of the pregnancy, and who are receptive to taking hormonal supplementation (estrogen and progesterone) in the first trimester. There are reports of healthy pregnancies in transgender men after cessation of testosterone treatment [25]. Further, with discontinuation of testosterone treatment, return of menses, if it occurs, takes place on average three months after cessation of treatment. This would potentially allow the transgender male to conceive with a male partner without reproductive assistance. Such a decision is extremely individualized and potentially one which most transgender males may be unlikely to make. However, presenting every option to a transgender patient or couple is the role of the provider in order to empower autonomous and informed decision-making.

Case Examples

Transgender Male (Transition from Female to Male) Presenting with a Female Partner

In the case of this couple, in order to have a child with his genetic material, the transgender male would have had to donate oocytes prior to transitioning or be willing to stop hormone therapy and undergo ovarian stimulation followed by oocyte retrieval. The female partner would be able to carry the pregnancy (in this scenario the female partner is acting as a gestational carrier), with the transgender male retrieved eggs and donor sperm. This treatment option is dependent on the gestational carrier laws in the state of residence and may vary in different countries.

The female partner may choose to undergo IUI or IVF using the same donor sperm so the offspring would share genetic material, allowing the children to be "half" biological siblings. Should the female partner be unable to carry a pregnancy, assuming the transgender male has not undergone a hysterectomy, the transgender male could carry the pregnancy. Oftentimes, the transgender male partner is unwilling to cease hormonal therapy and carry a pregnancy; however, this option should be presented to the couple so that they may make the most appropriate choice for them.

Transgender Male (Transition from Female to Male) Presenting with a Male Partner

When a transgender male presents with a male partner, both gametes are theoretically available or obtainable. Oocytes could be retrieved by stimulating the transgender male partner assuming normal ovarian reserve and could be used to create embryos with sperm from the male partner. If the couple desires fertility following transition, oocytes can be retrieved after the transition, should the transgender male be willing to undergo the necessary treatment. At times, the desire for fertility follows prior oocyte cryopreservation, which will require thawing of frozen eggs and performing IVF/ICSI with the male partner's sperm. The component of consideration here is the carrier. Should the transgender male be willing to cease hormonal treatment and carry a pregnancy, this is an option if hysterectomy was not performed. If this approach is not feasible, the couple may be able to select a gestational carrier, depending on the laws of the state/country.

Fertility Preservation in the Prepubertal Female

Fertility preservation in the prepubertal individual is an important area in which the clinician must be educated in order to properly advise patients and patients' family members. The physician must also stay current on the techniques and developments in this area as advances are made. Studies show that, even when thoroughly counseled, transgender youth do not utilize fertility preservation options. Recognizing the emotional distress that can accompany both infertility and being a transgender individual, the responsibility of the clinician is to mitigate this distress by working closely with transgender youth, educating and treating them in the way they are most comfortable. Involving a mental healthcare professional is an important component.

Transgender adolescents often desire treatment to suppress their natural pubertal transition to encourage the appearance of the desired gender. Recommendations for endocrine treatment in this population include suppressing puberty with GnRH agonists until approximately age 16, and then administering cross-sex hormones [26]. Because this treatment is potentially occurring on the cusp of puberty, fertility preservation must be considered.

Much of the research on prepubertal ovarian tissue/oocyte preservation has been done in cancer patients undergoing gonadotoxic treatment, which is chemotherapy that can affect the reproductive organs. Ovarian tissue freezing ("cryobanking") for fertility preservation has been performed for over 20 years. There are reports of live births following the transplantation of previously frozen ovarian tissue back into the patient's body, either in the pelvis or in a different area, such as the arm [27]. Portions of the ovary are removed and frozen for future use/transplantation. It has been performed in both prepubertal females as well as adults. This procedure has resulted in live births following reimplantation of the tissue [28, 29]. In a recent review of reported surgical techniques in fertility preservation for prepubertal and adolescent females, the authors concluded that there is no current consensus on operative technique for ovarian cortical tissue removal nor are there sufficient reports of outcomes in the pediatric population. Further research on operative technique and tissue harvesting is needed to determine the best approach for obtaining healthy ovarian follicles for future use [30]. Fasano et al. examined outcomes of immature eggs collected from ovarian tissue in adult and prepubertal patients. Oocyte maturation and freezing procedures after collection from frozen ovarian tissue were assessed according to patient age. A high number of eggs were collected in girls but there was a significantly higher percentage of degenerated or abnormal oocytes in this group (as compared with adults). Maturation rates were significantly lower in prepubertal than postpubertal girls [31]. The quality of eggs in this age group obtained by these methods is not known [32].

Role of the General OBGYN

Having an open discussion with transgender patients about their reproductive health allows for the opportunity for the patients to share their desires regarding family planning. Some patients may not wish to undergo the hormonal treatment required to obtain gametes as this could ultimately delay or offset gender affirming treatment. Since this could be traumatic for a patient, alternative options must be discussed. Physicians must be informed and be able to educate and be comfortable initiating a conversation concerning reproductive choices regardless of gender identity. The key is for the physician to be able to inform patients about their options, optimal timing, and the best way to meet their family building needs.

The Future

There have been isolated reports of successful pregnancy following uterus transplantation. Uterus transplantation may become an option in the future; however, to the best of our knowledge, this procedure has never been performed or attempted in a transgender female. Recent reports have confirmed successful breastfeeding of a transgender female, after her partner gave birth [33]. The treatment involved spironolactone to suppress testosterone, estradiol, and progesterone to mimic pregnancy, domperidone as a galactagogue, and a breast pump.

Conclusions

Caring for the transgender patient requires a multidisciplinary approach on social, medical, surgical, and legal levels. Given the relatively young age at which many patients begin their journey to transition, it is important to offer fertility preservation strategies for those that may want children in the future. Although there are currently no clearly established guidelines for the management of fertility preservation in male-to-female transgender patients, the well-established use of sperm cryopreservation in patients with genitourinary malignancies may be applied in these clinical scenarios as well. Sperm cryopreservation offers a viable, long-term, and well-researched avenue for maintaining fertility when planned prior to initiation of gender reassignment therapy. For female-to-male transgender patients, oocyte preservation procedures should be considered.

References

1. Gooren LJ, Giltary EJ, Bunck MC. Long-term treatment of transsexuals with cross sex hormones: extensive personal experience. J Clin Endocrinol Metab. 2008;93:19–25.
2. Dhejne C, Lichtenstein P, Boman M, Johansson AL, Langstrom N, Landem M. Long-term follow-up of transsexual persons undergoing sex reassignment surgery: cohort study in Sweden. PLoS ONE. 2011;6:e16885.
3. Judge C, O'Donovan C, Callaghan G, Gaoatswe G, O'Shea D. Gender dysphoria - prevalence and co-morbidities in an Irish adult population. Front Endocrinol. 2014;5:87.
4. Byne W, Bradley SJ, Coleman E, Eyler AE, Green R, Menvielle EJ, Meyer-Bahlburg HF, Pleak RR, Tompkins DA. American psychiatric task force on treatment of gender identity disorder. Report of the American psychiatric association task force on treatment of gender identity disorder. Arch Sex Behav. 2012;41:759–96.
5. Anger JT, Gilbert BR, Goldstein M. Cryopreservation of sperm: indications, methods and results. J Urol. 2002;170:1079–84.
6. Tanagho EA. Anatomy of the genitourinary tract. In: Smith's general urology, 17th ed. McGraw Hill Lange; 2008. p. 1–16.
7. Turek P. Male infertility. In: Smith's general urology, 17th ed. McGraw Hill Lange; 2008. p. 684–715.
8. Schneider F, Kliesch S, Schlatt S, Neuhaus N. Andrology of male-to-female transsexuals: influence of cross-sex hormone therapy on testicular function. Andrology. 2017;5:873–80.
9. Moore E, Wisniewski A, Dobs A. Endocrine treatment of transsexual people: a review of treatment regimens, outcomes, and adverse effects. J Clin Endocrinol Metab. 2003;88:3467–73.
10. Murray KS, James A, McGeady JB, et al. The effect of the new 2010 World Health Organization criteria for semen analyses on male infertility. Fertil Steril. 2012;98(6):1428–31.
11. Cooper TG, Noonan E, von Eckardstein S, Auger J, Baker HW, Behre HM, et al. World Health Organization reference values for human semen characteristics. Hum Reprod Update. 2010;16:231–45.
12. Polland A, Berookhim BM. Fertility concerns in men with genitourinary malignancies: treatment dilemmas, fertility options, and medicolegal considerations. Urol Oncol Semin Orig Invest. 2016;34:399–406.

13. van Casteren N, van Santbrink EJ, van Inzen W, Romijn JC, Dohle GR. Use rate and assisted reproduction technologies outcome of cryopreserved semen from 629 cancer patients. Fertil Steril. 2008;90:245–50.
14. Kuczynski W, Dhont M, Grygoruk C, Grochowski D, Wolczynski S, Szamatowicz M. The outcome of intracytoplasmic injection of fresh and cryopreserved ejaculated spermatozoa—a prospective randomized study. Hum Reprod. 2001;16:2109.
15. Clarke GN, de Liu Y, Baker HW. Recovery of human sperm motility and ability to interact with the human zona pellucida after more than 28 years of storage in liquid nitrogen. Fertil Steril. 2006;86:721–2.
16. Horne G, Atkinson AD, Pease EH, Logue JP, Brison DR, Lieberman BA. Live birth with sperm cryopreserved for 21 years prior to cancer treatment: case report. Hum Reprod. 2004;19:1448–9.
17. Hovay Y, Dan-Goor M, Yaffe H, Almagor M. Electroejaculation before chemotherapy in adolescents and young men with cancer. Fertil Steril. 2001;75:811–3.
18. Goldstein M. Surgical management of male infertility. In: Cambell-Walsh urology, 11th ed. Elsevier; 2015. p. 580–611.
19. Schlegel PN, Palermo GD, Alikani M, et al. Micropuncture retrieval of epididymal sperm with in vitro fertilization: importance of in vitro micro-manipulation techniques. Urology. 1995;46:238–41.
20. Vernaeve V, Verheyen G, Goosens A, Van Steirteghem A, Devroey P, Tournaye H. How successful is repeat testicular sperm extraction in patients with azoospermia? Hum Reprod. 2006;21:1551–4.
21. Berookhim BM, Schlegel PN. Azoospermia due to spermatogenic failure. Urol Clin North Am. 2014;41:97–113.
22. Honaramooz A, Behboodi E, Megee SO, et al. Fertility and germline transmission of donor haplotype following germ cell transplantation in immunocompetent goats. Biol Reprod. 2003;69:1260.
23. Hermann BP, Sukhwani M, Winkler F, et al. Spermatogonial stem cell transplantation into rhesus testes regenerates spermatogenesis producing functional sperm. Cell Stem Cell. 2012;11:715.
24. Parrington J, Coward K, Gadea J. Sperm and testis mediated DNA transfer as a means of gene therapy. Syst Biol Reprod Med. 2011;57:35.
25. Light AD, Obedin-Maliver J, Sevelius JM, Kerns JL. Transgender men who experienced pregnancy after female-to-male gender transitioning. Obstet Gynecol. 2014;124(6):1120–7.
26. Hembree WC, Cohen-Kettenis P, Delemarre-van de Waal HA, et al. Endocrine treatment of transsexual persons: an endocrine society clinical practice guideline. J Clin Endocrinol Metab. 2009;94:3132–54.
27. Jadoul P, Guilmain A, Squifflet J, Luyckx M, Votino R, Wyns C, Dolmans MM. Efficacy of ovarian tissue cryopreservation for fertility preservation: lessons learned from 545 cases. Hum Reprod. 2017;32(5):1046–54.
28. Donnez J, Silber S, Andersen CY, Demeestere I, Piver P, Meirow D, et al. Children born after autotransplantation of cryopreserved ovarian tissue. A review of 13 live births. Ann Med. 2011;43(6):437–50.
29. Dittrich R, Hackl J, Lotz L, Hoffmann I, Beckmann MW. Pregnancies and live births after 20 transplantations of cryopreserved ovarian tissue in a single center. Fertil Steril. 2015;103 (2):462–8.
30. Corkum KS, Laronda MM, Rowell EE. A review of reported surgical techniques in fertility preservation for prepubertal and adolescent females facing a fertility threatening diagnosis or treatment. Am J Surg. 2017;21(4):695–700.
31. Fasano G, Dechene J, Antonacci R, Biramane J, Vannin AS, Van Langedonckt A, Devreker F, Demeestere I. Outcomes of immature oocytes collected from ovarian tissue for cryopreservation in adult and prepubertal patients. Reprod Biomed Online. 2017;34(6):575–82.

32. Duncan FE. Egg quality during the pubertal transition-is youth all it's cracked up to be? Front Endocrinol (Lausanne). 2017;4(8):226.
33. Tamar R, Zil G. Case report: induced lactation in a transgender woman. Transgender Health. 2018;3(1).
34. Wein AJ, Kavoussi LR, Partin AW, Peters CA, editors. Campbell-Walsh urology, 11th ed. Philadelphia: Elsevier; 2016.

Chapter 12
Voice Changes in Transgender Care

Jean Sawyer

The human voice alone and in combination with visual appearance reflects aspects of an individual's identity, particularly, in relation to age and gender. Transgender individuals, or those whose gender identity differs from the sex assigned to them at birth, may seek hormonal and surgical interventions to facilitate changes in their visual appearance that correspond with their gender identity. Even if individuals alter their appearance, however, the human voice and communication-related behaviors may not follow suit. Thus, speech-language pathologists may provide voice and communication training that serves to facilitate authentic voice and communication consistent with an individual's gender identity.

The voice is comprised of the subsystems of respiration, phonation, and resonance. Respiration generates expiratory airflow from the lungs which acts as a power source for the vibration of the vocal folds. The vibrating vocal folds create a sound source which is further modified by the vocal tract or the area above the vocal folds consisting broadly of the head and neck. The voice is then articulated or shaped into meaningful sounds (i.e., speech) via movements of the lips, teeth, tongue, and other structures of the head and neck. Prosody of speech reflects the intent, emotions, or meaning of the speaker through variations in pitch, loudness, and rhythm across an utterance. Some of the anatomical structures used in speaking are depicted in Fig. 12.1.

J. Sawyer (✉)
Department of Communication Sciences and Disorders, Illinois State University
(This is a university and not a hospital), Normal, IL, USA
e-mail: jsawyer@ilstu.edu

L. Poretsky and W. C. Hembree (eds.), *Transgender Medicine*, Contemporary Endocrinology, https://doi.org/10.1007/978-3-030-05683-4_12

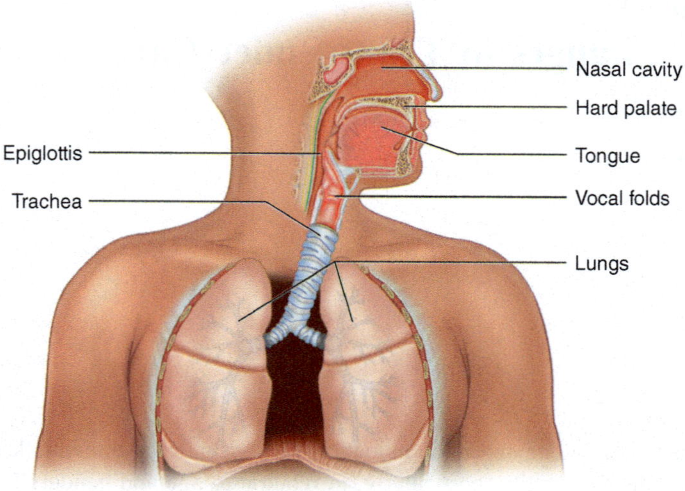

Fig. 12.1 Sagittal view of the oral cavity with a chest view of the lungs

Perceptions of Gender from Voice and Communication

Communication training targets for transgender individuals are based on a current understanding of the acoustic (measurable physical properties of sound) and auditory-perceptual (subjective perception of these physical properties) voice and speech features that are typically identified as more masculine or feminine. Research has indicated that aspects of voice (i.e., pitch, loudness, and intonation), resonance, speech (articulation), and prosody (rhythm, intonation, and stress) are significantly related to how a listener perceives the gender of a speaker [1, 2]. Language use and nonverbal forms of communication may also contribute to these perceptions, but are significantly more controversial [3].

Pitch and Intonation

One of the most investigated vocal markers of gender is the pitch of the voice. Pitch is the perceptual representation of the acoustic variable, fundamental frequency, or how many times the vocal folds fully open and close (i.e., vibrate) each second. The greater the number of vocal fold vibrations per second, the higher the perceived pitch of the voice. A typical female or male voice has a speaking fundamental frequency (SFF) of approximately 200 and 100 Hertz (Hz), respectively, with Hz indicating the number of vibratory cycles per second. Variability in pitch is a prosodic feature of the voice that is directly related to intonation, or the fluctuations in pitch that communicate the speaker's emotions or intent. Intonation is different, for example, when asking a question versus making a statement.

Investigations of gender identification based on intonation have been inconclusive. Hancock et al. [4] analyzed the intonation of recordings of transfeminine and transmasculine individuals and cismales and cisfemales describing a picture. Fourteen listeners rated the recordings on a scale of masculinity/femininity. No differences in intonation were found among the four speaker groups, but trends were found in gender identification for the transfeminine speakers. The transmasculine speakers passed as male, and six of the transfeminine speakers were rated as "ambiguous" in terms of masculinity/femininity. Five transfeminine individuals did not pass as female. Speakers with upward intonation and a larger range, measured in semitones, were identified as female. The transfeminine individuals who did not pass as female had more downward intonations than those who passed.

Gelfer and Schofield [5] found that transfeminine individuals who were reliably perceived as female had higher SFF and a higher maximum SFF (or highest upper frequency) than those who were perceived as male. Additionally, the prosodic feature of intonation tends to be more variable in female voices [6]. Thus, because individuals continuously change SFF across utterances, there is a range of frequencies that is likely perceived as within a female versus male range. Research findings indicate that SFF above 165 Hz and below 145 Hz may be especially important in perceiving an individual as female or male, respectively [2, 5, 7]. Voices that are produced within a range of 145–165 Hz, conversely, may depend on additional acoustic markers, like resonance, to facilitate gender identification by voice.

Resonance

While most research supports the raising of fundamental frequency in transfeminine individuals because it is the primary acoustic marker of gender in cisgender female speakers, speaking above 160 Hz is no guarantee that a speaker will be identified as female [5, 8, 9]. A few of the transfeminine participants in Gelfer and Schofield's [5] study, for example, had SFFs well above 160 Hz and were perceived as male. Mount and Salmon's [9] client had a SFF of 210 Hz but was perceived as male on the telephone. The client was not perceived as female until her vowel formant frequencies had increased to the female range via training to alter tongue placement.

The formant frequencies in the Mount and Salmon [9] study were a measure of resonance, which has been defined as the flow of air through the vocal tract [10]. Formant frequencies are sometimes called resonant frequencies and differ based on the size and shape of the vocal tract. Resonant frequencies are typically higher for ciswomen and children, and lower for cismales, due to the smaller vocal tracts anatomy of the former. A larger vocal tract will have lower resonant frequencies than a smaller one. Resonance is altered by changing the shape of the vocal tract by movement of the articulators. Moving the tongue more forward in the mouth or retracting the lips shortens the vocal cavity and raises resonant frequency. Protruding the lips will increase the size of the vocal cavity and lower the resonant frequency.

Resonance is typically measured by calculating the resonant frequencies of the vowels. Each resonant frequency is a formant, and the first three formant frequencies, F1, F2, and F3, characterize and differentiate the vowels. Different formant frequencies have been implicated in the perception of gender. Carew et al. [11] targeted resonance in a therapy for transfeminine individuals and found that all three formants rose after therapy, with the increase in F3 being statistically significant. SFF, though not formally targeted in the therapy, also rose, and participants perceived their voices as more feminine after treatment. Avery and Liss [12] found that F1 and F2 were higher in cismales whose voices were perceived as less masculine. In cismales, whose voices were perceived as more masculine, F1 and F2 were lower. Mount and Salmon [9] found that F2 correlated with listeners perceiving a voice as female, while Gunzburger [13] determined that increases in both F2 and F3 were necessary before a voice was perceived as feminine. Gelfer and Mikos [14] noted that both SFF and vowel formants were necessary to identify an individual's desired gender. Thus, a transfeminine individual is more likely to be rated as female if her SFF and vowel formants are within a cisfemale range than if either is in a cismale range [15]. A study that manipulated SFF and formants to determine their effects on perceived gender found that if both parameters were shifted, a person was perceived to be the opposite gender most of the time [16]. SFF alone distinguished gender better than the formant frequencies alone, but the two together are needed to specify gender consistently.

Voice Quality

Breathiness is an attribute of voice quality. The female voice has been described as more breathy than the male, and the voice is produced with an incomplete closure of the vocal folds posteriorly [17]. Breathiness has been assessed by measuring cycle-to-cycle variations in vocal fold vibration, or jitter and shimmer and by measuring air flow. Sorensen and Horii [18] found that the cismale voice has more shimmer and less jitter than the cisfemale voice. Owen and Hancock [15] found a moderately negative correlation between percent shimmer and femininity ratings for their transfeminine participants, but there was no relationship between jitter and femininity.

There have not been many studies that have examined gender identification and breathiness, and the effect of breathiness on voice perception is far from certain [8, 19]. One study of cisfemales found that breathier female voices were judged to be more feminine than voices that were not as breathy [20]. Thus, producing a breathier voice has been a target in some voice therapies for transfeminine individuals. Because a breathy voice quality may decrease vocal loudness, modifying

Table 12.1 Summary of vocal qualities which help identify a voice as masculine or feminine

Vocal parameter	Voice identified as masculine	Voice identified as feminine
Speaking fundamental frequency	Below 145 Hz	Above 165 Hz
Resonance	Lower formant frequencies	Higher formant frequencies
Intonation	Downward	Upward, larger range
Voice quality	Less breathy and more loud	More breathy and less loud

the voice to increase its perceived breathiness may be less efficient and lead to vocal fatigue [21]. A summary of vocal qualities that may be perceived as masculine or feminine is found in Table 12.1.

How Voice Changes Have Been Made in Two Populations

One of the most common professional goals in modifying the voice is to change the SFF so that the voice matches the gender of choice for the individual in terms of pitch. SFF change alone, however, does not mean that listeners are more likely to rate a speaker as male or female [5, 9]. One reason that SFF is not distinctive to gender is that there is overlap in the range that is perceived as male or female [22, 23].

Changes in SFF are not solely associated with voice satisfaction in the individual. Some transfeminine people have been reportedly satisfied with their voices even though they fell within typical female fundamental frequency range [24]. Conversely, possessing a fundamental frequency that is more characteristic of one's gender identity does not always lead to voice satisfaction. Hancock et al. [25] reported that one of their transmasculine participants was dissatisfied with his voice because it "did not reflect his 'true self'" (p. 2480), despite being within a typically masculine SFF range.

Modifications in SFF have been achieved through voice training, hormonal treatment in the case of transmasculine individuals, or surgery. Surgery has been designed to either increase or decrease SFF [19, 26]. Surgery to increase SFF for transfeminine individuals is more common, as transmasculine individuals usually achieve a lower pitch through hormonal treatment. Pitch-lowering surgery has been typically performed on males with voice disorders, such as mutational falsetto and dysphonia. The surgery lowers the pitch by reducing vocal fold tension through a resection of the cricothyroid cartilage [27]. SFF can be increased in transfeminine individuals surgically by increasing vocal fold tension, decreasing vocal fold mass, or shortening vocal fold length [21]. Figure 12.2 provides a comparison of the length of the male and female vocal folds. The most commonly used surgery to increase SFF for transfeminine individuals is cricothyroid approximation (CA).

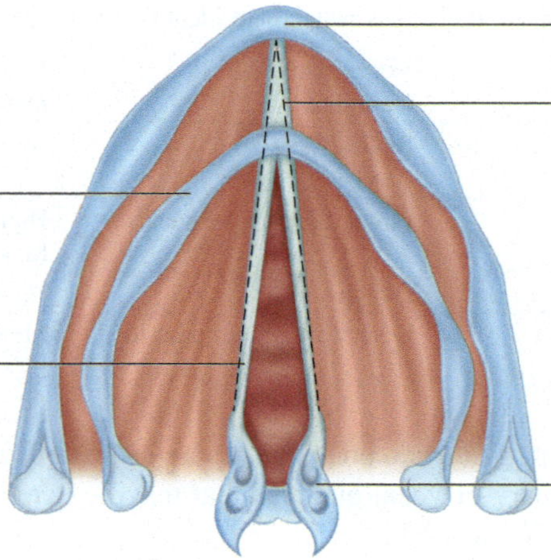

Fig. 12.2 Size comparison of the length of male and female vocal folds

The procedure decreases the distance between the cricoid and thyroid cartilages to tense and thin the vocal folds [28]. Because thinner and tenser vocal folds vibrate more quickly, the SFF will increase when these cartilages are permanently approximated [26, 29].

Voice training for transmasculine and transfeminine individuals may also facilitate SFF changes behaviorally, however, is not typically its sole focus [19, 30, 31]. Other voice training goals for transgender patients include changing resonance, intonation, and communication style [6, 32]. Methods of changing SFF and other aspects of communication are specific to gender. Hormonal treatment, for example, does not affect the voice in transfeminine people but does lower the fundamental frequency permanently in transmasculine individuals [33, 34]. Thus, transfeminine individuals are more likely to seek vocal training for help in making their voices congruent with their desired gender than are transmasculine individuals [19–21]. The challenges to changing the voice vary according to gender and the needs of the individual.

Voice Changes for Transmasculine Individuals

Research in transmasculine voice is incomplete, largely due to the common perception that testosterone treatment will make the voice masculine. As a result, transmasculine individuals are less likely to seek or to be referred for treatment than transfeminine individuals. Transmasculine individuals have been underrepresented in transgender voice literature, consequently. Reviews of literature on characteristics of the transmasculine voice indicate small sample sizes, variable or incomplete voice measures and methods [33, 35]. Several authors have documented treatment for transmasculine individuals, but there is little research as to what elements of vocal training are effective [21, 35].

As previously noted, testosterone treatment will lower SFF [25, 35, 36]. Treatment with testosterone thickens the vocal folds, resulting in lower pitch due to a slower rate of vocal fold vibration. These effects are similar to the results of hormonal changes in the male voice at puberty [33, 37, 38]. The changes in the voice are irreversible, even if testosterone supplementation ends [39]. Other ways to change the voice in transmasculine individuals include voice training, laryngeal surgery, and self-directed vocal change [33].

Testosterone treatment will lower fundamental frequency, but its effects are not uniform. The length of time for change in the voice to occur after initiating testosterone treatment varies. Gooren [40] reported a lowering of pitch within 6–10 weeks after hormone treatment was started. Nygren et al. [39] collected voice data for 50 transmasculine participants for 2 years and found that the decrease in frequency was complete within 12 month of testosterone treatment. There were inconsistencies in the study, however. Most (82%) of the participants did not complete the full protocol of voice measurements, and 12 of the 50 participants received voice training. In a survey of 16 participants, Van Borsel et al. [36] found that one participant perceived his voice had a lower vocal pitch a few days after the start of testosterone treatment. Over half the participants noted voice change after a "few months" (Van Borsel et al. [36], p. 430), and three noted a change after a year. Three said it took more than one year to notice a voice change. Hancock et al. [25] measured several acoustic features in seven transgender males' voices at 3, 6, 9, and 12 months after the initiation of testosterone treatment. Average fundamental frequency decreased for four individuals over a 6-month period, for one individual over a 3-month period, and for two individuals over a 12-month period. Table 12.2 provides a summary of how long it may take to notice voice change following testosterone treatment.

Testosterone treatment changes other parameters of voice besides pitch, and its effects on vocal function can be negative [25, 33]. Vocal fold mass increases through testosterone treatment, but the size of the vocal tract is not affected, which may lead to more feminine resonance patterns than a typical cismale. Adler et al. [41] have described this condition as an "entrapped FTM [female-to-male] vocality" (p. 162), which may result in a voice that is rough or hoarse. A voice that is

Table 12.2 Length of time before voice changes are reported after testosterone treatment

Study	Number of participants	Latency between testosterone treatment and Noticeable voice change
Gooren [40]	Expert opinion	6–10 weeks
Hancock et al. [25]	7	3 months to 1 year
Nygren et al. [39]	50	Within 12 months
Van Borsel et al. [36]	16	A few days to over 1 year

produced by thicker vocal folds due to a testosterone treatment, but a small vocal tract may sound similar to that of a pubescent male [39].

A reduction of power, or voice projection, and a reduction of vocal range after testosterone treatment has also been reported in a few studies. In a review of the literature on vocal function in transmasculine individuals, Azul et al. [35] found reports of a loss of high tones and monotone intonation. The longitudinal study of two participants in Van Borsel et al.'s [36] study revealed a markedly decreased pitch range. Van Borsel et al. [36] did not measure power. Nygren et al. [39] measured both power and range in their longitudinal study. Power, measured in sound pressure level and correlated with perceived vocal loudness, did not change over the course of testosterone treatment, but both power and range were found to be below normative values for healthy Swedish cismales. Hancock et al. [25] measured vocal pitch range in seven participants and found that group results generally decreased over time, but individual variation was wide, with four participants increasing their range, and three decreasing it. Azul et al. [35] looked at the individual data in Nygren et al. [39] study and found that 23 participants increased their pitch range, 12 showed a reduction, and 1 had no change. In a case study of a transmasculine individual who opted for surgery to lower SFF, the client's complaint was that testosterone treatment had not resulted in a lower pitch and that he was perceived as female on the telephone [41]. After surgery, his SFF decreased but complaints about an inability to raise pitch and a lack of vocal power led him to behavioral voice treatment.

The extent of change due to testosterone treatment is idiosyncratic. Cosyns et al. [34] examined the voices of 38 transmasculine individuals who had been on testosterone from 9 months to 22 years. The treatment was largely successful in reducing SFF, but not for 10% of the participants. Nygren et al.'s [39] longitudinal study found six participants (12%) had relatively higher pitch following a year of treatment. Their SFFs ranged from 143 to 170 Hz, while the mean for the group was 125 Hz. Van Borsel et al.'s [36] survey of transmasculine individuals revealed that two participants were not entirely pleased with their voices after testosterone training; one wanted a "heavier" (p. 430) voice and the other complained of vocal strain if he spoke at a lower pitch. Four participants, unsatisfied with the effects of testosterone on their voices, said they would be willing to undergo phonosurgery.

Perceptions of Voice While testosterone treatment usually has a pitch-lowering effect and many transmasculine individuals are satisfied with their voices, there is not only considerable variability in resulting voice changes, but also in individual perceptions of voice. Azul [42] suggested that the successful masculinization of the voice should take into account others' perceptions of the voice as well as the individual's attribution of gender to the voice. Interviews were conducted with 14 German-speaking transmasculine individuals to determine gender perceptions, including what gender they identified with and what gender they thought others attributed to them. While half the speakers perceived their voices as unambiguously male, others revealed themselves to be more gender-diverse, with more ambiguous voices. Three participants felt their voices were not masculine enough, and there was a mismatch between how the participants viewed their voices and how they perceived their listeners as viewing them.

The perception of voice as masculine does not always correlate with SFF. Van Borsel et al. [43] asked two groups of judges to rate audiovisual, visual-only, and audio-only speech samples of seven transmasculine individuals as to how "male" they were. Ratings were on a scale of 1–10, with 10 being "very male." The groups were speech-language pathologists and naïve listeners. The SFF of the speakers ranged from 140 to 190 Hz. Ratings across the three presentations were not different, but there was no correlation between the ratings and SFF. One of the participants in the Van Borsel et al. [36] study provides another example of the fluidity of gender identification and pitch. Participant S1 of the longitudinal study had an SFF of 155 Hz, which is close to the described 160 Hz threshold to be perceived as male. Even near the threshold, this participant's voice was perceived as male.

Voice Changes for Transfeminine Individuals

Transfeminine individuals may feel their voice betrays their sense of self and wish to speak in a voice that matches their desired gender [44]. As hormone treatment does not thin the vocal folds the way it thickens them in transmasculine individuals, transfeminine individuals will have to cope with the physiological barriers that work to prevent their voice from becoming more feminine. Longer, more massive vocal folds and a larger, longer vocal tract work together to produce lower SFF and resonant frequency that are more likely to be perceived as masculine [19, 24, 31]. Options to change the voice include self-treatment, voice treatment, or surgery. Self-treatment is not recommended, as it may damage the voice and lead to a voice disorder [19, 21]. It is not known how widespread self-treatment is, but there has been documentation of transfeminine patients coming in for vocal training with preexisting voice disorders [30].

Producing a voice that has a frequency that can be perceived as female, at a minimum of 155–165 Hz, is one of the priorities in behavioral treatment, and a desired outcome of phonosurgery [24, 45, 46]. Feminization of the voice is not achieved solely through a raised pitch alone, however. Working on resonance to increase formant frequencies contributes to the perception of a female voice [11, 30]. Vocal training for transfeminine individuals is not standardized, and speech-language pathologists work with patients to determine communication goals. Features of communication that are gender differentiated include articulation, vocal quality, intonation, word choice, and nonverbal communication [23, 30, 47]. Hancock and Garabedian [30] provided an overview of treatment techniques used over 5 years at a university clinic, and found goals for changing resonance and pitch, as well as teaching relaxation techniques, increasing intonation, and improving vocal hygiene and breath control. Goals were also written to help patients reduce phonotraumatic behaviors and practice feminine non-verbal communication and pragmatics.

There have been a few studies of treatment efficacy of vocal training for transfeminine individuals. The studies are not directly comparable due to different methodologies, measurements, and numbers of participants who completed the studies but overall, results show that vocal training is generally effective for raising pitch and resonance, and that those who have completed training are satisfied with their voices [11, 24, 31, 47, 48]. Not all studies included ratings of voice feminization or listeners' perception of voice, which would help determine treatment efficacy [30].

The outcomes of vocal training are variable. Long-term studies that have reassessed participants some time after their dismissal from vocal training have shown that some patients could increase SFF levels long after working directly with clinicians [24, 31, 47]. Other participants, however, had SFF revert to pretreatment levels over the long term. Dacakis [24] conducted a long-term maintenance check of 10 transfeminine clients, who were reexamined an average of 4.3 years after completing a voice treatment program that focused on increasing SFF. The number of therapy sessions ranged from 10 to 90, with a mean of 27 sessions. Voice measures were taken before treatment, at dismissal, and at follow-up, and participants also indicated their level of voice satisfaction. Voice and pitch satisfaction were high at discharge, as well as at follow-up. The mean SFF was 125.5 Hz before treatment, 168.8 Hz at discharge, and 146.5 Hz at follow-up, but there was variability in individual data. Four participants had a posttreatment SFF that was within 3 Hz of their pretreatment measure, and two participants maintained full treatment gains. Voice satisfaction did not fit with the acoustic measures of voice. Individual data showed that five participants had SFFs that would be regarded as masculine. A correlation indicated that the more therapy sessions participants competed, the better the maintenance of SFF after treatment.

Hancock and Garabedian [30] found a correlation between the gains made in fundamental frequency during treatment and the number of treatment sessions, implying that the longer a person is in treatment, the greater the gains in fundamental frequency. Their 25 participants attended an average of approximately 22 sessions, with a range of 2–77 sessions, and were able to increase SFF by an average of 48 Hz at the end of treatment.

Soderpalm et al. [31] assessed long-term outcomes of voice treatment in their transgender patients over an 11-year period. There were 16 transfeminine patients in the study who gave permission to publish their data. Participants rated their femininity on a 10-point visual analog scale, and voice measurements were made at baseline, during treatment, and at follow-up. Participants attended a mean of 17 sessions, with a range of 3 to over 45 sessions. Not all participants completed the research protocol and two chose to have phonosurgery. Results were variable, but at discharge, 5 of 12 patients had an SFF above 155 Hz. At follow-up, 10 patients had achieved 155 Hz on at least one of the visits. A trend towards increased SFF for those who completed more than 14 sessions of treatment was observed, but it was not significant. No differences in the ratings of femininity were noted across baseline, treatment, and follow-up.

One study of treatment efficacy focused on changing resonance, rather than fundamental frequency. Carew et al. [11] trained 10 transfeminine individuals to speak with the tongue more forward in the mouth and the lips more spread to increase resonant frequency over five sessions of therapy. Resonant frequency was significantly higher at the end of therapy compared to baseline, and an increase in SFF from an average of 119.4–133.3 Hz was observed. Twelve speech-language pathology students rated the voices on a 10-point rating scale, with 10 being "very feminine." The ratings were variable, with four participants being rated more feminine at the end of therapy, three having ratings that were either more masculine or unchanged, and three whose ratings too variable to categorize. All of the participant self-ratings were consistently more feminine at the end of therapy but were at odds with both the listener ratings and the SFF measures. The increase in SFF was spontaneous, as pitch training was not part of the therapy, but the increase was not enough to put the voices in a range that could be rated as feminine by observers.

One treatment outcomes study had three participants and a control group of two participants who did not receive therapy [48]. The treatment lasted 8–19 months and addressed pitch, pitch, articulation, and breathing techniques. Participants completed a self-rating of communicative impairment, and a "dysphonia index" was created which reflected the roughness, breathiness, and hoarseness of the voice. The voices of the participants in the control group were reanalyzed after 9 months. The pitch range diminished in the treatment group, due to a decrease in the production of voice at the lower frequencies. The frequencies in the pitch range for the treatment group were within the range of cisfemales at the end of therapy. The frequency range for the control group changed minimally over time, and one of the members had a range within that of cisfemales. Perceived communicative impairment only decreased in those individuals who received behavioral voice treatment.

The longitudinal studies of treatment outcomes help determine whether changes made in vocal treatment can be maintained. Measures of pitch, resonance, and patient perceptions of voice are one way to measure change, and listener perceptions are important, too. An increase in pitch or resonant frequencies do not necessarily mean the client will be perceived as feminine. It has been shown that isolated judgements of masculinity or femininity cannot predict gender identification, but measuring listener perceptions pre- and posttreatment is a good way to determine the social validity of treatment [5, 30]. Gelfer and Tice [47] went further to emphasize that ratings of femininity do not go far enough to determine the effectiveness of treatment. A rating of "very female," for example, may describe a voice that is still identified as male. Thus, gender identification is a better metric of successful therapy than a rating of masculinity or femininity.

Gelfer and Tice [47] wanted to determine the effectiveness of a pitch-raising therapy on gender identification. The voices of five transfeminine patients were measured acoustically prior to treatment, at the end of treatment, and 15 months posttreatment. For comparison, the study included five cismales and five cisfemales. Two groups of 26 college students were asked to listen to randomly ordered cisgender and transfeminine voices, indicate the perceived gender of the speaker, and rate the speaker's voice on a scale of masculinity and femininity. One group of listeners rated the transfeminine participants at the pretest and long-term posttest, and the other rated them at the pretest and at the immediate posttest at the end of therapy. All transfeminine participants were judged to be more feminine and less masculine at both posttests, but at the long-term posttest, most of the transfeminine speakers were perceived as male. There was considerable variability in the ratings. One of the participants was judged to be female only 9.6% of the time, while another was judged to be female 93.3% of the time. At the pretest, only 1.9% of the participants were perceived as female. This improved to 50.9% in the posttest and decreased in the long-term posttest to 33.1%. SFF decreased at the posttest as well. It was 119 Hz at the pretest, 178 Hz at the posttest, and 138 Hz at the long-term posttest. While listeners perceived the voices to be more feminine after therapy, both at the posttest and long-term posttest times, it was difficult for the listeners to identify gender based on audio samples of voice alone.

Surgical Considerations There are a variety of reasons that transfeminine individuals may choose phonosurgery to increase their pitch. Surgery means less effort expended on changing the voice and may reduce the risk of vocal trauma that may result from behavioral voice manipulations [19, 41]. It may be the case that there is not a skilled provider available for behavioral vocal training, or that progress in training has been minimal or limited [19]. Soderpalm et al. [31] indicated that one of the two transfeminine individuals who elected to have surgery was making progress on raising her pitch, but was impatient with the rate and degree of change. Even after successful behavioral treatment, if an individual is startled or awakened, or spontaneously laughs or yawns, the native masculine voice may appear [49, 50].

Transfeminine individuals typically choose CA as a surgical procedure, also known as type IV thyroplasty [26, 49]. CA creates vocal tension and produces a pitch increase over approximately 6–8 months [49]. Surgery can be repeated if the sutures become loosened over time [19]. After surgery, most individuals will experience a loss of their lower frequency range [49]. Additionally, during this surgery, the thyroid cartilage of the larynx may be shaved to reduce the prominence of the Adam's apple characteristic of males [46].

Surgery is not always effective in changing pitch, and there are some risks. There have been reported infections and scarring [19, 46]. Further, diminished vocal loudness, reduced vocal quality, and compromised swallowing and breathing may be consequences of surgery [19]. If the laryngeal cartilages have become ossified through age, the surgery cannot be performed [49]. Behavioral voice treatment is recommended post-surgery to help the patient adapt to the voice change and stabilize the voice [46].

CA has been reported to be largely effective in increasing pitch post-surgery. Gross [49] presented pre- and post-surgery data for 10 transfeminine individuals. Pitch was elevated in all patients, and habitual frequency averaged 116.9 Hz pre-surgery and 201 Hz post-surgery. A larger study of 67 patients in Germany reported that fundamental frequency was raised in 63 patients [46]. Two of the patients had no change in fundamental frequency, and two had a reduction in fundamental frequency. There were a few complications reported. One patient's wounds did not heal well, and she had to have a second operation. Some patients had postoperative hoarseness, which remitted before 4 weeks. Preoperatively, no one had a pitch within a female range, but postoperatively, 19 patients had voices in the female range. Vocal range decreased in 77% of the patients due to a loss of lower frequencies.

As mentioned above, a higher pitch does not mean that a person will be identified as female. Two CA efficacy studies included perceptions of others as to gender identity or degree of masculinity/femininity. The 14 patients in Brown et al.'s [51] study had variable results after surgery, as two showed no increase in the modal, or characteristic pitch post-surgery, and two others had large increases. Presurgery, the mean modal pitch was 142.07 Hz, and after surgery, it was 174.64 Hz. Voice recordings of the patients presurgery and 2 months post-surgery were played to 10 speech-language pathologists who labeled the voices as male or female. Modal pitch was highly correlated to judgments of the speakers as male or female, and 173 Hz was determined to be the midpoint of the ratings. Below 173 Hz, five listeners judged the participants as male, and above that, five listeners judged the patients as female.

Van Borsel et al. [26] asked 42 naïve listeners to rate audiovisual and audio recordings of nine transgender patients who had completed CA, along with nine cismale and cisfemale participants. The transfeminine individuals' voices had a mean average fundamental frequency of 118 Hz before surgery, and 169 Hz after surgery. The time post-surgery ranged from 1 to 124 months. CA raised the pitch in seven of the participants; there was no pre-operative data on fundamental frequency for two participants. Audio and audiovisual samples were rated on a visual analog 100-point scale of masculinity and femininity. The voices of the transfeminine participants were rated more feminine than the cismales, but not as feminine as the cisfemales. There was a significant correlation between average fundamental frequency and the degree of femininity. Judgments of femininity varied between male and female listeners, with the male judges rating the femaleness of the transgender individuals higher than the female judges. There was also a trend to score femaleness higher in the audiovisual mode than in the auditory mode, so physical appearance likely affected the judgments of femininity. Voice therapy after CA may be helpful in further facilitating perceptions of femaleness.

Long-term effects of CA surgery have not been widely reported. Soderpalm et al. [31] found at a second follow-up session that one of the two patients that had opted for CA had a decrease in the lowest pitch level. It had not decreased to the pre-operative level, and the patient expressed a lower level of satisfaction with the voice than she had post-surgery. The second patient with phonosurgery did not participate in follow-up, but was telephoned "some years" after the surgery. The phone call revealed that the higher pitch had not been maintained.

The Role of Perceptions in Voice Change Increasing pitch to a level that is within the range of cisfemale is an objective in both behavioral voice treatment and in surgical procedures. It is clear, however, that perceptions of femininity are not based on pitch alone, and quite likely other factors interact to influence the perception of femininity and gender identity, including resonance, intonation, word choice, and nonverbal communication [15, 19]. Physical presentation may contribute to gender identification and perceived femininity. To investigate the effect of appearance on ratings of femininity, Van Borsel et al. [52] asked two groups of raters, 22 speech-language pathology students and 22 naïve listeners, to rate the level of "femaleness" from three presentation samples from 14 transfeminine individuals. Presentations were visual-only (no voice), audio-only, and audiovisual, and were rated on a 10-point scale of masculinity/femininity. Ratings were assessed on a 10-point interval scale. Naïve listeners' ratings were no different from those of the more expert listeners. The degree of "femaleness" was correlated with fundamental frequency. The visual-only presentation was rated more feminine than the audiovisual presentation, and the audiovisual presentation was rated as more feminine than the audio-only, so appearance was important in the designation of femininity.

Just as pitch may not be an indicator of femininity, it may also not be a good indicator of patient satisfaction with the voice. McNeill et al. [38] examined the relationship between patient satisfaction and SFF and included a comparison of listeners' ratings of femininity. Twelve transfeminine individuals completed a quality of life questionnaire and rated the degree of happiness with their voice and their voice's level of femininity. Participants had completed between 2 and 30 months of voice therapy, with a mean of 12 months. The raters were a group of 15 speech-language pathologists and 40 naive listeners. The ratings between the two groups of listeners were strongly correlated, replicating Van Borsel et al.'s [52] findings. There was a strong correlation between the perception of femininity and SFF for the listeners, so participants with a higher SFF were rated as more feminine. Listeners' ratings of femininity were highly correlated with the transfeminine individuals' feelings about their voices. Happiness with the voice was not related to SFF, but self-perception of voice femininity was related to happiness with the voice. No relationship was found between the length of voice therapy and happiness with the voice. This study provided evidence that a client's perception of voice femininity may predict a listener's perceptions, and that measures of patient satisfaction may be more useful than measures of SFF in voice therapy.

Like McNeill et al. [38], Owen and Hancock [15] wanted to determine correlations between speaker-rated and listener-rated scales of femininity. Twenty transfeminine individuals made self-ratings and 25 naïve listeners rated audio samples on a VAS of masculinity/femininity. For the transfeminine individuals, self-ratings of femininity correlated positively with mean fundamental frequency and negatively with the range of the voice. So the higher the frequency and the smaller the range of semitones, the more feminine the voice was rated. Similar correlations were found in the listener ratings of femininity. The listeners' ratings of femininity were highly correlated with the speaker's self-ratings. Additionally, the longer the participant had been in voice treatment, the higher the rating of overall femininity. The findings of Owen and Hancock [15] give support to the use of self-rating and femininity rating scales in voice therapy.

Patient Satisfaction with Voice Change

As changes in voices are specific to gender, most studies that have examined satisfaction with transgender voice changes have typically focused on either transmasculine or transfeminine individuals. One study that examined both groups of transgender individuals examined the degree of vocal handicap in the voice [53]. Twenty-eight transfeminine and 20 transmasculine participants rated their voice on the Voice Handicap Inventory, a precursor of the Voice Handicap Index, which is a standard measure of the psychosocial consequences of voice disorders [54]. The median scores for transmasculine individuals were significantly lower than those for the transfeminine individuals, but neither group showed evidence of a voice handicap. Other studies focusing on voice satisfaction have revealed that both transmasculine and transfeminine individuals have experienced difficulty with voice changes [24, 25, 35, 38, 50, 55, 56].

Transmasculine Individuals' Satisfaction with Voice Change

For transmasculine individuals, while testosterone treatment lowers pitch, changes in pitch are not uniform and voice change can be problematic for some. In a survey of voice satisfaction in 16 individuals who had been on testosterone treatment for at least one year, Van Borsel et al. [36] found that eight had hoped for a faster change in their voice. Most (14) were satisfied with their voice, but three reported being addressed as a woman on social occasions and four were addressed as a woman on the telephone. Nygren et al. [39] found that most of the participants in their study were satisfied with their voice after 12 months of testosterone treatment. Twelve of the 50 participants reported difficulties with the voice, however, and sought voice training for vocal strain, fatigue, and instability. Some complained that their voice sounded young for their age, that they had insufficient vocal power, and were unable to lower their pitch to a satisfactory level. Participants completed a questionnaire addressing perceptions of the voice. Participants indicated the degree to which they agreed with statements about voice on a scale of 0–4, ratings that ranged from "never" to "always." Within 12 months of testosterone treatment, feelings of voice satisfaction and perceptions of being identified as a male on the telephone increased significantly. Over 24 months, levels of worry about the voice revealing the native sex decreased considerably. Hancock et al. [25] asked their participants to answer three questions about voice self-perceptions as a baseline measure before testosterone treatment and over a 12-month period of treatment. The questions addressed how much their voices reflected "the true me," how much they had to concentrate to make their voices sound like they wanted to, and how masculine their voices were. Before treatment, all seven participants felt their voices were more feminine, but after 3 months of treatment, all felt their voices sounded neutral or male. Each participant had a different timeline for reporting particular self-perceptions, but eventually all participants reported a decrease in feeling like their voice did not reflect the true self and indicated less effort put forth to modify the voice during verbal interactions.

One study of patient satisfaction examined gender-related problems with voice. Azul et al. [55] interviewed 14 German-speaking transmasculine individuals to learn about their desired gender attribution. All had been treated with testosterone. Listeners-rated audio recordings of the participants as to whether the speakers were men or women. The participants' self-perceptions of their voices were variable. Nine participants wished to be considered males, and two had no preference. None wished to be identified as female, and others preferred a nonbinary gender attribution. Nine participants wished for a lower pitch, although two in this group indicated they were generally satisfied with their voice. Seven participants reported difficulties with the control of their vocal gender presentation. One participant had a SFF that did not match the range for being identified as male gender. Four participants were not rated according to their gender preference by listeners. Seventy-nine percent of the participants presented with a gender-related voice problem, indicating many were having physical difficulty with their voices.

Determining the psychosocial problems with voice is helpful in being able to provide guidance to transgender individuals as to how to alleviate the problems. Azul et al. [35] recommend an instrument similar to the Transsexual Voice Questionnaire for Transfeminine People [57] be developed for transmasculine individuals. The Transsexual Voice Questionnaire measures psychosocial self-perceptions of voice. Such a tool for transmasculine individuals would give clinicians a systematic way to discover patients' self-evaluations of the voice, including its impact on daily life. To help transmasculine individuals achieve greater satisfaction with their voice, therapies should focus on patient preferences as well as the gender attributions of others.

Transfeminine Individuals' Satisfaction with Voice Change

For the most part, voice therapy or surgery leads to changes in the vocal pitch of transfeminine individuals. These changes do not always mean that a transfeminine person's voice will be perceived as being congruent with being female, but generally transfeminine individuals have been satisfied with voice change [24]. Neumann et al. [50] asked 28 transfeminine individuals who had completed CA surgery to evaluate their voices and subsequent vocal therapy. The evaluation was a questionnaire with a Likert scale of agreement or disagreement. Fourteen individuals were "satisfied or very satisfied" with voice therapy, and the same number of individuals was satisfied with their voices after surgery. Most felt their voice was more feminine after therapy. There was a strong correlation between how feminine the participants felt their voices were and their satisfaction with vocal therapy. Half of the participants had voice therapy before surgery, however, so for them, voice therapy was not sufficient in changing their voices. Some participants expressed disappointment, hoping to have had a higher pitch through surgery and voice therapy.

While voice therapy may raise pitch and increase a patient's satisfaction with the voice, there may be discrepancy between clinicians' and transfeminine individuals' perceptions of voice [36, 41]. The clinician may be keen to measure the voice acoustically and perceptually, and not take into account the client's level of satisfaction with voice changes [24, 57, 58]. Dacakis et al. [57] advocate adding self-measures of satisfaction to vocal therapy to help determine progress in therapy as well as determine when dismissal is indicated. A few scales have been developed to measure satisfaction with the voice.

Pasricha et al. [58] interviewed four focus groups of four transfeminine individuals each as a basis for designing the Functional Communicative Satisfaction Questionnaire (FCSQ). The topics for the focus groups included communicative situations, emotions, and communication groups. The strongest amount of dissatisfaction with the voice was when talking on the telephone, where there are no other indicators of gender besides the voice. Participants said it was difficult to maintain a feminine voice while they experienced emotion, such as anger and excitement. Likewise, maintaining a feminine voice was reportedly more difficult when talking to strangers, as opposed to family and friends. The time of day affected the use of a feminine voice as well, with evenings being more difficult. Participants reported being less satisfied with their voice as compared to other aspects of their communication (i.e., body language). They felt the voice was the feature that could most easily lead others to identify them as male.

Through the information gathered through the focus groups, Pasricha et al. [58] concluded that there were many situations where the ability to "pass" as female was strongly connected to communicative satisfaction. Pasricha et al. [58] used the outcomes of the focus groups to create the FCSQ, which could be used to determine which situations may be more important to be able to "pass" as female than others, and what aspects of communication contribute to being identified as female. The FCSQ has two 30-question scales. The first scale focuses on satisfaction with the voice, and the second scale has the same questions, but they are rated as to how important the issues are to the individual, ranging from a scale of "not at all important" to "very important."

Byrne et al. [59] explored transfeminine individual's perceptions of their pragmatic abilities (i.e., social communication), comparing a group of 21 individuals with 21 cisfemales' perceptions on the La Trobe Communication Questionnaire [60]. The pragmatic abilities were related to discourse. Examples of topics addressed were leaving out details, allowing others to assume the wrong impressions from a conversation, changing speaking style depending upon the situation, and knowing when to talk and when to listen. The participants rated the questions on a scale of 1–4, ranging from never or rarely to usually or always. The transfeminine group rated satisfaction with communication from extremely dissatisfied to extremely satisfied. Results indicated that the cisgender group rated their pragmatic abilities more positively than the transfeminine group did. The perception of the speaker's voice was a better predictor of communication satisfaction than pitch. A regression analysis revealed that three factors which were associated with communication satisfaction were satisfaction with the voice, the self-perception of pragmatic ability, and the length of time since starting the gender reassignment program. The factor that accounted for the most variance in communication satisfaction was satisfaction with the voice.

The Transgender Self-Evaluation Questionnaire (TSEQ) [61] was developed to measure voice handicap, and thus assess the quality of life in transgender individuals. Hancock et al. [56] used the measure to determine the quality of life of 20 transfeminine individuals. Participants were recorded describing a picture and asked to rate the likability and femininity of their voices. Five cismales and five cisfemales were also recorded describing the picture. Twenty naïve participants then listened to the 30 voices and rated them according to likability and femininity. TSEQ scores were correlated with likeability ratings more strongly than ratings of femininity. Ratings of likeability and femininity had a strong positive correlation. No relationship between femininity and likeability was found for the listeners, however.

The TSEQ was reassessed by Dacakis et al. [57] and became The Transsexual Voice Questionnaire for Male-to-Female Transsexuals (TVQ). One of the reasons the TVQ was developed was to characterize the health of transfeminine individuals according to the International Classification (ICF) of Functioning, Disability and Health framework [62]. The categories of activity, participation, and psychosocial wellbeing are part of the ICF framework and have been adopted in the TVQ. The 35 transfeminine individuals who participated in the psychometric evaluation of the TVQ reported the most problems with vocal functioning. They specifically indicated problems in psychosocial wellbeing related to voice [57]. Participants indicated that their voice made them feel "less feminine" and had an impact on self-identity. Participants reported the areas of participation and activity were less problematic and that the voice did not prevent them from talking to acquaintances, nor did it prevent them from "living as a woman."

Risks of Self-Treatment

Transgender individuals might wish to change their voice by themselves, through help from the internet or by talking to friends or watching YouTube videos. Lowering or raising pitch can mean using excessive muscle tension, which puts individuals at a risk for a voice disorder. Trying to change habitual pitch may result in vocal edema and voice strain [24]. It is recommended that transgender individuals seek the help of speech-language pathologists in order to modify their voices safely.

Transgender individuals may come to voice treatment with a vocal disorder. Hancock and Garabedian [30] noted that 38% of their transfeminine clients had disordered voices. Four of seven displayed mild-to-moderate dysphonia, two had vocal strain, and one had been diagnosed by an otolaryngologist with a voice disorder. Soderpalm et al. [31] reported that half of their patients showed moderate to pronounced supraglottal constriction while phonating, and reported vocal fatigue and soreness in the throat, likely due to having tried to adopt a different voice before therapy. It is probably not uncommon that transmasculine individuals try to change their voices before testosterone treatment. Van Borsel et al. [36] reported that 6 of the 16 transmasculine participants had tried to change their voices by speaking at a lower pitch level before treatment.

Transmasculine individuals may not seek voice treatment due to the frequency lowering caused by testosterone. Testosterone treatment, though, does not always lead to an acceptable lowering of pitch for the individual, who may compensate with laryngeal muscle tension and high impact closure of the vocal folds [41]. A typical strategy is a harsh glottal attack. Other strategies might include imitation of other voices, changing resonance by not opening the jaw sufficiently, and backward tongue positioning [35]. These effortful phonatory behaviors may alter the vocal fold mucosa, resulting in vocal fold edema or lesions [10, 63]. In addition to excessive muscular activity to change pitch, transgender individuals may engage in other behaviors that lead to trauma to the vocal folds, such as smoking, voice overuse, excessive throat clearing [63].

For transfeminine individuals, changing the pitch requires considerable changes to habitual voice production, so there is a potential for damaging the voice through self-guided change [19]. Attempts to "push the voice upward" may lead to dysphonia or a compromised voice quality, rather than producing a feminine voice [46, 48].

Barriers to Successful Vocal Treatment

Transgender individuals may be reluctant to seek medical care, as they may fear discrimination or a lack of empathy from caregivers, and may have had previous negative experiences [64]. Soderpalm et al. [31] pointed out that even after receiving services, transgender individuals may not return for follow-up visits. The authors pointed out, that patients may have been eager to leave their past lives, and going back to a provider was a reminder of past experiences.

Transgender individuals are also likely to experience bias in health care services [64–67]. Transgender individuals have reported negative experiences with health care providers, including feeling judged, being ridiculed, and being refused service [67]. Transgender health care is not regularly covered by health insurance, and providers may not be knowledgeable about transgender health care or the need to respect identity or confidentiality [65]. Even if providers are aware of transgender health needs, they may not be capable of providing competent care [68]. Providers must not only be supportive of transgender individuals but also be knowledgeable about how to help them achieve a satisfying life in the role of their preferred gender [21]. In the case of transfeminine individuals, for example, speech-language pathologists will be more successful in helping them be perceived as female if they work on both resonance and pitch, rather than on either solely [16]. For transmasculine individuals, speech-language pathologists should not assume that testosterone treatment leads to satisfactory voice change [25, 55]. Additionally, providers should not assume that transgender individuals are a homogenous group wishing to conform to a binary standard of gender. Helping the transgender individual find a comfortable gender expression is advocated by the World Professional Association for Transgender Health (WPATH) ([69], pp. 52–54). Competent care means knowing the terminology relating to transgender clients, understanding the diversity of gender identity and expression, and being knowledgeable about the physical, social, and emotional issues that affect care [21]. In interviews with 253 transgender individuals about their experiences with health care providers, Pitts et al. [67] found that health care providers who had a positive impact were knowledgeable about the barriers transgender individual face in healthcare and were sensitive to gender diversity.

Kelly and Robinson [64] explored the attitudes of 192 lesbian, gay, bisexual and transgender (LGBT) individuals toward speech-language pathologists and audiologists and their perceptions of bias in these professionals. Most (162) had sought professional services. The transgender participants in the study who had sought services were transfeminine individuals seeking voice therapy, and all disclosed they were transfeminine in treatment. Less than half of the other participants disclosed their membership in the LGBT community, however, and the majority felt their providers were biased toward heteronormative behavior.

Sawyer et al. [70] investigated the perceptions of both speech-language pathologists and LGBT individuals. Eighty-eight LGBT individuals completed surveys asking them about their knowledge of and interest in speech-language pathology services. For the 88 participants in the LGBT group, 27 identified as transgender and 12 as transsexual. Most of the participants (91%) indicated they had not worked with a speech-language pathologist. Fifty-seven percent knew that speech-language pathologists could help transgender individuals with voice and communication training; others thought that practice was limited to working with people who had articulation errors. Those who had received services were self-referred, and only four participated in therapy due to gender transitioning. Reasons for not seeking therapy varied. Cost of therapy was listed as a factor by some individuals as a reason for not seeking services, and others indicated availability of "trans-friendly" service providers was limited. Some indicated they did not know how treatment could help them. Five participants, one of whom was working on voice-related gender changes, indicated they had negative experiences with their speech-language pathologist.

The few studies that have investigated speech-language pathologists' perceptions have shown that there are biases toward transgender individuals and a lack of competence or confidence in serving this population. A survey of knowledge and attitudes of 279 speech-language pathologists in the United States, Australia, Canada, and New Zealand revealed that while there was little discomfort in working with people who are lesbian, gay, bisexual, transgender or queer (LGBTQ), practitioners professed a lack of knowledge as to how to serve this population [71].

Only about half, for example, were able to describe transgender voice therapy, and of those, fewer than 15 mentioned vocal quality or vocal hygiene. Their lack of knowledge may have stemmed from not having any coursework in their graduate programs that addressed transgender vocal treatment. Additionally, the group displayed more negative feelings toward transgender individuals than towards homosexual subgroups. The transgender population has been reported as being highly socially stigmatized by health care providers when compared to other sexual minority groups [65]. Hancock and Haskin's [71] results point to an urgent need to provide clinicians with more education about transgender individuals and more coursework about effective assessment and treatment.

Sawyer et al. [70] surveyed 288 speech-language pathologists residing in the state of Illinois about their familiarity with, and service to the LGBT community. Many of the respondents showed confusion over the terms used with LGBT clients. Thirty-eight percent of the participants indicated they had no idea what the acronym LGBT stood for, and only 28% could correctly define the term "transgender." Most (69%) felt that providing voice training was within the scope of practice for speech-language pathologists, and over half (62%) indicated they had not had any information about providing transgender care during their educational training. Over half of the participants reported being "uncomfortable" in assessing and treating a transgender client. Only 12 participants had ever treated a transgender client.

The American Speech–Language–Hearing Association (ASHA) [72], the accrediting body for speech–language pathologists in the United States, requires speech–language pathologists to be culturally competent with the population they serve, and discriminating against any population is a violation of the ethics code. ASHA's Office of Multicultural Affairs puts transgender voice care into its website of cultural and linguistic diversity (https://www.asha.org/Practice/multicultural/) and has a Special Interest Group on culturally and linguistically diverse populations. ASHA does not mandate curricular requirements for working with transgender population in graduate programs, however [73]. Preparing individuals to be competent clinicians for transgender individuals involves teaching them skills, but also cultural competence. To be culturally competent, individuals must be willing to examine their own biases and beliefs [64, 74]. Speech–language pathologists need to work to learn the needs of transgender individuals and increase their competence. There is also a need to educate transgender individuals and other service providers about the services speech-language pathologists can provide [64, 70]. Medical professionals should be able to refer transgender individuals to speech-language pathologists to assist their clients in attaining the voice that matches their desired gender.

References

1. Leung Y, Oates J, Pang Chan S. Voice, articulation, and prosody contribute to listener perceptions of speaker gender: a systematic review and meta-analysis. J Speech Lang Hear R. 2018;61:266–97.
2. Gelfer MP, Bennett QE. Speaking fundamental frequency and vowel formant frequencies: effects on perception of gender. J Voice. 2013;27(5):556–66.
3. Hancock AB, Stutts HW, Bass A. Perceptions of gender and femininity based on language: implications for transgender communication therapy. Lang Speech. 2015;58(3):315–33.
4. Hancock A, Colton L, Douglas F. Intonation and gender perception: applications for transgender speakers. J Voice. 2014;28(2):203–9.
5. Gelfer MP, Schofield KJ. Comparison of acoustic and perceptual measures of voice in male-to-female transsexuals perceived as female versus those perceived as male. J Voice. 2000;14(1):22–33.
6. Oates JM, Dacakis G. Voice change in transsexuals. Venereology. 1997;10(3):178–87.
7. Spencer LE. Speech characteristics of male-to-female transsexuals: a perceptual and acoustic study. Folia Phoniatr Logop. 1988;40(1):31–42.
8. Hardy TL, Boliek CA, Wells K, Dearden C, Zalmanowitz C, Riegera JM. Pretreatment acoustic predictors of gender, femininity, and naturalness ratings in individuals with male-to-female gender identity. Am J Speech-Lang Pat. 2016;25:125–37.
9. Mount KH, Salmon SJ. Changing the vocal characteristics of a postoperative transsexual patient: a longitudinal study. J Commun Disord. 1988;21(3):229–38.
10. Andrews M. Manual of voice treatment: pediatrics through geriatric. 3rd ed. Boston: Allyn & Bacon; 2006.
11. Carew L, Dacakis G, Oates J. The effectiveness of oral resonance therapy on the perception of femininity of voice in male-to-female transsexuals. J Voice. 2007;21(5):591–603.
12. Avery JD, Liss JM. Acoustic characteristics of less-masculine-sounding male speech. J Acoust Soc Am. 1996;99(6):3738–48.
13. Gunzburger D. Acoustic and perceptual implications of the transsexual voice. Arch Sex Behav. 1995;24(3):339–48.
14. Gelfer MP, Mikos VA. The relative contributions of speaking fundamental frequency and formant frequencies to gender identification based on isolated vowels. J Voice. 2005;19(4): 544–54.
15. Owen K, Hancock AB. The role of self-and listener perceptions of femininity in voice therapy. Int J Transgenderism. 2010;12:272–84.
16. Hillenbrand JM, Clark MJ. The role of fundamental frequency and formant frequencies in distinguishing the voices of men and women. Atten Percept Psychophys. 2009;71(5):1150–66.
17. Södersten M, Hertegård S, Hammarberg B. Glottal closure, transglottal airflow, and voice quality in healthy middle–aged women. J Voice. 1995;9(2):182–97.
18. Sorensen D, Horii Y. Frequency and amplitude perturbation in the voices of female speakers. J Commun Disord. 1983;16(1):57–61.
19. Davies S, Papp VG, Antoni C. Voice and communication change for gender nonconforming individuals: giving voice to the person inside. Int J Transgenderism. 2015;16(3):117–59.
20. Van Borsel J, Janssens J, De Bodt M. Breathiness as a feminine voice characteristic: a perceptual approach. J Voice. 2009;23(3):291–4.
21. Davies S, Goldberg JM. Clinical aspects of transgender speech feminization and masculinization. Int J Transgenderism. 2006;9(3–4):167–96.
22. Wiltshire A. Not by pitch alone: a view of transsexual vocal rehabilitation. Natl Student Speech Lang Hear Assoc J. 1995;22:53–7.
23. Wolfe VI, Ratusnik DL, Smith FH, Northrop G. Intonation and fundamental frequency in male-to-female transsexuals. J Speech Hear Disord. 1990;55(1):43–50.
24. Dacakis G. Long-term maintenance of fundamental frequency increases in male-to-female transsexual. J Voice. 2000;14(4):549–56.

25. Hancock AB, Childs KD, Irwig MS. Trans male voice in the first year of testosterone therapy: make no assumptions. J Speech Lang Hear R. 2017;60(9):2472–82.
26. Van Borsel J, Van Eynde E, De Cyupere G, Bonte K. Feminine after cricothyroid approximation? J Voice. 2008;22(3):379–84.
27. Nakamura K, Tsukahara K, Watanabe Y, Komazawa D, Suzuki M. Type 3 thyroplasty for patients with mutational dysphonia. J Voice. 2014;27(5):650–4.
28. de Bruin MD, Coerts MJ, Grevan AJ. Speech therapy in the management of male-to-female transsexuals. Folia Phoniatr Logop. 2000;52(5):220–7.
29. Isshiki N, Morita H, Okamura H, Hiromoto M. Thyroplasty as a new phonosurgical technique. Acta Otolaryngol. 1974;78:451–7.
30. Hancock A, Garabedian L. Transgender voice and communication treatment: a retrospective chart review of 25 case. Int J Lang Commun Disord. 2013;48(1):54–65.
31. Soderpalm E, Larsson A, Almquist SA. Evaluation of a consecutive group of transsexual individuals referred for vocal intervention in the west of Sweden. Logop Phoniatr Vocol. 2004;29(1):18–30.
32. Pickering J, Baker L. A historical perspective and review of the literature. In: Adler RK, Hirsch S, Mordaunt M, editors. Voice and communication therapy for the transgender/transsexual client: a comprehensive clinical guide. 2nd ed. San Diego: Plural; 2012. p. 1–34.
33. Azul D. Transmasculine people's vocal situations: a critical review of gender-related discourses and empirical data. Int J Lang Commun Disord. 2015;50(1):31–47.
34. Cosyns M, Van Borsel J, Wierckx K, Dedecker D, Van de Peer F, Daelman T, et al. Voice in female-to-male transsexual persons after long-term androgen therapy. Laryngoscope. 2014;124(6):1409–14.
35. Azul D, Nygren U, Södersten M, Neuschaefer-Rube C. Transmasculine people's voice function: a review of the currently available evidence. J Voice. 2017;31(2):261.e9–23.
36. Van Borsel J, De Cuypere G, Rubens R, Destaerke B. Voice problems in female-to-male transsexuals. Int J Lang Commun Disord. 2000;35(3):427–42.
37. Hollen H, Green R, Massey K. Longitudinal research on adolescent voice change in males. J Acoust Soc Am. 1994;96:2646–54.
38. McNeill EJM, Wilson JA, Clark S, Deakin J. Perception of voice in the transgender client. J Voice. 2008;22(6):727–33.
39. Nygren U, Nordenskjöld A, Arver S, Södersten M. Effects of voice fundamental frequency and satisfaction with voice in trans men during testosterone treatment—a longitudinal study. J Voice. 2016;30(6):766.e23–34.
40. Gooren L. Hormone treatment of the adult transsexual patient. Horm Res. 2005;64(suppl 2):31–6.
41. Adler RK, Constansis AN, Van Borsel J. Female-to-male transgender/transsexual considerations. In: Adler RK, Hirsch S, Mordaunt M, editors. Voice and communication therapy for the transgender/transsexual client: a comprehensive clinical guide. 2nd ed. San Diego: Plural; 2012. p. 154–85.
42. Azul D. Gender-related aspects of transmasculine people's vocal situations: insights from a qualitative content analysis of interview transcripts. Int J Lang Commun Disord. 2016;51(6): 672–84.
43. Van Borsel J, De Pot K, De Cuypere G. Voice and physical appearance in female-to-male transsexuals. J Voice. 2009;23(4):494–7.
44. Adler RK, Christianson A. Psychosocial issues. In: Adler RK, Hirsch S, Mordaunt M, editors. Voice and communication therapy for the transgender/transsexual client: a comprehensive clinical guide. 2nd ed. San Diego: Plural; 2012. p. 69–94.
45. Colton RH, Casper JK, Leonard R, editors. Understanding voice problems: a psychological perspective for diagnosis and treatment. 3rd ed. Baltimore: Lippincott Williams & Wilkins; 2006.
46. Neumann K, Welzel C. The importance of the voice in male-to-female transsexualism. J Voice. 2004;18(1):153–67.

47. Gelfer MP, Tice RM. Perceptual and acoustic outcomes of voice therapy for male-to-female transgender individuals immediately after therapy and 15 months later. J Voice. 2013;27(3):335–47.
48. Mészáros K, Vitez LC, Szabolcs I, Goth M, Kovacs L, Gorombel Z, Hacki T. Efficacy of conservative voice treatment in male-to-female transsexuals. Folia Phoniatr Logop. 2005;57:111–8.
49. Gross M. Pitch-raising surgery in male-to-female transsexuals. J Voice. 1999;13(2):246–50.
50. Neumann K, Welzel C, Gonnermann U, Wolfradt U. Satisfaction of MtF transsexuals with operative voice therapy: a questionnaire-based preliminary study. Int J Transgenderism [Internet]. 2002 [cited 2018 May 15]; [2018 May];6(4). Available from: http://atria.nl/ezines/web/ijt/9703/numbers/symposion/ijtvo06no04_02.html.
51. Brown M, Perry A, Cheesman AD, Pring D. Pitch change in male-to-female transsexuals: has phonosurgery a role to play? Int J Lang Commun Disord. 2000;35:129–36.
52. Van Borsel J, De Cuypere G, Van den Berghe H. Physical appearance and voice in male-to-female transsexuals. J Voice. 2001;15(4):570–5.
53. T'Sjoen G, Moerman M, Van Borsel J, Feyen E, Rubens R, et al. Impact of voice in transsexuals. Int J Transgenderism. 2006; 9(1):1–7.
54. Jaconson B, Johnson A, Grywalski C, Silbergleit A, Jacobson G, Benninger M, et al. The voice handicap index (VHI): development and validation. Am J Speech-Lang Pat. 1997;6:66–70.
55. Azul D, Arnold A, Neuschaefer-Rube C. Do transmasculine speakers present with gender-related voice problems? Insights from a participant-centered mixed-methods study. J Speech Lang Hear Res. 2018;61(1):25–39.
56. Hancock AB, Krissinger J, Owen K. Voice perceptions and quality of life of transgender people. J Voice. 2010;25(5):553–8.
57. Dacakis G, Davies S, Oates JM, Douglas JM, Johnston JR. Development and preliminary evaluation of the transsexual voice questionnaire for male-to-female transsexuals. J Voice. 2013;27(3):312–20.
58. Pasricha N, Dacakis G, Oates J. Communicative satisfaction of male-to-female transsexuals. Logop Phoniatr Vocol. 2008;33:25–34.
59. Byrne LA, Dacakis G, Douglas JM. Self-perceptions of pragmatics communications abilities in male-to-female transsexuals. Adv Speech Lang Pathol. 2003;5(1):15–25.
60. Douglas JM, O'Flaherty CA, Snow PC. Measuring perception of communicative ability: the development and evaluation of the La Trobe communication questionnaire. Aphasiology. 2000;14(3):251–68.
61. Davies S, Goldberg JM. Trans care gender transition: changing speech. Vancouver Coastal Health, Transcend Transgender Support and Education Society and Canadian Rainbow Health Coalition; 2006.
62. World Health Organization. ICF: international classification of functioning, disability and health. Geneva, Switzerland: World Health Organization; 2001.
63. Adler RK, Antoni C. Vocal health and phonotrauma. In: Adler RK, Hirsch S, Mordaunt M, editors. Voice and communication therapy for the transgender/transsexual client: a comprehensive clinical guide. 2nd ed. San Diego: Plural; 2012. p. 139–52.
64. Kelly RJ, Robinson GC. Disclosure of membership in the lesbian, gay, bisexual, and transgender community by individuals with communication impairments: a preliminary web-based survey. Am J Speech Lang Pathol. 2011;20(2):86–94.
65. Bockting W, Robinson B, Benner A, Scheltema K. Patient satisfaction with transgender health services. J Sex Marital Ther. 2004;30(4):277–94.
66. Lombardi E. Varieties of transgender/transsexual lives and their relationship with transphobia. J Homosex. 2009;56(8):977–92.
67. Pitts M, Couch M, Croy S, Mitchell A, Mulcare H. Health service use and experiences of transgender people: Australian and New Zealand perspectives. Gay Lesbian Issues Psychol. 2009;5(3):167–76.

68. Turner K, Wilson WL, Shirah MK. Lesbian, gay, bisexual and transgender cultural competency for public health practitioners. In: Shankle MD, editor. The handbook of lesbian, gay, bisexual, and transgender public health: a practitioner's guide to serve. New York: Harrington Park Press; 2006. p. 59–83.
69. World Professional Association for Transgender Health. Standards of care for the health of transsexual, transgender, and gender non-conforming people (Version 7). Minneapolis, MN: Author. [cited 23 Mar 2018]. Retrieved from http://wpath.org (2001).
70. Sawyer J, Perry JL, Dobbins-Scaramelli A. A survey of the awareness of speech services among transgender individuals and speech language pathologists. Int J Transgenderism. 2014;15(3–4):146–63.
71. Hancock A, Haskin G. Speech-language pathologist' knowledge and attitude regarding lesbian, gay, bisexual, transgender, and queer (LGBTQ) populations. Am J Speech Lang Pathol. 2015;24(2):206–21.
72. American Speech-Language Hearing Association. Code of ethics [Ethics]. [cited 8 Feb 2018]. Available from: http://asha.org/policy (2010).
73. American Speech-Language-Hearing Association. Standards for accreditation of graduate education programs in audiology and speech-language pathology. Rockville, MD: Author. [cited 9 Feb 2018]. Retrieved from http://asha.org/academic/accreditation/accredmanual/section3.htm (2008).
74. Sue DW. Multidimensional facets of cultural competence. Couns Psychol. 1998;9(1):1–7.

Chapter 13
HIV Infection in Transgender Persons

Ladan Ahmadi, Angelica Nocerino and Daniel Puneky

Introduction

Transgender persons are disproportionately affected by HIV compared to the general population. In this chapter, we hope to shed light on the true burden of HIV on this marginalized population. We will review the factors that contribute to the high prevalence of HIV among transgender persons, in particular, high-risk sexual behaviors and substance abuse. Additionally, we will discuss the unique socioeconomic and psychosocial barriers that predispose this population to poor outcomes related to HIV prevention and treatment. We will also explain the contribution of transphobia in healthcare systems to the poor outcomes across the continuum of HIV care. This chapter will highlight challenges for transgender persons living with HIV, and attempt to offer solutions to overcome some of the obstacles. The choice of antiretroviral therapy with concomitant use of gender-affirming therapies will be discussed in detail.

L. Ahmadi (✉) · A. Nocerino · D. Puneky
Department of Internal Medicine, Lenox Hill Hospital, Northwell Health, New York, NY, USA
e-mail: lahmadi@northwell.edu

A. Nocerino
e-mail: anocerino@northwell.edu

D. Puneky
e-mail: dpuneky@northwell.edu

L. Poretsky and W. C. Hembree (eds.), *Transgender Medicine*, Contemporary Endocrinology, https://doi.org/10.1007/978-3-030-05683-4_13

Epidemiology

Global HIV Prevalence

HIV was first recognized in a small group of men who have sex with men (MSM) in 1981. Since then, the epidemic has grown globally. As of 2016, the number of people worldwide estimated to be infected with the virus is approximately 36.7 million for a global prevalence of approximately 0.8% [1]. Certain populations with higher burdens of disease have been well characterized throughout the literature focusing both on geography (sub-Saharan Africa, Southeast Asia, Latin America, and the United States) and on sexual identity and behaviors (MSM, sex workers, intravenous drug users (IVDU), and prisoners).

In the United States, the CDC estimates that there are over 1.1 million people living with HIV, with 1 in 7 of those unaware of their diagnosis [2]. While the overall number of annual infections is thought to have declined by 18% from 2008 to 2014, there were still 39,782 new infections reported to the CDC in 2016 alone. The most highly affected group is MSM, who accounted for 67% of new infections in 2016. Furthermore, African-American MSM made up a disproportionate share of that number.

As the acceptance of the transgender community grows in the US and worldwide, there is an increasing need to understand the burden of HIV on these individuals. To date, studies of HIV in the transgender population are limited, but the picture they paint is dire.

Challenges in Assessing HIV Prevalence in Transgender Individuals

While it is clear that, compared to the general population, prevalence of HIV infection is increased in the transgender community, it is not as well characterized as in other populations. This is due to logistical difficulties in studying this at-risk population. Cross-sectional population-based studies are severely limited because most national agencies do not collect gender identity information. Even when gender identity information is collected, there is risk of inaccuracy in the recording of the correct gender identity [2]. Due to this limitation, there is a reliance on convenience and snowball sampling to identify and study transgender populations, while acknowledging their inherent flaws. Sample sizes are typically small, resulting in insufficient power from which to make significant conclusions. Furthermore, researchers frequently target locations where transgender individuals are known to congregate. These locations include bars, clubs, and healthcare facilities that target sexual and gender minority populations. This may lead to sampling from a subgroup with a different level of risk than the general transgender population.

There are significant behavioral differences between transmen and transwomen that lead to different prevalence between these two populations. As such, they must be studied separately. In fact, the majority of research to date has been in trans-women, and only recently have there been studies focusing on the transmale population. This is likely due to the perception of transwomen's heightened risk of HIV acquisition due to sexual behaviors including number of partners and sexual practices similar to MSM. Recent, small studies show that HIV risk may also be elevated in certain groups of transmen who have sex with men, and additional studies are necessary to better characterize prevalence and risk factors in this group [3, 4].

HIV Prevalence in Trans-women

The majority of studies of prevalence in transwomen are limited to small geographic regions, mainly major urban areas such as Boston, Chicago, Los Angeles, San Francisco, and New York City, with a few additional studies at the state or regional level. Given the limited sample areas, the true burden of disease is likely underestimated. Based on a 2008 nationwide meta-analysis, the demonstrated prevalence of positive HIV testing in transwomen is 27.7%, while HIV positive status was self-reported by only 11.8% of transwomen [5]. The prevalence in this population is higher than the prevalence of HIV infection in MSM in the US, which was reported to be 15.35% (95% CI 14.82–15.98%) in 2010 [6].

In a more recent review, Poteat et al. published a broad range of self-reported HIV prevalence in transwomen of 2.0–29.9% [7]. They also found that laboratory-confirmed HIV prevalence was even higher in certain community samples in San Francisco and New York City, 35.0 and 40.1%, respectively. In a 2013 review, Baral et al. found that transwomen ages 15–49 were at significantly increased risk of HIV infection in both the US (OR = 34.21% (95% CI 31.22–37.48)) and worldwide (OR = 48.78% (95% CI 31.19–76.28)), as compared to the general population [8]. They also found a similar prevalence of 21.7% (95% CI 18.4–25.1) in the US population studied, while the worldwide prevalence was 19.1% (95% CI 17.4–20.7). While these results are startling, there are large variances when considering subpopulations, particularly by race and geographic region.

Outside of the areas already mentioned, the southeastern region of the United States has been greatly affected by HIV in both MSM and transfemale populations. Self-reported prevalence in this region is as high as 60% in locations such as Atlanta, GA [9]. In this study, the majority of participants (83.7%) were African-American with HIV prevalence as high as 63%. Even more concerning is that 40% of the participants were either not taking antiretroviral therapy or had poor adherence.

On a global scale, prevalence varies widely by region and, in some areas, by country. In sub-Saharan Africa, overall HIV prevalence in transwomen is approximately 25%. Higher prevalence is seen in various areas, for example, prevalence in

Lesotho is 59%, Gambia is 50%, and Senegal is 39% [10]. The transfemale population in many South American countries is also affected with HIV prevalence as high as 33.5% (95% CI 28.3–38.8) in Argentina and 33.1% (95% CI 26.7–39.4) in Brazil. Other South American countries are similarly though not quite as strongly affected [8]. Prevalence varies widely among countries in Asia. Reported HIV prevalence in transwomen in Pakistan is 2.2%, Cambodia is 5.9%, Thailand is 12.5%, Indonesia is 26.1%, and in India as high as 43.7% [8, 11]. While prevalence varies widely by both global region and individual country, it is clear that there is a significant burden of disease throughout the transfemale population worldwide.

HIV Prevalence in Trans-men

Owing to the assumption of lower risk and prevalence of HIV in transmen as compared to transwomen, there is a paucity of evidence on burden of disease and risk factors in this population. To date, research has focused predominantly on transwomen.

A study of transgender individuals in Ontario, Canada found elevated HIV risk factors in transmen who have sex with men. While there were no self-reported HIV diagnoses in this population, rates of testing in the prior year were only 18%. Rates of ever receiving an HIV test were less than 50%. The result of HIV testing was not recorded as part of the study, so true HIV prevalence was not calculated [12]. In the US, a study in Boston, MA identified a number of factors leading to increased HIV risk in the transmen who have sex with men including: having three or more sexual partners in the prior 6 months, condomless anal or vaginal sex with a cisgender male in the prior 6 months, and lifetime sexually transmitted infection (STI) diagnosis. In this study, the rate of HIV testing in the prior 6 months was only 40% [13]. Unfortunately, the result of HIV testing was not included in this study either. In a San Francisco, California-based study, HIV infection rates between transmen and transwomen receiving care in STI clinics from 2006 to 2009 were comparable at 10 and 11%, respectively [14]. A 2006–2010 study of HIV in transgender individuals in New York City, 6% of new diagnoses were among transmen [15].

These studies highlight the need for additional research to fully define the prevalence of HIV in the transmale population and develop risk-reduction strategies for this population.

Risk Factors for HIV Transmission

Transgender persons are at increased risk for acquisition of HIV infection owing to an intersection of various behavioral and biological factors. These factors include types of sexual activity, trading sex for money, shelter, drugs, higher rates of incarceration, social and societal stigma, as well as higher rates of depression, drug use, and other factors.

The greatest risk factor for HIV transmission in transwomen is unprotected receptive anal intercourse [5]. From a purely virologic perspective, efficiency of HIV transmission is dependent on properties of the virus itself as well as the method of exposure. When considering sexual routes of transmission, receptive anal intercourse is the most efficient method of viral transmission with a significantly higher per act risk than receptive vaginal intercourse or insertive intercourse of any type [16]. Additionally, risk may be further increased by the presence of other STIs including chlamydia, gonorrhea, syphilis, and herpes simplex infection [17]. When considering risk of HIV transmission in receptive neovaginal intercourse, there is insufficient research to quantify risk.

From a behavioral standpoint, there are a variety of reasons why transwomen are more likely to participate in unprotected receptive anal intercourse. For some transwomen, there may be external pressure from a committed sex partner to engage in unprotected intercourse in order to maintain the relationship. Studies show that transwomen experience pressure to engage in unprotected intercourse for fear of being replaced with a cisgender partner [18]. For other individuals, participating in unprotected sex with men may provide affirmation of their chosen gender [19]. Some transwomen who engage in sex work are coerced into engaging in unprotected sex because clients may offer extra compensation for condomless sex acts. This extra money can be necessary to meet basic needs or to improve access to gender-affirming therapies (i.e., hormonal therapy) [20].

Because stigma and discrimination by employers make obtaining and/or keeping a job difficult for transwomen, sex work is common among these individuals. Rates of ever participating in sex work are as high as 75% in transwomen in Tijuana, Mexico [21], and 68% in black transwomen in Atlanta, GA [22]. When other sources of income are unavailable, transwomen may turn to sex work to meet their basic needs. In addition to leading to higher numbers of unprotected sex acts, sex work also leads to a higher number of sexual partners, which also increases risk for transmission of HIV and other STIs.

Increased HIV prevalence is independently tied to prevalence of other STIs. In a 2016 study in Cambodia, HIV prevalence was significantly greater for individuals with STIs in the prior 12 months. Risk was even greater in individuals who had a genital ulceration or sore at the same time, as compared to those who did not [11]. The reason for the increased prevalence is two-fold: the same behaviors that increase risk of STIs also increase the risk of HIV transmission, and active STIs independently increase the risk of HIV infection by increasing local inflammation and recruiting additional CD4 cells susceptible to HIV infection to the area [23].

Historically, incarceration has been considered a risk factor for HIV infection. The first case of AIDS in an incarcerated individual was reported in 1983, just 1 year after the first reports of AIDS in MSM [24]. High rates of HIV in prisoners are likely not related to HIV infection while incarcerated, but rather the concentration of substance abusers and sex workers who are imprisoned or pass through the prison system. A 1997 estimate put the percentage of the HIV positive population of the US who passed through the prison system in that year at 20–26% [16]. Transgender individuals are at risk of incarceration given the high rates of substance use and sex work as previously described. In a 2012 cross-sectional study of transwomen in Chicago, IL and Los Angeles, CA, Brennan et al. demonstrate that incarceration was associated with increased risk of HIV infection in this population [25]. Using a convenience sample from the National Transgender Discrimination Survey, Reisner et al. found that 19.3% of transwomen in the sample had been incarcerated. They also showed that the risk of having ever been incarcerated was significantly higher in Black transwomen as compared to their Caucasian counterparts (ARR 3.26 (95% CI 2.24–4.75)) [26].

In the US, African-American race is associated with increased risk of HIV transmission, particularly in the southern states, an association that does not spare the transgender community. The high seroprevalence in this population increases the likelihood of exposure to the virus [4, 7]. In a San Francisco-based study, African-American race was the single largest risk factor for HIV infection (AOR 5.81 (95% CI 2.82–11.96)) [27]. In addition to high seroprevalence in this population, African-American race is associated with added discrimination that leads to accumulation of HIV risk factors already discussed, including: unemployment, incarceration, sex work, and abuse [22]. This is particularly important when considered within the context of prevalence of racial groups within the transgender community. African-American comprise 16% of the transgender population as compared to 13% of the general US population. While the majority of the transgender population is composed of Non-Hispanic Whites (55%), African-American are overrepresented within the transgender community as compared to the general population. This serves to further highlight the increased burden of HIV disease in the African-American minority [28].

Social and mental disorders are common among transgender individuals and lead to increased HIV risk. A 2017 study in sub-Saharan Africa found an elevated odds ratio (OR 1.48 (95% CI 1.21–1.81)) for HIV infection in transwomen and cis-MSM who also had positive depression screens [10]. Poteat et al. identified mental health as one of the most common syndemic factors with HIV infection [7]. In 2016, a study of transwomen in Chicago, IL and Boston, MA showed that 41.5% of participants had one or more mental health or substance dependence disorder. The most common diagnoses identified were major depressive episode, suicidality, generalized anxiety disorder, posttraumatic stress disorder, alcohol dependence, and non-alcohol psychoactive substance use [29].

Substance use is a well-described risk factor for HIV infection, especially IV drug use through sharing of needles [30]. While education and needle exchange programs have decreased the frequency of transmission via this modality, there continue to be new outbreaks of HIV in this subpopulation in different localities throughout the world [31]. This increased risk translates also to transgender individuals. In a study of Black and Latina transwomen in Chicago, IL, Houston, TX and Los Angeles County, CA, as many as 16% reported ever injecting illicit drugs in their lifetime [32]. In a San Francisco study, nonhormonal injection drug use was associated with increased adjusted odds ratio of HIV infection (AOR 2.69 (95% CI

1.56–4.62)) [27]. When considering hormone injection, there is conflicting evidence of HIV transmission risk. A Cambodian study showed increased risk of HIV infection in transwomen who injected gender-affirming hormones (AOR 4.4 (95% CI 1.1–17.3)) [11], but significant increased risk was not seen in the group of transwomen in San Francisco mentioned previously (AOR 1.67 (95% CI 0.94–2.97)). The risk from sharing needles for hormone injection is an area that deserves further scrutiny.

It should now be clear that the prevalence of HIV in transwomen is high, owing to a complex risk profile for HIV infection. Risk factors include sexual behaviors especially condomless anal intercourse, any psychoactive substance use, injection drug use, Black/African-American race, employment status, sex work, mental health, and social and societal stigma. These disparities will be described in greater detail later on. Furthermore, there is lack of recognition of elevated risk in transmen who have sex with men. Both transmen and transwomen should be rigorously screened for HIV and other STIs, and be targeted for appropriate education, prevention, and care.

HIV-Related Health Disparities in Transgender People

We established the high prevalence of HIV infection among adult transgender persons and outlined the contributing factors leading to this high prevalence in Sect. 14.1. Despite the high HIV prevalence, transgender persons are less likely to exercise prevention modalities for HIV or know their HIV status. Those living with HIV also experience poorer health outcomes across the HIV care continuum. Studies have shown that HIV positive transgender persons are less likely to be linked to care, retained in care, receive and adhere to antiretroviral therapy (ART) or achieve sustainable HIV viral suppression compared to HIV positive cisgender persons [33–36].

There are multiple factors contributing to health disparities in transgender persons, many of which are discussed in detail in earlier chapters of this book. Health disparities among transgender persons are important and preventable contributors to higher rates of HIV infection, and are major contributing factors to relatively poor outcomes in those who become infected with HIV.

What follows is a non-exhaustive list of factors contributing to HIV-related health disparities among transgender persons. These factors act together, many simultaneously occurring, or syndemic, to contribute to the higher rate of HIV infection and to potentially lead to poorer health outcomes associated with HIV infection in transgender persons [36–38]. We have grouped these factors into three categories: socioeconomic factors, psychosocial and behavioral factors, and social and healthcare-related stigmatization. It is important to acknowledge the interplay between these categories and how one feeds on the other to place the transgender person in a disadvantageous and marginalized group with major impacts on health including HIV-related health and outcomes.

Socio-Economic Factors

Poverty and economic inequality are contributing factors in the HIV epidemic [39]. Poverty leads to development of socially marginalized communities and HIV hot spots and increases the individual's chance of risky behavior [39, 40]. **Minimal legal employment opportunities** and poverty have both been identified as risk factors for sexually transmitted infections including HIV among the transgender population [39, 41, 42]. In a survey conducted in Massachusetts between 2007 and 2009, it was found that the transgender adult respondents were 3.2 times more likely to be unemployed and 3.1 times more likely to be living at less than or equal to 100% poverty than non-transgender adults [43]. Another survey submitted as a report in 2013 by Human Rights Campaign (HRC) Deputy Communications Director called *A Broken Bargain: Discrimination, Fewer Benefits, and More Taxes for LGBT Workers* concluded that the rate of unemployment in the transgender workers surveyed was twice as much as cisgender worker, it was also discovered that many who worked were underemployed and were more likely to have an annual household income under $10,000. Poverty and minimal legal employment opportunities contribute to the high prevalence of **unstable housing** in transgender persons as well [41, 44, 45]. Transwomen who have unstable housing or are homeless have higher rates of substance use and risky sexual behaviors, especially unprotected serodiscordant receptive anal intercourse [41]. Housing instability also contributes to poor HIV-related health outcomes [44]. In an attempt to escape poverty and unstable housing, many transwomen engage in HIV risk behaviors, including **sex work** [41]. Economic inequality and discrimination specific to transgender people are important contributing factors to transgender women's engagement in sex work to earn money [27, 41]. Another noteworthy socioeconomic factor impacting HIV prevalence and outcomes in transgender minorities—especially Latinas in United States—is immigration **documentation status**. Legal authorization to live in the US is not only a barrier for HIV testing and treatment but also a key risk factor for HIV infection [46]. In a study of transgender Latinas between 18- and 29-years-old, it was found that "obtaining legal documentation to live in the United States can protect against HIV infection risk among undocumented transgender Latinas by affirming their identity, making it easier to avoid controlling sexual partners, and providing access to greater employment opportunities and public services" [46].

Psychosocial and Behavioral Factors

Minority stress theory suggests that sexual minorities, including transgender persons, suffer increased prevalence of more health problems due to social stressors, most notably due to the impact of stigma on various aspects of life [47]. The collective impact of stressors can be a potential contributing factor to higher rates of

mental illness in this population [37, 47]. Multiple studies have shown that transgender persons have higher risks of depression and anxiety, and between 26.0 and 43.0% attempt suicide in their lifetime [27, 48, 49]. There is a syndemic relationship between mental health and other health outcomes including HIV infection. Studies have shown a higher rate of HIV prevalence in individuals receiving mental health services in the US [37, 50]. According to Substance Abuse and Mental Health Services Administration (SAMHSA) in 2014, the rate of **substance use disorders** in general population was 8.4%. The rate of substance use disorders in transgender persons is much higher, with estimates between 25 and 28% [51, 52]. The National Survey on Drug Use and Health (NSDUH) in 2015 reported that sexual minority adults including transgender persons were more likely to have used alcohol, illicit drugs, marijuana, or misused pain relievers in the past year [53]. The relationship between substance use disorder and HIV infection is well established. Illicit drug use can increase risk of HIV infection via the sharing of needles or other paraphernalia. Illicit drug use also increases risky sexual behavior due to impaired judgment. There are multiple common links between mental health, substance abuse, and HIV infection and the co-occurrence of this triad is so common that many agencies and healthcare centers focus on comprehensive services located in one setting to address all three components in an attempt to improve linkage, retention, and health outcomes associated with these challenging illnesses. Another psychosocial and behavioral factor that impacts the transgender person's approach to both testing and treatment of HIV is **mistrust of social services and healthcare providers**. This has been shown to be due to either conspiracy beliefs [37, 54], in response to transphobia within the healthcare system, or in some cases due to gender insensitivity and forced care [55].

Social and Healthcare-Related Stigmatization and Transphobia

Transphobia in healthcare settings has a major impact on the transgender person's medical experience and leads to decreased access to HIV-related prevention and care [56, 57]. Transphobia is exaggerated in HIV-infected transgender persons due to collection of stigmatized social identities, namely, HIV status and gender identity [5, 57]. Transgender women of color are most affected by this stigmatization [5]. Transphobia in the delivery of social and healthcare services may, in extreme cases, manifest as denial of services by providers [46, 58–60]. HIV-related stigma also impacts organization of care as evidenced by low levels of engagement of transgender persons in healthcare research [57, 61]. Figure 13.1 is adopted from an article on the topic by Dr. Ashley Lacombe-Duncan who argues that the intersectional analysis of the depicted factors helps to understand and improve this experience of social exclusion [57]. **Societal stigma** and **internalized stigma** have also been shown as factors associated with HIV vulnerability and lower

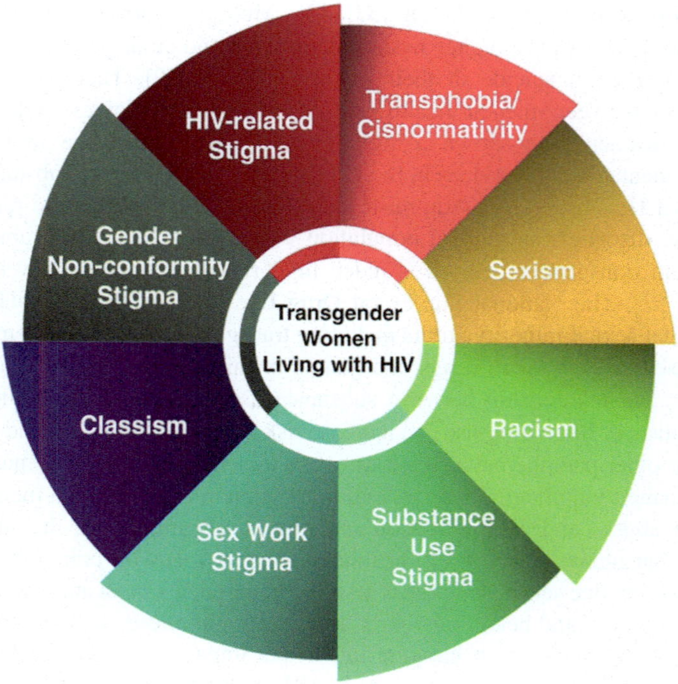

Fig. 13.1 Intersecting stigmas influencing access to HIV-related health care for transgender women—adapted from Lacombe-Duncan perspective published [57]

engagement and retention rates in HIV-related care [41, 62]. Adequate **social and tangible support** is an important factor contributing to effective and enduring engagement in HIV care as well [37, 63]. Tangible support is defined as "having persons available to help out and offer practical assistance in times of need" [37], and has shown to impact linkage and adherence in HIV-infected individuals [63, 64]. Studies show that compared to cisgender men and women, transwomen have the lowest degree of tangible social support [37, 63]. **Family-based stigma and rejection** seem to be important contributors to the reduced support system of transgender persons and contributes significantly to rates of homelessness, substance use, depression, and suicide attempt in this population [65]. In a secondary analysis of the 2015 data from the National Transgender Discrimination Survey of 3458 individuals who self-identified as transgender or gender nonconforming, health risks by reported family support were examined. Odds of drug and alcohol use to cope with transgender-related discrimination was significantly increased with increasing level of family rejection even after controlling for age, race, and other socioeconomic factors [65]. Suicide attempts were reported in 42.3% of the sample [65]. The researchers concluded that "Family rejection related to gender identity is an understudied interpersonal stressor that may negatively affect health outcomes for transgender and gender nonconforming individuals" [65].

Summary

In conclusion, as listed above, there are multiple, interwoven, co-occurring factors that work together to create a perfect storm of HIV-related health disparities in transgender persons. The approach to prevent new HIV infections and to improve the health outcomes for those already infected is multifaceted. Any solution must include interventions to deal with socioeconomic disadvantages, such as addressing the housing insecurity [45] and implementing anti-discrimination laws to name a few. Psychosocial and behavioral factors should address resilience building and empowerment [57] as well as supporting and expanding healthcare systems that provide mental health, substance use, and HIV services in a transgender friendly environment, with providers that are trained to provide culturally sensitive, unbiased care to this population in a comprehensive manner.

Special Programs of National Significance (SPNS) in transgender care by the Health Resources and Services Administration (HRSA) in the United States is an example of a multifaceted approach implemented and studied to improve the HIV-related health outcomes. HRSA funded this project from 2012 to 2017. The funds supported multiple demonstration projects at different clinical sites to design, implement, and evaluate novel interventions to improve HIV care outcomes in transgender women of color, who, as pointed out before, are the most affected by the HIV epidemic in transgender community in both the US and internationally [8, 66]. The funded demonstration projects used different interventions including community outreach, transcompetency training, transcompetent HIV medical care, non-HIV trans-related healthcare services, social network engagement, and establishment of community advisory boards among others [66]. The interventions of this initiative addressed many of the barriers discussed above for the HIV-infected transgender community. The outcome results of this project may give us a road map toward better understanding and caring for transgender persons along the HIV care continuum from prevention strategies to effective, sustainable interventions toward HIV control in those infected.

Screening Transgender Persons for HIV and Other STIs

As discussed previously, many of the behaviors that increase the risk of HIV infection in transgender persons also increase the risk of sexually transmitted infections (STIs) such as multiple sexual partners, condomless intercourse, sex work, mental health, and substance abuse disorders. Data on STI prevalence in the transgender population are limited. There are a number of small studies in various countries that show elevated rates [67–71]. Although all transgender persons in the US can be affected, non-White transgender individuals carry a disproportionate burden of STIs [72].

Formal guidelines for STI testing in asymptomatic transgender persons are lacking. The CDC recommends testing based on anatomy and sexual behaviors as assessed by the clinician, but does not put forth any formal recommendations for routine screening for asymptomatic STIs in transgender persons [73]. The WHO does recommend routine screening for asymptomatic STIs in transwomen and transmen who have sex with men, although the strength of these recommendations vary depending on the organism being tested and the modality used [74].

As previously discussed, transwomen, transmen who have sex with men, and MSM tend to participate in similar sexual behaviors [5, 75, 76]. Given the similarities in risk between these groups, it is reasonable to apply STI screening guidelines based on sexual practices rather than identity. As such, at least yearly screening for asymptomatic STIs should be done as follows: syphilis, HIV in those who have had more than one partner since their most recent HIV test, urethral gonorrhea and chlamydia in those who have had insertive intercourse in the prior year, rectal gonorrhea and chlamydia in those who have had receptive anal intercourse in the prior year, and pharyngeal gonorrhea and chlamydia in those who have had receptive oral intercourse in the prior year [73]. This testing is recommended regardless of condom usage. In accordance with CDC guidelines, the preferred testing modality for urethral gonorrhea and chlamydia testing is by urine nucleic acid amplification test (NAAT). For pharyngeal and rectal testing, NAAT of swab specimens from pharynx and rectal area is the test of choice [77]. Those patients who have known exposures or present with symptoms consistent with an STI should also be tested. Additionally, it is recommended to test every 3–6 months in patients with increased risk, including those who have multiple sexual partners, or who have partners with multiple sexual partners [73].

Viral hepatitis can also be transmitted via sexual behaviors. The CDC recommends one-time screening for hepatitis B in all MSM, followed by vaccination if not immune. Those tested positive should be referred to a provider who is experienced in the treatment of hepatitis B. Due to the high risk of sexually transmitted hepatitis C infection in patients with HIV infection, screening is recommended in patients who are newly diagnosed with HIV, and in those with chronic HIV infection [78]. Cost-effective screening in asymptomatic HIV positive individuals relies on two screening methods. Liver function testing (LFT) is cost-effective and recommended at least every 6 months. In areas where prevalence of hepatitis C is greater than 1.25 cases/100 person-years, LFTs should be checked every 3 months. Both should be coupled with yearly hepatitis C antibody serologies in asymptomatic patients [79]. Screening is also recommended in patients who have ever used IV drugs as this is the predominant method of transmission [80]. To our knowledge there have been no studies to date of prevalence of viral hepatitis in transgender persons but given the similarities in risk in transwomen and transmen who have sex with men as compared to MSM, we recommend following the guidelines for MSM in these groups.

The most effective means of prevention of hepatitis A and hepatitis B is immunization. Immunization for hepatitis A is recommended for MSM, people who use IV drugs, and anyone with chronic liver disease in whom there is no documentation of immunity. Hepatitis B vaccination is part of the recommended childhood vaccination schedule in the US since 1994. For those born prior to 1994, the recommendation for immunization is for high-risk populations including MSM, people who use IV drugs, and anyone with multiple sexual partners unless there is confirmed documentation of immunity. Again, given the similar risk profile in transwomen and transmen who have sex with men, we recommend immunization for hepatitis A and hepatitis B for both of these groups. Consideration for immunization should also be given for transmen who use IV drugs or have multiple sexual partners, regardless of whether or not they have sex with men [81].

In summary, while recommendations specific to transgender persons are minimal and evidence is severely limited, both worldwide and in the US, we believe that testing for HIV and other STIs remains a very important part of the primary care of transgender individuals. These groups are at high risk for acquisition of HIV and other STIs due to a high prevalence of risky sexual behaviors. All patients with signs and symptoms concerning for infection with HIV or STIs should be tested. In addition, screening for asymptomatic STIs in transwomen, transmen who have sex with men, and other transmen with identified risk factors should be performed at least yearly and more frequently in those with significantly increased risk. Screening and treatment of asymptomatic infection will lead to improvement in the health of this special population and lead to a decrease in transmission of these diseases.

HIV Prevention, Pre-exposure Prophylaxis, and Nonoccupational Post-exposure Prophylaxis in Transgender Persons

What is Pre-exposure Prophylaxis (PrEP)?

Traditionally, HIV prevention has focused on abstinence from sex, condom usage during sexual acts, needle exchange programs, and postexposure prophylaxis (PEP) following high risk exposures with antiretroviral medications, and more recently, treatment as prevention in those who are HIV infected as a means to decrease transmission. One of the newest developments in HIV prevention is the introduction of pre-exposure prophylaxis (PrEP). A co-formulation of tenofovir disoproxil fumarate (TDF) and emtricitabine (FTC) in a fixed-dose combination pill that is taken once a day by individuals at high risk of HIV infection is currently the only United States Food and Drug Administration (FDA) drug approved for PrEP. It is intended to be used in conjunction with safer sexual practices. Studies of additional drugs and formulations are currently underway, and other options for PrEP may be available in the future [82].

TDF/FTC was approved by the FDA for PrEP in 2012 based on favorable data from two large, randomized, double-blind, placebo-controlled clinical trials:

Pre-exposure prophylaxis for HIV prevention (iPrEx) and antiretroviral prophylaxis for HIV prevention in heterosexual men and women (Partners PrEP Trial) [83]. The Centers for Disease Control and Prevention (CDC) quickly endorsed the use of PrEP but stipulated that it required consistent usage. They recommended usage as part of a larger package of preventative services including risk-reduction education, access to condoms, and interventions for prevention, early diagnosis, and treatment of other STIs [84]. The CDC did not publish formal guidelines for the usage of PrEP until 2014 [85]. Early adoption was slow, but education of providers and strategic advertising has increased the number of at-risk persons on PrEP, with the goal to decrease the number of new HIV infections.

Efficacy

Large, randomized, double-blind, placebo-controlled clinical trials have proven efficacy of PrEP in MSM and serodiscordant heterosexual couples [86, 87]. While efficacy was not studied specifically in the transgender population, transwomen were included in the iPrEx trial. A 2015 subgroup analysis of this group of transwomen showed that PrEP is efficacious in transwomen if they are adherent to the daily regimen. There were a total of 339 transwomen included in the iPrEx trial. In the modified intent-to-treat analysis, there were a total of 21 seroconversions in transwomen, 11 of which were in the treatment group. Of those 11 seroconversions, however, none had detectable drug levels in plasma or peripheral blood mononuclear cells at the time of their seroconversion. Incidence of HIV infection in transwomen was 0 (95% CI not calculable) if drug was detected, as compared to 4.9/100 PY (95% CI 0-0.8) if drug was not detected [88]. The overall results from the trial showed a relative risk reduction of 92% (95% CI 70–99; $p < 0.001$) in all study participants who had detectable drug levels [86].

While evidence shows that PrEP is highly efficacious, there are concerns that individuals on PrEP may become infected with a viral strain that is resistant to one or both of the antiretroviral drugs used in PrEP. To date, there are only two documented cases of patients—both MSM—with verified medication adherence becoming infected with a strain of HIV that is at least partially resistant to both of the antiviral agents in PrEP. In both of these cases, there is evidence that each patient became infected with HIV virus with transmitted resistance mutations against both TDF and FTC [89, 90].

Barriers to Use of PrEP in Transgender Persons

The most important barriers to widespread use of PrEP in high-risk transgender persons center around awareness of PrEP, access to PrEP-related services, and challenges with adherence due to factors described in the HIV-related disparities section of this chapter. For example, fear of stigma in healthcare centers, mental illness, housing instability, distrust of healthcare services, and fear of interaction of PrEP with medications used for gender-affirming therapy [91].

While many of these disparities have been addressed previously, it is important to consider the interaction of PrEP with gender-affirming hormonal therapy. For transwomen, there is substantial concern about taking other medications that may interact with and decrease efficacy of their hormonal regimen. This may lead to a direct decrease in PrEP adherence. The subgroup analysis of transwomen in iPrEx showed a decreased likelihood to have detectable ARV drug levels in transwomen on hormones as compared to those not on hormonal therapy [88]. Furthermore, in the previously cited San Francisco survey transwomen expressed outright lack of interest in taking a PrEP regimen if it would interfere with hormonal therapy [91].

Although there are studies underway to evaluate the interactions of PrEP and gender-affirming hormonal therapy in transwomen, to date there have been no prospective studies of interactions between TDF/FTC and gender-affirming hormonal therapy in transwomen or transmen [92]. There have, however, been studies of TDF and FTC in combination with hormonal contraceptive therapy. While estrogens and progestins are extensively metabolized in the liver, TDF and FTC are prodrugs that are converted to their active forms intracellularly. They undergo minimal biotransformation via the CYP system and are primarily excreted unchanged in the urine. A 2009 study of TDF concurrently administered with norgestimate ethinyl estradiol showed no change in hormone levels while taking TDF [93]. A 2016 review of the pharmacology of PrEP in transwomen failed to identify any theoretical or experimental evidence of drug interactions between TDF/FTC and estradiol, progestins, or spironolactone; however, there is still ample room for prospective study in this area [94].

Who Should Receive PrEP?

To date, the study of PrEP has not focused on the transgender population leading to a lack of representation in the current CDC and World Health Organization (WHO) guidelines. While recognizing these limitations, it is still reasonable to extrapolate indications for use in transgender individuals based on the risk factors for HIV transmission that are shared among transwomen, MSM, and transmen who have sex with men.

The WHO recommends initiation of oral PrEP in all individuals with substantial risk of HIV infection, which they define as an incidence of greater than 3 per 100 person-years [95]. The CDC guideline is somewhat more narrow, and is based on provider assessment of risk factors for each patient in the context of HIV prevalence within their community or demographic [85]. As mentioned previously, this guideline does not specifically mention transgender persons, making it necessary for clinicians to extrapolate how to apply these guidelines to transgender persons without a large body of empiric evidence. It is reasonable to apply these guidelines to transwomen and transmen who have sex with men with consideration of the specific HIV risk factors that we have discussed earlier in this chapter.

Based on the recommendations for MSM, we propose that PrEP should be used in transmen and transwomen without acute or chronic HIV infection, who are not in a monogamous partnership with a known HIV negative partner, who have had any male sexual partner in the past 6 months, and/or who have one or more significant risk factors, which include any condomless anal sex in the past 6 months, any vaginal sex with one or more partners of unknown HIV status who are at substantial risk of HIV infection (defined as illicit drug use or a bisexual male partner), any STI diagnosis within the past 6 months, any IV drug use with sharing of injection or drug preparation equipment in the past 6 months, been in a methadone, buprenorphine, or suboxone treatment program in the past 6 months, or in an ongoing relationship with an HIV positive partner. The CDC also recommends screening for increased risk based on use of alcohol and non-injection illicit substances (alcohol use before sexual activity, amyl nitrite, stimulants, etc.) which may affect sexual risk behaviors, although they do not formally recommend PrEP use based on these risk factors alone [85].

FDA drug labeling identifies one absolute contraindication for TDF/FTC use as PrEP: unknown or positive HIV-1 status. Additionally, because of renal clearance of the drugs, patients with a calculated creatinine clearance less than 60 mL/min should not be started on PrEP. Because TDF has been associated with bone mineral density loss, any pathologic fracture or risk factors for osteoporosis and bone loss should be considered relative contraindications to PrEP [96].

How to Appropriately Prescribe PrEP in Transgender Persons

The goal of PrEP is to reduce morbidity, mortality, and cost of HIV infection by decreasing acquisition of the disease. To this end, the CDC has recommended a number of subgoals: prescribing safe and effective medication regimens, educating patients on their regimen to maximize use, provide support with medication adherence, provide HIV risk reduction and prevention services to minimize HIV exposure, and monitor for HIV infection, medication toxicities, and risk behaviors [85].

At present, there are no formal guidelines for prescribing PrEP to transgender patients. The prescribing and care of transgender PrEP patients should be comparable to the care of cisgender PrEP patients, with modifications made based on the biologic sex of the patient, their individual risk factors, and special consideration to barriers and adherence as discussed previously.

For patients who are deemed to have elevated risk for HIV infection and who would benefit from PrEP use, there are a number of steps that must be taken to identify individuals who may be harmed from initiation of PrEP. First, counseling on PrEP use and misuse should be given to clarify any misconceptions and to assess the likelihood of adherence with therapy. For transwomen and transmen on gender-affirming hormone therapy, concerns about possible interaction with PrEP drugs should be discussed [97]. Drug interactions between antiretroviral therapy and gender-affirming hormone therapy will be discussed in detail later in this chapter. After making the decision that PrEP would be appropriate and acceptable to a transgender patient, HIV testing should be performed and negative results confirmed prior to initiation of therapy. The CDC recommends a negative HIV test (preferably point of care fourth-generation antigen–antibody test) within 1 week before initiating therapy. Risk of recent HIV infection and possibility of acute HIV infection should also be assessed. Patients who have a recent potential exposure (e.g., condom breakage during sex with an HIV positive partner, condomless sex for money, injection drug use with shared equipment, etc.) may require more rigorous screening prior to initiation of PrEP, especially in the setting of nonspecific signs or symptoms of viral infection. In these patients, it is reasonable to repeat testing at a later date and/or consider performing HIV RNA testing to rule out acute HIV infection. Only after a negative HIV test has been confirmed should a 30-day prescription for TDF/FTC be provided [85, 98].

In addition to HIV testing, other baseline laboratory testing should be performed and confirmed prior to initiating therapy. Urinalysis and calculated creatinine clearance should be assessed to rule out chronic kidney disease that would make PrEP contraindicated. STI screening (gonorrhea, chlamydia, and syphilis) should be performed and infections treated given shared infection risk and increased risk of HIV transmission with active STI infection [17]. Hepatitis A, B (HBsAg, anti-HBs, anti-HBc IgG or total), and C serologies, and liver enzymes should be checked as there is risk of co-infection with these viruses. Chronic hepatitis B infection deserves special consideration as TDF and FTC are also effective against hepatitis B virus, and discontinuation of these medications in HIV-infected patients has resulted in reactivation of the disease. For those with positive hepatitis B antigen, quantitative HBV DNA should be tested and the patient should be referred to a clinician familiar with treatment of hepatitis B [99].

Following initiation of PrEP, patients should follow-up at 30 days for assessment of medication tolerability and adherence. Repeat renal function testing can be sent at this time in patients with borderline renal function at baseline. Risk-reduction counseling should also be reinforced at this visit, as well as any other patient concerns [98]. HIV testing is not necessary during this visit unless there is concern for acute HIV infection that was previously unrecognized. If all is well, a 60-day refill of PrEP can be given.

At the next follow-up, the patient should be assessed for signs and symptoms of acute HIV infection. Regardless of the presence of symptoms, HIV testing should be repeated. Again, medication tolerability and adherence should be assessed. Support should be given for medication adherence and risk-reduction behaviors [85, 98].

After the initial period, patients should return at least every 3 months for assessment of signs and symptoms of acute HIV infection and repeat HIV testing, assessment of signs or symptoms of other STIs (gonorrhea, chlamydia, and syphilis) with testing as appropriate, assessment of medication tolerability and adherence, support with medication adherence and risk-reduction counseling, and refill of PrEP prescription. In addition, calculated creatinine clearance, urinalysis, and STI testing should be performed every 6 months. Finally, need to continue PrEP for HIV prevention should be reassessed at least once a year, but can be assessed at each visit [85, 98].

Prescribing PrEP at this point, where the only option is combination of Tenofovir and Emtricitabine, does not require comprehensive knowledge of HIV medicine and can be performed by any provider with a reasonable amount of education in PrEP prescribing practices. This is important because a study of barriers to PrEP acceptability in transwomen found that adding additional appointments and medical monitoring to an already busy schedule would decrease tolerability [91]. Transwomen reported greater willingness to take PrEP if it was included in their usual transgender care [97]. This bundling of trans-related services may not only increase the willingness to take PrEP, but also increase knowledge of and access to PrEP for transgender persons by offering it in a trans-friendly environment with gender-affirming policies and procedures [100].

Appropriate Discontinuation of PrEP

In patients on PrEP, there are several important indications for discontinuation of PrEP. These include new HIV infection, calculated creatinine clearance less than 50 mL/min while on PrEP, failure to comply with HIV testing requirements, and those no longer at risk for HIV infection [85].

PrEP should be immediately discontinued for any patient who tests positive for HIV infection while on PrEP. Supplemental testing should be sent in accordance with the CDC recommended HIV testing algorithm [101]. Assessment of interruptions in therapy or adherence should be performed and documented. Consultation with a clinician experienced in HIV care should be obtained for consideration of initiation of full antiretroviral treatment with at least three antiretroviral medications. Only if supplementary testing does not confirm infection should PrEP be resumed [102].

In patients who fail to comply with HIV testing requirements, who are poorly compliant with regular follow-up, or who have ongoing poor adherence with the PrEP medication regimen, clinicians should identify and discuss barriers and possible modifications that would improve compliance with care. The risk versus benefits of continuing PrEP in the setting of poor adherence should also be discussed. Consideration should be given to discontinuing PrEP if patients continue to have poor adherence with testing and medications despite attempts at barrier modification [85, 102].

Finally, patients who are no longer at risk of HIV infection can safely discontinue PrEP. However, the subpopulation of PrEP patients who are chronically infected with hepatitis B deserves special consideration. Acute flares of hepatitis B due to reactivation have been triggered by discontinuation of TDF/FTC in patients infected with HIV. To date, there have been no reports of acute flares of hepatitis B in individuals without HIV infection who have discontinued PrEP. However, patients should be monitored by a clinician experienced in hepatitis B management so that prompt recognition and appropriate treatment can be initiated [85].

Nonoccupational Post-exposure Prophylaxis for HIV

It is possible, even likely, that transgender patients will approach their provider with concerns regarding known or possible sexual, injection drug use, or other nonoccupational exposure to HIV infection. While safe sexual practices, safe injection drug practices, and PrEP are the preferred methods of risk reduction for HIV acquisition, postexposure prophylaxis for HIV (PEP) is a viable option to reduce the risk of HIV infection in the appropriate setting.

Postexposure prophylaxis for HIV has been used for years but due to ethical considerations has never been studied in prospective randomized controlled clinical trials. PEP is divided into occupational and nonoccupational uses. Occupational PEP (oPEP) is defined as the practice of providing antiretroviral therapy (ART) to healthcare workers who sustain exposure to blood or body fluids from a known HIV-infected patient to reduce the risk of infection. Nonoccupational PEP (nPEP) is defined as the practice of providing ART after exposure to blood, genital secretions, and other body fluids that might contain HIV to reduce the likelihood of infection [103].

A 1997 case–control study of the use of single drug oPEP with the drug zidovudine represents the best efficacy data for the use of PEP. That study showed an 81% reduction in the odds of HIV transmission among healthcare workers with percutaneous exposure to HIV (95% CI = 48–97%) [104]. Formal 2005 CDC guidelines for the use of oPEP are available and should be referred to in the event of HIV exposure in the healthcare setting [105]. The quality of evidence for nPEP is poor and relies almost entirely on observational and case studies. Despite the limited data for use of nPEP, the CDC produced 2005 guidelines for its use and released an update in 2016, which is the basis of our discussion here [106].

Determining the appropriateness of use of nPEP is based primarily on three factors: demonstrated HIV negative status of the exposed individual, risk of HIV acquisition, and time since exposure. PEP is indicated only for HIV-uninfected people, and it is possible that the potentially exposed person may have undiagnosed HIV infection. As such, all potentially exposed individuals should be screened for HIV infection with a rapid third-generation Ab or fourth-generation Ag/Ab test within 1 hour if available. In the event that results of HIV testing are unavailable during the initial evaluation, it is reasonable to assume HIV negative status pending results of the test so as not to delay initiation of therapy. If results are subsequently positive for HIV infection, PEP should be discontinued [106]. Patients should then be referred to an experienced HIV provider for initiation of ART. When screening for HIV during the initial evaluation, patient should also be screened for other STIs including gonorrhea, chlamydia, and syphilis, which should be treated if infection is present [107]. Other testing at the initial evaluation should include CBC, BUN, creatinine, LFTs, and pregnancy test if applicable.

For patients who are confirmed to be HIV negative—or those with pending results—it is important to assess the risk of HIV acquisition based on the type of exposure. Nonoccupational PEP is indicated for high risk exposures. High risk exposures are defined as exposure of vagina, rectum, eye, mouth, other mucosal membranes, non-intact skin, or percutaneous contact to blood, semen, vaginal secretions, rectal secretions, breast milk, or body fluid visibly contaminated with blood. Conversely, there is negligible risk of HIV transmission through exposure of the prior mentioned sites to urine, nasal secretions, saliva, sweat, or tears unless visibly contaminated with blood, and nPEP is not recommended for these low exposures [106]. Although not part of the CDC recommendations, the New York State Department of Health defines an intermediate risk exposure group and recommends case-by-case evaluation. This group is defined as oral–vaginal, oral–rectal, and both receptive and insertive penile–oral contact with or without ejaculation. nPEP is not necessary in this group unless additional risk factors are present, such as know high HIV viral load in the source patient, oral mucosa that is not intact, blood exposure, or presence of genital ulcerative disease or other STI. Patients can be safely counseled that nPEP is not necessary for exposures from kissing, oral–oral contact without mucosal damage, human bites without blood, exposure to solid bore needles, and mutual masturbation without skin breakdown or blood exposure [107].

Animal models demonstrate that efficacy of PEP is time dependent. PEP is less effective the longer the amount of time that has elapsed since exposure to HIV, and is unlikely to be effective if initiated more than 72 h following exposure [108]. For this reason, during the initial evaluation, it is important to verify a time line of potential exposure, and to counsel patients on the diminishing returns of therapy when significant time has passed since exposure.

Nonoccupational PEP can be initiated in individuals who are determined or assumed to be HIV negative pending test results, who have experienced a high risk exposure, and who have been exposed within the previous 72 h. For those in whom nPEP is indicated, counseling regarding medication side effects, duration of therapy, and importance of adherence should be provided. The preferred regimen for nPEP with a calculated creatinine clearance greater than 60 is a three-drug regimen containing fixed-dose combination TDF/FTC 300–200 mg with either raltegravir 400 mg twice a day or dolutegravir 50 mg once daily. For those patients with a calculated creatinine clearance less than 60, TDF/FTC can be replaced with zidovudine and lamivudine with doses adjusted based on creatinine clearance. Raltegravir and dolutegravir do not require adjustment for level of renal function. Duration of therapy with either regimen for nPEP is 28 days [106]. Regardless of whether or not nPEP is indicated, patients should be counseled on HIV risk-reduction behaviors. They should also be referred to a provider experienced in HIV care for follow-up.

Nonoccupational PEP necessitates close follow-up for assessment of medication adherence and toxicities. Patients should be reevaluated in 3 days, either in person or by phone and then weekly while taking nPEP. Repeat serum liver enzymes, BUN, creatinine, and CBC should be checked at weeks 2 and 4. HIV testing should be repeated on week 4. If HIV testing remains negative at 4 weeks, patients can return at week 12 for final HIV testing [107]. If negative at week 4, it is reasonable to consider initiation of PrEP in patients who are eligible based on the previously described criteria. Patients who refuse PrEP or in whom PrEP is not indicated, can be discharged from care if week 12 HIV testing is negative.

Summary

In summary, PrEP is a safe, effective method of HIV prevention that has the potential to decrease the blight of HIV in at-risk transgender persons. While it has not been extensively studied in the trans-population, subgroup analysis from studies that included trans as part of other groups shows benefit in transwomen and transmen who have sex with men. Limited studies show that while knowledge of PrEP in the trans-population is low, when educated on its benefits there is significant interest as well as high acceptability. While further study of PrEP in the trans-population is warranted, incorporation into regular transgender care—including education on the lack of interaction between PrEP and gender-affirming hormone therapy—would likely increase acceptability of and adherence to the regimen by bypassing barriers to care in this unique population. For those patients not receiving PrEP who experience a known HIV exposure, nPEP is a viable option to reduce the risk of HIV acquisition.

Approach to New HIV Infection in Transgender Persons

Due to the high prevalence of HIV in the transgender population, it is important that clinicians who treat transgender persons be aware of the natural history of HIV and methods of diagnosis. It is also vital that clinicians are aware of appropriate counseling and linkage to care with an experienced HIV practitioner. Furthermore, clinicians should have a high suspicion for acute HIV infection for patients who present with history of risk behaviors or known exposure and symptoms of the acute retroviral syndrome.

Natural History and Methods of Diagnosis of HIV Infection

The natural history of HIV infection is inoculation followed by an acute retroviral syndrome that can be mild and disregarded by the recently infected person or severe enough to lead to seeking medical care in some. What follows if undiagnosed is a chronic, relatively asymptomatic period during which CD4+ T cells are depleted that finally culminates in symptomatic severe immunodeficiency. This final stage of infection is known as the acquired immune deficiency syndrome (AIDS). The estimated mean time of progression from infection to AIDS without treatment is approximately 11 years [109].

The natural history of the disease informs laboratory testing algorithms for HIV infection. Following infection, there is an "eclipse" period lasting approximately 7–10 days in which virus is undetectable in blood [110]. After this period, PCR for viral RNA becomes positive. At approximately 14 days there is sufficient circulating viral p24 antigen to be detected by currently available fourth-generation immunoassays. Detectable levels of antibodies to the virus appear only after 20–45 days [111]. The delay between infection and detectability is called the "window period," in which HIV antibody testing may be falsely negative.

The most recent recommendations from the CDC favor screening for HIV with a highly sensitive and specific fourth-generation immunoassay that tests for the presence of p24 antigen in addition to HIV-1/2 antibodies. It is also acceptable to use a third-generation HIV-1/2 antibody immunoassay if the fourth-generation test is not available; however, clinicians should be aware that there is a longer window period—up to 3 months—with this test owing to the lack of testing for the p24 antigen [112].

Patients may also present with signs and symptoms consistent with the acute retroviral syndrome. The symptoms are nonspecific, present in 50–90% of acutely infected individuals and may include one or more of the following: fever, malaise, lymphadenopathy, rash, headache, arthralgias, and myalgias. Atypical findings (encephalitis, nerve palsies, chest pain, acute renal insufficiency, pancytopenia, etc.) may also be present alone or as part of a syndrome [113]. Patients with high risk behaviors or known exposure, who present with any of these symptoms, should be suspected of acute HIV infection. In those suspected of acute HIV infection, testing with fourth-generation antigen/antibody testing should be performed promptly. A negative fourth-generation test in this setting should be followed by virologic testing for HIV RNA. Alternatively, it is reasonable to test with a third-generation antibody test with concurrent HIV RNA testing [112].

Following a positive result on a screening test, patients should be informed that they have a preliminary positive result, and confirmatory testing should be sent to a certified laboratory. Confirmatory testing consists of an HIV-1/2 differentiation immunoassay, Western blot, or indirect immunofluorescence assay. It is important to be aware that the fourth-generation antigen/antibody testing can be positive earlier than the confirmatory testing in some patients with acute infection. In the setting of a positive antigen/antibody test and negative confirmatory test, HIV RNA testing should be sent to verify the presence or absence of HIV infection [112].

HIV Diagnosis Counseling in Transgender Persons

Though the stigma surrounding HIV-infected individuals has declined over time, there remains considerable stigma attached to HIV infection, because of the history of HIV and the AIDS crisis. In the case of transgender patients, this stigma is even stronger, and a new diagnosis often places significant stress on patients. Following a positive test result, all patients must be provided with the result of their test. They should also be provided with appropriate diagnosis counseling to address specific concerns regarding the diagnosis as well as emotional and social support. Patients should be counseled regarding the consequences of a positive test, what discrimination they may face, and what resources are available for support [114]. This is of particular importance in transgender persons because they already face significant stigma as a result of their gender identity [10]. In addition, they should be informed of the reportable nature of the disease and the need for both retrospective and prospective partner notifications.

In addition to psychosocial counseling, patients with a new diagnosis should be counseled regarding the medical implications of the diagnosis and their need for establishment of ongoing care. As previously described, there are numerous factors (fear of discrimination, lack of financial means, homelessness, etc.) that lead to decreased access to medical care or low willingness to use the healthcare system among the transgender population. Patients should be counseled on the chronic and treatable nature of HIV if they remain in care [112]. Patients should also be counseled on methods to prevent/reduce disease transmission, including abstinence and correct, consistent condom use. Finally, it is of the utmost importance to link newly diagnosed patients to a provider experienced in HIV care for initiation of antiretroviral therapy.

Partner Notification in Transgender Persons

Partner notification is vital to link potentially exposed or infected partners to testing resources and treatment to prevent further spread of infection. Patients should be encouraged to notify sexual partners regarding their diagnosis. This also applies to any partners with whom they have shared needles or injection equipment, either for injectable drugs or hormone injections [112, 114]. The area of partner notification for HIV in transgender persons has not been rigorously studied.

Theoretically, the fear of being replaced by an alternate partner, loss of housing, and the high prevalence of sex work that we have discussed in prior sections may create barriers to willingness to notify partners. A study of both transwomen and

MSM in Lima, Peru showed that only 52.5% of persons with either HIV or other STI infection would notify their partner. Likeliness to notify was higher in stable partners, but lower in casual and commercial partners. In qualitative analysis of the study, the examiners found that likeliness to notify partners of HIV infection was lower in all groups. The reported reasons were fears of interpersonal violence, social exclusion, and societal stigma [115]. This area is deserving of further study, given the high prevalence of HIV in this population.

We recommend encouraging patients to disclose their diagnosis with any sexual partners who may have been exposed. As part of that process, we recommend psychosocial assessment to determine if there are any barriers to or risks of partner notification for individual patients. Assessment should include screening for housing status, domestic abuse, sex work, and number of both stable and casual or commercial partners. Any identified barriers should also be intervened upon as necessary as they may also be associated with a decreased likelihood to enter into regular medical care. In the event that a patient is unwilling to notify their partner, information should be forwarded to a local partner notification service, if available, for confidential notification and linkage to testing. Furthermore, any partners who may have been exposed in the prior 72 h should be considered for postexposure prophylaxis [112]. Assessment of need for and providing nonoccupational post-exposure prophylaxis for HIV has been discussed previously in this chapter.

Referral to an Experienced HIV Provider

As previously stated, it is of paramount importance that patients newly diagnosed with HIV infection are referred to an experienced HIV provider. HIV medicine remains a quickly evolving field and the medications used in management are numerous, complex, and frequently have interactions with other medications. As such, it is outside the scope of a practitioner to manage HIV without appropriate credentials and expertise, or without the assistance of an experienced HIV provider. We recommend that clinicians find and maintain a network of local HIV providers and HIV resources.

There are numerous barriers to HIV care for transgender persons including number of medical appointments, negative healthcare experiences related to stigma, and concern for drug–drug interactions with a prioritization for gender-affirming therapies over HIV treatment, which will be described in upcoming sections. When possible, HIV care should be coupled with transgender care to circumvent these obstacles. Centers that are able should utilize an on-site HIV provider for co-management of HIV and transgender care [116]. While there are no prospective trials, an on-site comprehensive care approach may increase adherence with follow-up and treatment, while simultaneously increasing tolerability for patients. When it is not feasible to have an HIV provider on-site, it is important to use other methods to keep an open dialog between transgender persons and HIV providers to address patient concerns including any conflicts in treatment plans.

In the US, the American Academy of HIV Medicine credentials providers, and maintains a directory of certified HIV providers which can be found at https://providers.aahivm.org/referral-link-search?reload=timezone.

HIV Cascade of Care for Transgender

The HIV care continuum or cascade of care describes the number of people who are living with HIV at each stage of care, starting from all infected persons and moving toward those who are diagnosed, linked to care, and achieve viral suppression. This model for HIV care was developed in order to monitor the progress of testing, linkage, and treatment of HIV [117]. As of 2016, the World Health Organization (WHO) estimates that there are over 36.7 million individuals living with HIV worldwide, yet only 25.5 million are aware of their diagnosis. Of those who are diagnosed with HIV, only 19.5 million are on ART, with approximately 16 million achieving viral suppression [118]. In 2013, the WHO set a goal to diagnose 90% of HIV-infected persons, treat 90% of those diagnosed, and achieve viral suppression in 90% of those treated by the year 2020. This is referred to as "90-90-90." Figure 13.2 shows the estimated number of people at each level of HIV care continuum in 2016, with the area in red representing the remaining population needed to reach the 90-90-90 goal.

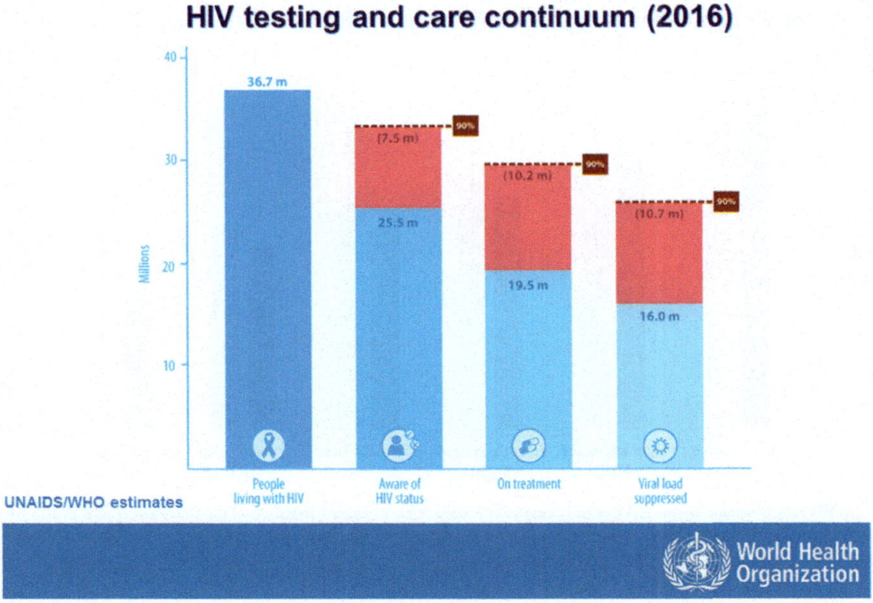

Fig. 13.2 The global estimate for the HIV cascade of care according to the World Health Organization [118]

While there is evidence that HIV greatly impacts the transgender community, the cascade of care for the transgender community is not clearly understood on a global level. The reason for this gap in knowledge is possibly due to lack of a systematic method to record and share information on gender identity in most health systems. For example, often times, transwomen are grouped together with MSM making it even more difficult to interpret the disaggregated data [119]. Thus, the care continuum among the transgender community may be underreported. To date, there have been small region-specific studies analyzing the HIV care continuum among transgender communities in Rio de Janeiro, Brazil and San Francisco, United States of America.

Jalil et al. studied a sample of 345 transwomen living in Rio de Janeiro, Brazil from 2015 to 2016. Of the 345 transwomen, 141 had HIV (40.9%), with 77.5% of HIV-infected individuals aware of their diagnosis. Approximately 62.2% of individuals were on antiretroviral therapy (ART), with only 35.4% achieving viral suppression (Fig. 13.3) [119]. A second study was conducted among 314 transwomen living in San Francisco in 2010, with a HIV prevalence of 39%. Of those who were HIV positive, 77% were linked to care, yet only 65% were on ART, of which 44% achieved viral suppression [45].

These studies, although scant, help fill in some of the gaps in understanding the true global cascade of care among the transgender community. These findings show evidence that there is a high prevalence of HIV in the transgender community, with modest use of ART, and lower than desired rates of virologic suppression. These findings emphasize the need to implement policies aimed at improving access to testing, linkage to care, and providing services to ensure retention in care among the transgender population [45, 118–120]. More studies are needed both globally and in

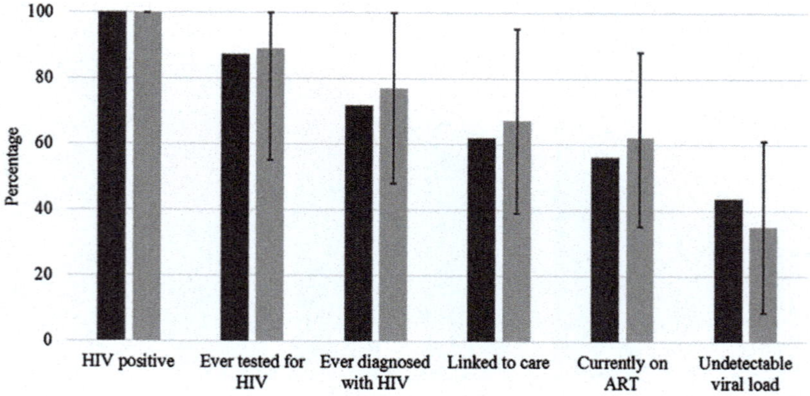

The HIV care continuum among HIV-positive transgender women in Rio de Janeiro, Brazil ($N = 141$). Crude percentages in dark grey, respondent-driven sampling weighted population estimates in light grey, error bars represent 95% confidence intervals for population estimates.

* $N = 138$ for denominator with undetectable viral load due to missing data.

Fig. 13.3 The HIV cascade of care among transwomen in Rio de Janeiro, Brazil, as adopted from Jalil et al. [119]

the United States to shed light on the epidemiologic characteristics of HIV infection in transgender people.

Choice of Antiretroviral Therapy in Transgender Persons

Goals of Therapy

The goals of antiretroviral therapy (ART) have evolved over the course of the past three decades. In 1987, the United States Food and Drug Administration (FDA) approved the first antiretroviral drug, zidovudine (AZT), a nucleoside reverse-transcriptase inhibitor (NRTI). The use of one medication, however, was not effective at maintaining viral suppression and led to resistance [121]. Over the years that followed, more medications were approved by the FDA, with the introduction of protease inhibitors (PIs) in 1995. By 1997, effective combination therapy to achieve sustained virologic suppression with NRTIs and PIs became the standard of care [122–124]. To date, there are now over 30 drugs approved for use in HIV treatment [125].

Over the decades since the availability of effective antiretroviral therapies, the pendulum has moved frequently on the appropriate timing for the initiation of therapy. Previously, CD4-guided treatment was the standard of care for the initiation of therapy, based on CD4 counts of 200 or 350 [126, 127]. Currently, the most updated recommendation is treatment for all HIV-infected individuals, regardless of CD4 count. This recommendation is based on two major studies, the Strategic Timing of Antiretroviral Therapy (START) as well as the Strategies for Management of Antiretroviral Therapy (SMART). In the START trial, a multi-continental study, 4685 HIV positive adults with a CD4 count >500 were randomized to start therapy immediately or to defer until CD4 count <350. The primary endpoints were AIDS-related events, non-AIDS-related events, or death from any cause. The primary endpoints occurred in 42 individuals in the immediate imitations group, in contrast to 96 patients in the deferred-initiation group, with a hazard ratio of 0.43. The conclusion of this study was that the initiation of ART regardless of CD4 count provided a net benefit as compared to deferring treatment to a certain CD4 count [128].

Antiretroviral therapy has revolutionized the care of all HIV-infected individuals, with the main goal of suppressing HIV RNA to undetectable levels in order to enhance the immune function of infected individuals and prevent the clinical progression of HIV disease [129]. By suppressing viral load and increasing CD4 count, ART decreases the morbidity and mortality associated with HIV, as well as decreases the risk of transmission of HIV [130]. In addition to reducing opportunistic infections, the SMART trial proved that ART decreases the incidence of death secondary to HIV-related comorbid conditions [131]. In the SMART trial, 5472 participants were randomly assigned to receive ART regardless of CD4 count or to defer therapy until CD4 count was <250. This study concluded that immediate ART decreased the risk of opportunistic disease, and death from any cause including cardiovascular, renal, and hepatic disease. Further studies have also shown that the introduction of ART has also reduced the incidence of infection-related cancers, such as Kaposi sarcoma and lymphoma [128, 132]. There have also been studies that have shown that ART decreases the risk of non-AIDS defining malignancies, such as liver, breast, colorectal, and lung cancer [133].

Multiple clinical studies have made evident these life-sustaining goals of ART. Walensky et al. examined how treatment has influenced survival benefits. Through the use of national surveillance data, efficacy data, and probability models, it was concluded that as of 2006 ART has saved at least 3 million years of life in the United States [134]. In 2010, the HIV Cohorts Analyzed Using Structural Approaches to Longitudinal data (HIV-CASUAL) Collaboration Study included 62,760 HIV-infected individuals from five European countries [135]. During the follow-up period of 3 years, there were approximately 2039 deaths. When comparing individuals on therapy to those who were not, it was demonstrated that ART halved the mortality rate of HIV positive patients [135].

Based on these landmark studies, ART is recommended for all individuals living with HIV, regardless of gender identity, sexual orientation, age, and race. These life-sustaining goals are universal and apply to transgender persons as well.

Treatment as Prevention

In addition to improving the health of infected individuals, another major benefit of ART is that it plays a major role in the prevention of HIV transmission. The lower the concentration of the HIV virus in an individual's blood and genital secretions, the decreased is the likelihood of transmission to others, including sexual partners, intravenous (IV) drug users sharing needles, and mother to child transmission during pregnancy and breastfeeding [136].

The results from the 2011 HIV Prevention Trials Network (HPTN052) confirmed the notion that treatment can be used to prevent transmission of HIV. This study was conducted in nine countries and included 1763 discordant couples, in which one partner was HIV positive and the other partner was seronegative. A large majority of the individuals in the study were heterosexual, with CD4 counts ranging from 350 to 550. The partners who were HIV positive were randomly assigned to receive ART immediately or to wait until the CD4 count declined to 250. The final analysis revealed 39 cases of HIV transmission, with 28 cases being linked to the infected partner, with only one occurring in the early-therapy group. This study provided evidence that early initiation of ART reduced the risk of transmission to seronegative partner by 96% [137]. This landmark study promoted the universal importance of treatment as a means of prevention.

There have, however, been very limited studies that have analyzed the effect of treatment as a means of HIV prevention in the transgender community. Historically, it has been difficult to engage the transgender community in clinical trials and research, due to barriers we have previously described [138]. More studies are needed in order to better target transgender-specific interventions in the goal of treatment as prevention.

Preferred ARV Regimen in Transgender Persons

The choice of antiretroviral therapy for transgender individuals does not differ from non-transgender individuals, as long as consideration is given to drug–drug interaction for those concomitantly on hormone or other gender-affirming therapy. Below, we discuss first-line recommendations for preferred therapy and later discuss considerations regarding hormone therapy.

The HIV life cycle can be categorized into seven separate steps: (1) binding, (2) fusion, (3) reverse transcription, (4) integration, (5) replication, transcription, and translation, (6) assembly, and (7) budding and maturation. There are currently six classes of antiviral medications, each with different mechanisms of action directed to inhibit the HIV life cycle. When drugs from different groups are combined, the HIV virus can be disrupted at multiple stages of replication, as seen in Fig. 13.4 [139].

Chemokine receptor inhibitors (CCR5) such as maraviroc inhibit the binding or attachment of the HIV virus to the cell. Fusion or entry inhibitors (EI), such as enfuvirtide (T-20) inhibit the fusion of the HIV envelope and CD4 membrane and thus prevent HIV from entering the cell. Nucleoside reverse-transcriptase inhibitors (NRTIs) act as competitive substrate inhibitors of reverse transcriptase, with examples including zidovudine (AZT), emtricitabine (FTC), lamivudine (3TC), and abacavir (ABC). Nucleotide reverse-transcriptase inhibitors also act as competitive inhibitors of reverse transcriptase, with tenofovir disoproxil fumarate (TDF), and tenofovir alafenamide (TAF) being the most commonly prescribed drugs. Non-nucleoside reverse-transcriptase inhibitors (NNRTIs) act as noncompetitive inhibitors of reverse transcriptase. This class of medication can be classified as first-generation drugs, which include nevirapine (NVP) and efavirenz (EFV), and second-generation drugs, which include etravirine (ETR) and rilpivirine (RPV) [140]. Integrase nuclear strand transfer inhibitors (INSTIs) inhibit the enzyme integrase, blocking the insertion of viral DNA into the DNA of the host CD4 cell. Examples include elvitegravir (EVG) and dolutegravir (DTG). Protease inhibitors (PIs) competitively inhibit the cleavage of the Gag-Pol polyproteins in HIV-infected cells, which inhibit the maturation and budding of the virus. Example of PIs includes darunavir (DRV) and atazanavir (ATV) [141].

Since the advent of AZT in 1987, there have been multiple studies to assess the most appropriate drug regimen to suppress HIV viral load. Clinical studies have proven that monotherapy is associated with high rates of virological failure, and is thus not recommended [121, 142]. In 1997, in a double-blinded study, 97 HIV-infected individuals were randomized to receive monotherapy, dual therapy, or

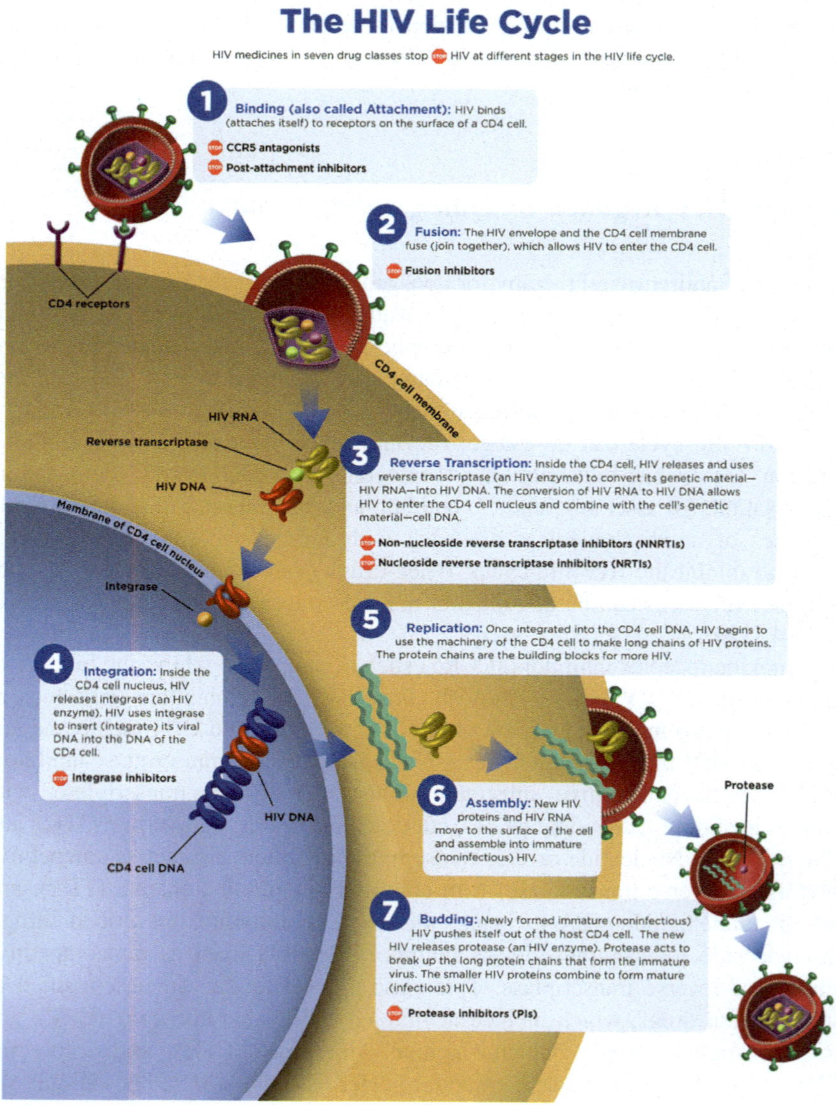

Fig. 13.4 The HIV life cycle and the targets for the six classes of drugs [139]

triple therapy. The three-drug group experienced the greatest decline in viral load over the longest period of time. Since this landmark study, the preferred recommendation for ART includes the combination of three or more ARV drugs from two classes [124]. As of 2016, the World Health Organization (WHO) recommends starting two NRTIs plus a NNRTI or an INSTI [143]. The 2016 International Antiviral Society-USA (IAS-USA) and the 2017 U.S Department of Health and

Human Services (USDHHS) guidelines recommend integrase-based regimens as initial therapy for most people with HIV. Under certain clinical situations, alternative regimens such as combinations of NRTIs with a boosted PI or a NNRTI may be more appropriate [144, 145].

The global recommendation for ART may vary depending on cost, availability of medications, and an individual's comorbidities [146]. The exact timing of medication initiation has also been debated throughout the years. As described earlier, according to all three guidelines published by US DDHS, IAS-USA, and WHO, presently it is recommended to start ART as soon as possible after diagnosis, regardless of CD4 count [147]. Acknowledging the guidelines and multiple studies that have proven that early initiation of ART improves short- and long-term outcomes and decreases morbidities and mortalities due to HIV infection, we need to point out that there are many other factors that may delay the initiation of ART like availability, affordability, some acute illnesses, and patient acceptance, to name a few.

Interactions with Hormonal Therapies

Both ART and hormone therapy (HT) can improve the quality of life for transgender persons, yet drug–drug interactions need to be assessed and taken into account before drugs are prescribed. Studies have reported HT use in anywhere from 27 to 93% of transwomen [146]. Studies have also shown that up to 40% of transwomen were not taking ART because of concerns regarding drug interactions with HT [33]. Thus, it is imperative for both providers and patients to discuss drug–drug interactions and any concerns and barriers patients may have to treatment.

Masculinizing hormone therapy consists of testosterone, which is available in oral (testosterone undecanoate), parenteral (testosterone enanthate or cypionate or undecanoate), and transdermal forms (gel or patch). Testosterone is metabolized in the liver by glucuronosyltransferases and sulfotransferases [148]. Testosterone has been used safely with ART with no reported drug interactions. This evidence is based on studies in which testosterone, prescribed for reasons such as hypogonadism and erectile dysfunction, was used concomitantly with ART without any evidence of drug interactions [149–151].

Feminizing hormone therapy consists of three classes of medications: estrogen, antiandrogens, and gonadotropin-releasing hormone (GnRH) agonists. Estrogen is available in oral (17 beta-estradiol valerate), transdermal (estradiol patch), and parenteral routes (estradiol valerate, estradiol cypionate). Antiandrogen, examples including spironolactone, finasteride, and cyproterone acetate, acts as competitive inhibitor of the androgen receptor and inhibit testicular steroidogenesis. GnRH agonists inhibit gonadotropin secretion and suppress testicular testosterone production, and include leuprolide and goserelin [152].

To date, we are not aware of any clinical studies examining the interaction of feminizing hormone therapy in transgender persons and antiretroviral therapy.

There have been many studies, however, that have analyzed the interactions of oral contraceptives containing estrogen and progesterone with ART. These studies can be extrapolated to understand the potential interactions between feminizing hormone therapy and ART. It is important to use caution when applying these studies to transgender women, who would have to take estrogen doses 3–4 times that of what is recommended for contraceptive purposes [153].

When discussing drug interactions, it is important to understand how each drug is metabolized. Estradiol is metabolized via hydroxylation into catechol estrogens through the cytochrome P450 enzymes and is a P-glycoprotein/ABCB1 substrate. In the liver, estradiol is metabolized into 2-hydroxyestradiol by CYP1A2, CYP3A4, and CYP2CP and also metabolized into estrone by CYP2CP, CYP2C19, and CYP2C8 via 17β-hydroxy dehydrogenation [154]. Thus, any medication that may affect the aforementioned cytochrome enzymes can result in a drug interaction.

Ritonavir and cobicistat are strong inhibitors of cytochrome P450 enzymes, especially CYP3A4, and due to this property are used rather commonly as a booster of other ART, mostly PIs and some integrase inhibitors. Due to the same CYP inhibitory properties, these boosters may increase the levels of estradiol when used concomitantly [146, 153]. On the other hand, some NNRTIs can induce the CYP3A4 system. Thus, the levels of estradiol, a CYP3A4 substrate, may be decreased when combined with these NNRTIs [153]. Thus, for the transgender person who is prescribed these medications as part of their ART, hormone levels need to be monitored and adjusted accordingly. Table 13.1 is adapted from a comprehensive literature review by Radix et al. published in 2016 and summarizes the interaction of most currently available ART with ethinyl estradiol which is the most commonly used estrogen in oral contraceptives.

NRTIs do not impact the cytochrome P450 system. They are converted intracellularly by hydrolysis through non-CYP enzymes. Thus, this class of medications is not expected to have any effect on the metabolism of hormonal therapy or hormone levels. Clinical studies have confirmed this and to date, no clinically significant drug interactions have been reported between currently used NRTIs and hormonal therapy [94]. Further studies have identified that zidovudine combined with contraceptive therapy has no effect on CD4 count and viral load [155]. No interactions have been noted between estradiol and the chemokine receptor inhibitors such as maraviroc [153]. INSTIs, such as raltegravir and dolutegravir, are also substrates of BCRP/ABCG2 enzymes. There have also been no described drug interactions with this class of medication and estradiol.

In some instances, estradiol may impact ART level with potential to cause virologic failure. There are some studies that point to decrease efficacy of amprenavir, unboosted fosamprenavir, and stavudine when used with ethinyl estradiol [146, 156]. These medications are not part of preferred ART regimen anymore and their use in the US and worldwide are limited. Considering the possible interaction outlined above, their concomitant use with feminizing hormones should be discouraged.

Conjugated equine estrogens are not recommended for feminizing hormone therapy because of the toxicities associated with its use, including thrombogenicity

Table 13.1 Interactions between antiretroviral therapy and ethinyl estradiol

Effect on ethinyl estradiol levels (AUC)	Antiretroviral	Change
Increase	Atazanavir [72]	AUC ↑ 48%
	Etravirine [89]	AUC ↑ 22%
	Fosamprenavir [72]	Cmin ↑ 32%
	Rilpivirine [72, 90]	AUC ↑ 0–14%, Cmax ↑ 17%
Decrease	Atazanavir/ritonavir [72, 84]	AUC ↓ 19%, Cmax ↓ 16% and Cmin ↓ 37%
	Darunavir/ritonavir [86]	AUC ↓ 44%, Cmin ↓ 62%, Cmax ↓ 32%
	Fosamprenavir/ritonavir [84]	AUC ↓ 37%, 28% ↓ Cmax and 34%
	Lopinavir/ritonavir [72, 87]	AUC ↓ 42%, Cmax ↓ 41% ↓ 58%
	Nevirapine [72, 88]	AUC ↓ 29%
	EVG/c/TDF/FTC [72]	AUC ↓ 25%, Cmin ↓ 44%
	Tipranavir/ritonavir [72]	AUC ↓ 37–48%
No effect	Dolutegravir [72, 97]	
	Efavirenz [94]	
	Maraviroc [91]	
	Raltegravir [72, 92]	
	Tenofovir [94]	
	Zidovudine [95]	
No data	Abacavir	
	Atazanavir/cobicistat	
	Darunavir/cobicistat	

Adapted from a literature review by Radix et al. JIAS 2016 [146]

and cardiovascular risk [157]. Yet, this class of medication has been used in the past for feminizing hormone therapy and there are cases in which it still may be used. Thus, understanding any drug interactions with ART is imperative. Conjugated equine estrogen is an inhibitor of CYP1A2 and a major substrate of CYP3A4. Conjugated estrogen can interact with NNRTIs, which are CYP3A4 inducers. Thus, NNRTIs may decrease the concentration of the conjugated estrogen. There are no reported drug interactions between this class of medications and boosted or non-boosted PIs, entry inhibitors, or NRTIs [158].

Antiandrogens, such as spironolactone, undergo extensive hepatic metabolism including deacetylation by esterases followed by glucuronidation [94]. There are no known drug interactions between antiandrogens and boosted or non-boosted PIs, NRTIs, NNRTIs, or INSTIs. The metabolism and transport effects of GnRH are unknown. GnRH agonists are known to be QTc-prolonging agents, and this therapy needs to be monitored when combined with ritonavir and NNRTIs, another QTc-prolonging agent.

To summarize, it is important to note that antiretroviral therapy is not a contraindication for hormone therapy. Masculinizing hormone therapy can safely be combined with ART. Combination of some feminizing hormone therapy with some antiretroviral agents, however, requires close follow-up, as estradiol may interact with boosted PIs and NNRTIs. QTc needs to also be monitored when GnRH agonists are combined with boosted PIs and NNRTIs. It is encouraging to point out that to date there is no evidence of drug interaction between available unboosted integrase inhibitors (raltegravir, dolutegravir, and bictegravir) and gender-affirming medications. Considering that integrase-based regimens for treating HIV infection are currently preferred in most cases, it may be reasonable to use integrase-inhibitor-based therapy as a first choice, when possible, for transgender persons who are also on hormone therapy. Hormone therapy is best provided in the context of HIV care. Providers should use treatment with hormones as a means to discuss antiretroviral therapy and link patients to care [146].

Adherence

Importance of Adherence and Development of Resistance

Medication adherence is of utmost importance for viral suppression. Lack of medication adherence is directly linked to the development of drug resistance. Skipping medications allows the virus to multiply and increases the risk of viral mutations leading to drug resistance. Mutated virus may not be inhibited by ART, and will continue to replicate despite therapy. This in turn leads to treatment failure. Drug-resistant HIV can be spread to other people, and thus infected individuals may have drug resistance before even starting ART [159].

Multiple studies have shown that transgender women have lower adherence to medication compared to non-transgender males and non-transgender females [160]. Baguso et al. analyzed 295 individuals living with HIV in San Francisco. The study concluded that 72.4% of cisgender men and 23.1% of cisgender women achieved viral suppression, compared to only 4.5% of transgender women [161]. The conclusions from this study are also in agreement with Wiewel et al. who compared adherence among transgender persons compared with MSM in New York City from 2006 to 2011. Transgender women were likely to be linked to care, but less likely to adhere to medication and achieve viral suppression as compared to MSM [162].

There are many barriers to engage and retain HIV-infected transgender persons in care, which may explain the lower level of adherence to ART. These barriers and health disparities were discussed in earlier sections.

Conclusion

As we have shown throughout this chapter, prevalence of HIV is significantly increased in the transgender community as compared to both the general population and MSM. This is particularly true in transwomen and transmen who have sex with men. In addition, transgender persons suffer from the intersection of multiple socioeconomic, psychosocial, and behavioral disparities including transphobia in health care, which lead to poor performance at all levels of HIV cascade of care. It is important that providers who care for transgender patients be aware of the prevalence of HIV, risk factors for acquisition of HIV infection, and the barriers that these individuals face in obtaining and remaining in care. Additionally, providers must be aware of the options for HIV prevention, including the use of PrEP in high risk individuals. Finally, it is important to reiterate the greater acceptability of obtaining HIV care commensurately with transgender care, and the ability to improve outcomes when care is obtained together. With improved recognition of the barriers that transgender patients face, increased preventative services based on risk factors, and systematic improvement in the manner in which HIV and transgender care is delivered, it should be possible to reduce the prevalence of HIV in the transgender community and improve the HIV-related health outcomes of this at-risk population.

References

1. UNAIDS. Global factsheet. 2016. http://aidsinfo.unaids.org/. Accessed Feb 2018.
2. CDC. HIV surveillance. 2018. https://www.cdc.gov/hiv/library/reports/hiv-surveillance.html/.
3. Reisner SL, Murchison GR. A global research synthesis of HIV and STI biobehavioural risks in female-to-male transgender adults. Glob Public Health. 2016;11(7–8):866–87.
4. Clark H, Babu AS, Wiewel EW, Opoku J, Crepaz N. Diagnosed HIV infection in transgender adults and adolescents: results from the national HIV surveillance system, 2009–2014. AIDS Behav. 2017;21(9):2774–83.
5. Herbst JH, Jacobs ED, Finlayson TJ, et al. Estimating HIV prevalence and risk behaviors of transgender persons in the United States: a systematic review. AIDS Behav. 2008;12(1):1–17.
6. Beyrer C, Baral SD, van Griensven F, et al. Global epidemiology of HIV infection in men who have sex with men. Lancet. 2012;380(9839):367–77.
7. Poteat T, Scheim A, Xavier J, Reisner S, Baral S. Global epidemiology of HIV infection and related syndemics affecting transgender people. J Acquir Immune Defic Syndr. 2016;72 (Suppl 3):S210–9.
8. Baral SD, Poteat T, Strömdahl S, Wirtz AL, Guadamuz TE, Beyrer C. Worldwide burden of HIV in transgender women: a systematic review and meta-analysis. Lancet Infect Dis. 2013;13(3):214–22.
9. Salazar LF, Crosby RA, Jones J, Kota K, Hill B, Masyn KE. Contextual, experiential, and behavioral risk factors associated with HIV status: a descriptive analysis of transgender women residing in Atlanta, Georgia. Int J STD AIDS. 2017;28(11):1059–66.

10. Poteat T, Ackerman B, Diouf D, et al. HIV prevalence and behavioral and psychosocial factors among transgender women and cisgender men who have sex with men in 8 African countries: a cross-sectional analysis. PLoS Med. 2017;14(11):e1002422.
11. Chhim S, Ngin C, Chhoun P, et al. HIV prevalence and factors associated with HIV infection among transgender women in Cambodia: results from a national integrated biological and behavioral survey. BMJ Open. 2017;7(8):e015390.
12. Scheim AI, Bauer GR, Travers R. HIV-related sexual risk among transgender men who are gay, bisexual, or have sex with men. J Acquir Immune Defic Syndr. 2017;74(4):e89–96.
13. Reisner SL, White Hughto JM, Pardee D, Sevelius J. Syndemics and gender affirmation: HIV sexual risk in female-to-male trans masculine adults reporting sexual contact with cisgender males. Int J STD AIDS. 2016;27(11):955–66.
14. Stephens SC, Bernstein KT, Philip SS. Male to female and female to male transgender persons have different sexual risk behaviors yet similar rates of STDs and HIV. AIDS Behav. 2011;15(3):683–6.
15. Hygiene NDoHaM. HIV among people identified as transgender in New York City, 2012–2016. 2016. https://www1.nyc.gov/assets/doh/downloads/pdf/dires/hiv-aids-in-msm.pdf. Accessed Feb 2018.
16. Baggaley RF, White RG, Boily MC. HIV transmission risk through anal intercourse: systematic review, meta-analysis and implications for HIV prevention. Int J Epidemiol. 2010;39(4):1048–63.
17. Bernstein KT, Marcus JL, Nieri G, Philip SS, Klausner JD. Rectal gonorrhea and chlamydia reinfection is associated with increased risk of HIV seroconversion. J Acquir Immune Defic Syndr. 2010;53(4):537–43.
18. Poteat T, German D, Flynn C. The conflation of gender and sex: gaps and opportunities in HIV data among transgender women and MSM. Glob Public Health. 2016;11(7–8):835–48.
19. Melendez RM, Pinto R. 'It's really a hard life': love, gender and HIV risk among male-to-female transgender persons. Cult Health Sex. 2007;9(3):233–45.
20. Gama A, Martins MRO, Mendão L, Barros H, Dias S. HIV infection, risk factors and health services use among male-to-female transgender sex workers: a cross-sectional study in Portugal. AIDS Care. 2018;30(1):1–8.
21. Salas-Espinoza KJ, Menchaca-Diaz R, Patterson TL, et al. HIV prevalence and risk behaviors in male to female (MTF) transgender persons in Tijuana, Mexico. AIDS Behav. 2017;21(12):3271–8.
22. Siembida EJ, Eaton LA, Maksut JL, Driffin DD, Baldwin R. A comparison of HIV-related risk factors between black transgender women and black men who have sex with men. Transgender Health. 2016;1(1):172–80.
23. Levine WC, Pope V, Bhoomkar A, et al. Increase in endocervical CD4 lymphocytes among women with nonulcerative sexually transmitted diseases. J Infect Dis. 1998;177(1):167–74.
24. Wormser GP, Krupp LB, Hanrahan JP, Gavis G, Spira TJ, Cunningham-Rundles S. Acquired immunodeficiency syndrome in male prisoners. New insights into an emerging syndrome. Ann Intern Med. 1983;98(3):297–303.
25. Brennan J, Kuhns LM, Johnson AK, et al. Syndemic theory and HIV-related risk among young transgender women: the role of multiple, co-occurring health problems and social marginalization. Am J Public Health. 2012;102(9):1751–7.
26. Reisner SL, Bailey Z, Sevelius J. Racial/ethnic disparities in history of incarceration, experiences of victimization, and associated health indicators among transgender women in the U.S. Women Health. 2014;54(8):750–67.
27. Clements-Nolle K, Marx R, Guzman R, Katz M. HIV prevalence, risk behaviors, health care use, and mental health status of transgender persons: implications for public health intervention. Am J Public Health. 2001;91(6):915–21.
28. Flores AR, Brown TNT, Herman JL. Adults who identify as transgender are more racially and ethnically diverse than the U.S. general population. Los Angeles, CA: The Williams Institute; 2016.

29. Reisner SL, Biello KB, White Hughto JM, et al. Psychiatric diagnoses and comorbidities in a diverse, multicity cohort of young transgender women: baseline findings from project lifeskills. JAMA Pediatr. 2016;170(5):481–6.
30. Des Jarlais DC, Friedman SR. HIV infection among intravenous drug users: epidemiology and risk reduction. AIDS. 1987;1(2):67–76.
31. Des Jarlais DC, Kerr T, Carrieri P, Feelemyer J, Arasteh K. HIV infection among persons who inject drugs: ending old epidemics and addressing new outbreaks. AIDS. 2016;30 (6):815–26.
32. Denson DJ, Padgett PM, Pitts N, et al. Health care use and HIV-related behaviors of Black and Latina transgender women in 3 US metropolitan areas: results from the transgender HIV behavioral survey. J Acquir Immune Defic Syndr. 2017;75(Suppl 3):S268–75.
33. Braun HM, Candelario J, Hanlon CL, et al. Transgender women living with HIV frequently take antiretroviral therapy and/or feminizing hormone therapy differently than prescribed due to drug-drug interaction concerns. LGBT Health. 2017;4(5):371–5.
34. Mizuno Y, Frazier EL, Huang P, Skarbinski J. Characteristics of transgender women living with HIV receiving medical care in the United States. LGBT Health. 2015;2(3):228–34.
35. Sevelius JM, Saberi P, Johnson MO. Correlates of antiretroviral adherence and viral load among transgender women living with HIV. AIDS Care. 2014;26(8):976–82.
36. Lemons A, Beer L, Finlayson T, McCree DH, Lentine D, Shouse RL. Characteristics of HIV-positive transgender men receiving medical care: United States, 2009–2014. Am J Public Health. 2018;108(1):128–30.
37. Kalichman SC, Hernandez D, Finneran S, Price D, Driver R. Transgender women and HIV-related health disparities: falling off the HIV treatment cascade. Sex Health. 2017;14 (5):469–76.
38. Singer M, Clair S. Syndemics and public health: reconceptualizing disease in bio-social context. Med Anthropol Q. 2003;17(4):423–41.
39. Pellowski JA, Kalichman SC, Matthews KA, Adler N. A pandemic of the poor: social disadvantage and the U.S. HIV epidemic. Am Psychol. 2013;68(4):197–209.
40. El-Sadr WM, Mayer KH, Hodder SL. AIDS in America—forgotten but not gone. N Engl J Med. 2010;362(11):967–70.
41. Fletcher JB, Kisler KA, Reback CJ. Housing status and HIV risk behaviors among transgender women in Los Angeles. Arch Sex Behav. 2014;43(8):1651–61.
42. Nuttbrock L, Hwahng S, Bockting W, et al. Lifetime risk factors for HIV/sexually transmitted infections among male-to-female transgender persons. J Acquir Immune Defic Syndr. 2009;52(3):417–21.
43. Conron KJ, Scott G, Stowell GS, Landers SJ. Transgender health in Massachusetts: results from a household probability sample of adults. Am J Public Health. 2012;102(1):118–22.
44. Dowshen N, Matone M, Luan X, et al. Behavioral and health outcomes for HIV+ young transgender women (YTW) linked to and engaged in medical care. LGBT Health. 2016;3 (2):162–7.
45. Santos GM, Wilson EC, Rapues J, Macias O, Packer T, Raymond HF. HIV treatment cascade among transgender women in a San Francisco respondent driven sampling study. Sex Transm Infect. 2014;90(5):430–3.
46. Palazzolo SL, Yamanis TJ, De Jesus M, Maguire-Marshall M, Barker SL. Documentation status as a contextual determinant of HIV risk among young transgender Latinas. LGBT Health. 2016;3(2):132–8.
47. Frost DM, Lehavot K, Meyer IH. Minority stress and physical health among sexual minority individuals. J Behav Med. 2015;38(1):1–8.
48. Grossman AH, D'Augelli AR. Transgender youth and life-threatening behaviors. Suicide Life Threat Behav. 2007;37(5):527–37.
49. Budge SL, Adelson JL, Howard KA. Anxiety and depression in transgender individuals: the roles of transition status, loss, social support, and coping. J Consult Clin Psychol. 2013;81 (3):545–57.

50. Blank MB, Himelhoch SS, Balaji AB, et al. A multisite study of the prevalence of HIV with rapid testing in mental health settings. Am J Public Health. 2014;104(12):2377–84.
51. Clements-Nolle K, Marx R, Katz M. Attempted suicide among transgender persons: the influence of gender-based discrimination and victimization. J Homosex. 2006;51(3):53–69.
52. McCabe SE, West BT, Hughes TL, Boyd CJ. Sexual orientation and substance abuse treatment utilization in the United States: results from a national survey. J Subst Abuse Treat. 2013;44(1):4–12.
53. Medley G, Lipari RN, Bose J, Cribb DS, Kroutil LA, McHenry G. Sexual orientation and estimates of adult substance use and mental health: results from the 2015 national survey on drug use and health. Substance Abuse and Mental Health Services Administration; 2016.
54. Dale SK, Bogart LM, Wagner GJ, Galvan FH, Klein DJ. Medical mistrust is related to lower longitudinal medication adherence among African-American males with HIV. J Health Psychol. 2016;21(7):1311–21.
55. Kosenko K, Rintamaki L, Raney S, Maness K. Transgender patient perceptions of stigma in health care contexts. Med Care. 2013;51(9):819–22.
56. Cruz TM. Assessing access to care for transgender and gender nonconforming people: a consideration of diversity in combating discrimination. Soc Sci Med. 2014;110:65–73.
57. Lacombe-Duncan A. An intersectional perspective on access to HIV-related healthcare for transgender women. Transgender Health. 2016;1(1):137–41.
58. Stotzer RL, Silverschanz P, Wilson A. Gender identity and social services: barriers to care. J Soc Serv Res. 2013;39(1):63–77.
59. Kattari SK, Walls NE, Whitfield DL, Langenderfer Magruder L. Racial and ethnic differences in experiences of discrimination in accessing social services among transgender/gender-nonconforming people. J Ethn Cult Divers Soc Work. 2017;26(3):217–35.
60. Bradford J, Reisner SL, Honnold JA, Xavier J. Experiences of transgender-related discrimination and implications for health: results from the Virginia transgender health initiative study. Am J Public Health. 2013;103(10):1820–9.
61. Andrasik MP, Yoon R, Mooney J, et al. Exploring barriers and facilitators to participation of male-to-female transgender persons in preventive HIV vaccine clinical trials. Prev Sci. 2014;15(3):268–76.
62. Ganju D, Saggurti N. Stigma, violence and HIV vulnerability among transgender persons in sex work in Maharashtra, India. Cult Health Sex. 2017;19(8):903–17.
63. Cook CL, Canidate S, Ennis N, Cook RL. Types and delivery of emotional support to promote linkage and engagement in HIV care. Patient Prefer Adherence. 2018;12:45–52.
64. Kelly JD, Hartman C, Graham J, Kallen MA, Giordano TP. Social support as a predictor of early diagnosis, linkage, retention, and adherence to HIV care: results from the steps study. J Assoc Nurses AIDS Care. 2014;25(5):405–13.
65. Klein A, Golub SA. Family rejection as a predictor of suicide attempts and substance misuse among transgender and gender nonconforming adults. LGBT Health. 2016;3(3):193–9.
66. Rebchook G, Keatley J, Contreras R, et al. The transgender women of color initiative: implementing and evaluating innovative interventions to enhance engagement and retention in HIV care. Am J Public Health. 2017;107(2):224–9.
67. Dasarathan S, Kalaivani S. Study of prevalence of sexually transmitted infections/human immunodeficiency virus and condom use among male-to-female transgender: a retrospective analysis from a tertiary care hospital in Chennai. Indian J Sex Transm Dis. 2017;38(1):43–6.
68. Keshinro B, Crowell TA, Nowak RG, et al. High prevalence of HIV, chlamydia and gonorrhoea among men who have sex with men and transgender women attending trusted community centres in Abuja and Lagos, Nigeria. J Int AIDS Soc. 2016;19(1):21270.
69. Green N, Hoenigl M, Morris S, Little SJ. Risk behavior and sexually transmitted infections among transgender women and men undergoing community-based screening for acute and early HIV infection in San Diego. Med (Baltimore). 2015;94(41):e1830.
70. Pickering JM, Whitworth JA, Hughes P, et al. Aetiology of sexually transmitted infections and response to syndromic treatment in southwest Uganda. Sex Transm Infect. 2005;81(6):488–93.

71. Hope-Rapp E, Anyfantakis V, Fouéré S, et al. Etiology of genital ulcer disease. A prospective study of 278 cases seen in an STD clinic in Paris. Sex Transm Dis. 2010;37(3):153–8.
72. McFarland W, Wilson EC, Raymond HF. HIV prevalence, sexual partners, sexual behavior and HIV acquisition risk among trans men, San Francisco, 2014. AIDS Behav. 2017;21 (12):3346–52.
73. CDC. Special populations—2015 STD treatment guidelines. 2015. https://www.cdc.gov/std/tg2015/specialpops.htm.
74. WHO. Prevention and treatment of HIV and other sexually transmitted infections among men who have sex with men and transgender people. WHO; 2011. http://www.who.int/hiv/pub/guidelines/msm_guidelines2011/en/.
75. Sevelius J. "There's no pamphlet for the kind of sex I have": HIV-related risk factors and protective behaviors among transgender men who have sex with nontransgender men. J Assoc Nurses AIDS Care. 2009;20(5):398–410.
76. Reisner SL, Perkovich B, Mimiaga MJ. A mixed methods study of the sexual health needs of New England transmen who have sex with nontransgender men. AIDS Patient Care STDS. 2010;24(8):501–13.
77. CDC. Recommendations for the laboratory-based detection of Chlamydia trachomatis and Neisseria gonorrhoeae. MMWR Recomm Rep. 2014;63(RR02):1–19.
78. Garg STL, Grasso C, Mayer KH. Prevalent and incident hepatitis C infection among HIV-infected men who have sex with men engaged in primary care in a Boston community health center. Clin Infect Dis. 2013;56(10):1480–7.
79. Linas BP, Wong AY, Schackman BR, Kim AY, Freedberg KA. Cost-effective screening for acute hepatitis C virus infection in HIV-infected men who have sex with men. Clin Infect Dis. 2012;55(2):279–90.
80. CDC. Guidelines for viral hepatitis surveillance and case management. 2005.
81. CDC. Viral hepatitis—2015 STD treatment guidelines. 2018. https://www.cdc.gov/std/tg2015/hepatitis.htm.
82. AIDSinfo. Pre-exposure prophylaxis (PrEP) understanding HIV/AIDS. 2018. https://www.ncbi.nlm.nih.gov/pubmed/. Accessed Feb 2018.
83. AIDSinfo. FDA approves first drug for reducing the risk of sexually acquired HIV infection. 2018. https://aidsinfo.nih.gov/news/1254/fda-approves-first-drug-for-reducing-the-risk-of-sexually-acquired-hiv-infection.
84. CDC. FDA approves drug for HIV prevention. 2018. https://www.cdc.gov/nchhstp/newsroom/2012/fda-approvesdrugstatement.html. Accessed Feb 2018.
85. CDC. Preexposure prophylaxis for the prevention of HIV in the United States—2014: a clinical practice guideline. 2014. https://www.cdc.gov/hiv/pdf/prepguidelines2014.pdf. Accessed Feb 2018.
86. Grant RM, Lama JR, Anderson PL, et al. Preexposure chemoprophylaxis for HIV prevention in men who have sex with men. N Engl J Med. 2010;363(27):2587–99.
87. Baeten JM, Donnell D, Ndase P, et al. Antiretroviral prophylaxis for HIV prevention in heterosexual men and women. N Engl J Med. 2012;367(5):399–410.
88. Deutsch MB, Glidden DV, Sevelius J, et al. HIV pre-exposure prophylaxis in transgender women: a subgroup analysis of the iPrEx trial. Lancet HIV. 2015;2(12):e512–9.
89. Knox DC, Anderson PL, Harrigan PR, Tan DH. Multidrug-resistant HIV-1 infection despite preexposure prophylaxis. N Engl J Med. 2017;376(5):501–2.
90. Mascolini M. Infection with multidrug-resistant HIV while adherent to TDF/FTC PrEP. Chicago, IL: HIV Research for Prevention; 2016.
91. Sevelius JM, Keatley J, Calma N, Arnold E. 'I am not a man': trans-specific barriers and facilitators to PrEP acceptability among transgender women. Glob Public Health. 2016;11 (7–8):1060–75.
92. CHRP. UCSD: PrEP linkage adherence & pharmacology in transgender persons. 2018. http://www.californiaaidsresearch.org/files/award-abstracts/prevention-and-linkage-to-care/ucsd-prep-trans.html.

93. Kearney BP, Mathias A. Lack of effect of tenofovir disoproxil fumarate on pharmacokinetics of hormonal contraceptives. Pharmacotherapy. 2009;29(8):924–9.
94. Anderson PL, Reirden D, Castillo-Mancilla J. Pharmacologic considerations for preexposure prophylaxis in transgender women (1999). J Acquir Immune Defic Syndr. 2016;72(Suppl 3): S230–4.
95. WHO. Guideline on when to start antiretroviral therapy and on pre-exposure prophylaxis for HIV. WHO. 2015.
96. Gilead. Truvada prescribing information package insert. 2018. https://www.accessdata.fda.gov/drugsatfda_docs/label/2016/021752s047lbl.pdf. Accessed Feb 2018.
97. Sevelius JM, Deutsch MB, Grant R. The future of PrEP among transgender women: the critical role of gender affirmation in research and clinical practices. J Int AIDS Soc. 2016;19 (7 Suppl 6):21105.
98. Institute NA. PrEP to prevent HIV acquisition guideline—AIDS institute clinical guidelines. 2017. https://www.hivguidelines.org/prep-for-prevention/prep-to-prevent-hiv/.
99. Liaw YF, Chu CM. Hepatitis B virus infection. Lancet. 2009;373(9663):582–92.
100. Poteat T, Malik M, Scheim A, Elliott A. HIV prevention among transgender populations: knowledge gaps and evidence for action. Curr HIV/AIDS Rep. 2017;14(4):141–52.
101. CDC. 2018 quick reference guide: recommended laboratory HIV testing algorithm for serum or plasma specimens. 2018. https://stacks.cdc.gov/view/cdc/50872/cdc_DS1_50872.pdf.
102. Institute NA. Discontinuing PrEP. 2017.
103. Smith DK, Grohskopf LA, Black RJ, et al. Antiretroviral postexposure prophylaxis after sexual, injection-drug use, or other nonoccupational exposure to HIV in the United States: recommendations from the U.S. Department of Health and Human Services. MMWR Recomm Rep. 2005;54(RR-2):1–20.
104. Cardo DM, Culver DH, Ciesielski CA, et al. A case-control study of HIV seroconversion in health care workers after percutaneous exposure. Centers for Disease Control and Prevention Needlestick Surveillance Group. N Engl J Med. 1997;337(21):1485–90.
105. Kuhar DT, Henderson DK, Struble KA, et al. Updated US Public Health Service guidelines for the management of occupational exposures to human immunodeficiency virus and recommendations for postexposure prophylaxis. Infect Control Hosp Epidemiol. 2013;34 (9):875–92.
106. CDC. Updated guidelines for antiretroviral postexposure prophylaxis after sexual, injection drug use, or other nonoccupational exposure to HIV. Atlanta, GA; 2016.
107. Institute NA. PEP for non-occupational exposure to HIV guideline—AIDS institute clinical guidelines. 2014. https://www.hivguidelines.org/pep-for-hiv-prevention/non-occupational/.
108. Otten RA, Smith DK, Adams DR, et al. Efficacy of postexposure prophylaxis after intravaginal exposure of pig-tailed macaques to a human-derived retrovirus (human immunodeficiency virus type 2). J Virol. 2000;74(20):9771–5.
109. Smit C, Geskus R, Walker S, et al. Effective therapy has altered the spectrum of cause-specific mortality following HIV seroconversion. AIDS. 2006;20(5):741–9.
110. Konrad BP, Taylor D, Conway JM, Ogilvie GS, Coombs D. On the duration of the period between exposure to HIV and detectable infection. Epidemics. 2017;20:73–83.
111. CDC. Laboratory testing for the diagnosis of HIV infection: updated recommendations. 2018. https://stacks.cdc.gov/view/cdc/23447/cdc_23447_DS1.pdf.
112. CDC. HIV infection: detection, counseling, and referral—2015 STD treatment guidelines. 2018. https://www.cdc.gov/std/tg2015/hiv.htm.
113. Braun DL, Kouyos RD, Balmer B, Grube C, Weber R, Günthard HF. Frequency and spectrum of unexpected clinical manifestations of primary HIV-1 infection. Clin Infect Dis. 2015;61(6):1013–21.
114. Institute NA. Post-testing counseling, notification, and domestic violence screening. 2013. https://www.hivguidelines.org/adult-hiv/testing-diagnosis/provider-guide-to-hiv-testing-quick-reference-card/.
115. Clark JL, Perez-Brumer AG, Segura ER, Salvatierra HJ, Sanchez J, Lama JR. Anticipated notification of sexual partners following STD diagnosis among men who have sex with men

and transgender women in Lima, Peru: a mixed methods analysis. PLoS ONE. 2016;11(9): e0163905.
116. Sevelius JM, Patouhas E, Keatley JG, Johnson MO. Barriers and facilitators to engagement and retention in care among transgender women living with human immunodeficiency virus. Ann Behav Med. 2014;47(1):5–16.
117. Gardner EM, McLees MP, Steiner JF, del Rio C, Burman WJ. The spectrum of engagement in HIV care and its relevance to test-and-treat strategies for prevention of HIV infection. Clin Infect Dis: An Official Publication of the Infectious Diseases Society of America. 2011;52 (6):793–800.
118. WHO. Global cascade of care, 2016. 2016. http://www.who.int/hiv/data/en/.
119. Jalil EM, Wilson EC, Luz PM, et al. HIV testing and the care continuum among transgender women: population estimates from Rio de Janeiro, Brazil. J Int AIDS Soc. 2017;20 (1):21873.
120. NYDOH. HIV among people identified as transgender in New York City, 2012–2016. 2017. http://www1.nyc.gov/site/doh/data/data-sets/epi-surveillance-slide-sets.page.
121. Fischl MA, Richman DD, Grieco MH, et al. The efficacy of azidothymidine (AZT) in the treatment of patients with AIDS and AIDS-related complex. A double-blind, placebo-controlled trial. N Engl J Med. 1987;317(4):185–91.
122. USDHHS. A timeline of HIV and AIDS. 2016. https://www.hiv.gov/hiv-basics/overview/history/hiv-and-aids-timeline.
123. Hammer SM, Squires KE, Hughes MD, et al. A controlled trial of two nucleoside analogues plus indinavir in persons with human immunodeficiency virus infection and CD4 cell counts of 200 per cubic millimeter or less. AIDS Clinical Trials Group 320 Study Team. N Engl J Med. 1997;337(11):725–33.
124. Gulick RM, Mellors JW, Havlir D, et al. Treatment with indinavir, zidovudine, and lamivudine in adults with human immunodeficiency virus infection and prior antiretroviral therapy. N Engl J Med. 1997;337(11):734–9.
125. Imamichi T. Action of anti-HIV drugs and resistance: reverse transcriptase inhibitors and protease inhibitors. Curr Pharm Des. 2004;10(32):4039–53.
126. Scaling up antiretroviral therapy in resource-limited settings: guidelines for a public health approach. Executive summary. IAPAC Mon. Apr 2002;8(6):168–75.
127. Richardson ET, Grant PM, Zolopa AR. Evolution of HIV treatment guidelines in high and low-income countries: converging recommendations. Antiviral Res. 2014;103:88–93.
128. Lundgren JD, Babiker AG, Gordin F, et al. Initiation of antiretroviral therapy in early asymptomatic HIV infection. N Engl J Med. 2015;373(9):795–807.
129. Palella FJ Jr., Delaney KM, Moorman AC, et al. Declining morbidity and mortality among patients with advanced human immunodeficiency virus infection. HIV outpatient study investigators. N Engl J Med. 1998;338(13):853–60.
130. Wilson EMP, Sereti I. Immune restoration after antiretroviral therapy: the pitfalls of hasty or incomplete repairs. Immunol Rev. 2013;254(1):343–54.
131. El-Sadr WM, Lundgren J, Neaton JD, et al. CD4+ count-guided interruption of antiretroviral treatment. N Engl J Med. 2006;355(22):2283–96.
132. Borges AH, Neuhaus J, Babiker AG, et al. Immediate antiretroviral therapy reduces risk of infection-related cancer during early HIV infection. Clin Infect Dis: An Official Publication of the Infectious Diseases Society of America. 2016;63(12):1668–76.
133. Silverberg MJ, Abrams DI. Do antiretrovirals reduce the risk of non-aids defining malignancies? Curr Opin HIV AIDS. 2009;4(1):42–51.
134. Walensky RP, Paltiel AD, Losina E, et al. The survival benefits of AIDS treatment in the United States. J Infect Dis. 2006;194(1):11–9.
135. Ray M, Logan R, Sterne JA, et al. The effect of combined antiretroviral therapy on the overall mortality of HIV-infected individuals. AIDS (London, England). 2010;24(1):123–37.
136. Mayer KH. Antiretroviral therapy for HIV prevention: present status and future prospects. Am J Public Health. 2010;100(10):1867–76.

137. Cohen MS, Chen YQ, McCauley M, et al. Prevention of HIV-1 infection with early antiretroviral therapy. N Engl J Med. 2011;365(6):493–505.
138. Mayer KH, Grinsztejn B, El-Sadr WM. Transgender people and HIV prevention: what we know and what we need to know, a call to action. J Acquir Immune Defic Syndr (1999). 2016;72(Suppl 3):S207–9.
139. USDHHS. The HIV life cycle. 2017. https://aidsinfo.nih.gov/understanding-hiv-aids/fact-sheets/19/73/the-hiv-life-cycle.
140. Usach I, Melis V, Peris JE. Non-nucleoside reverse transcriptase inhibitors: a review on pharmacokinetics, pharmacodynamics, safety and tolerability. J Int AIDS Soc. 2013;16(1).
141. FDA. FDA-approved HIV medicines. 2018. https://aidsinfo.nih.gov/understanding-hiv-aids/fact-sheets/21/58/fda-approved-hiv-medicines.
142. Pirrone V, Thakkar N, Jacobson JM, Wigdahl B, Krebs FC. Combinatorial approaches to the prevention and treatment of HIV-1 infection. Antimicrob Agents Chemother. 2011;55(5):1831–42.
143. WHO guidelines approved by the guidelines review committee. In: Consolidated guidelines on the use of antiretroviral drugs for treating and preventing HIV infection: recommendations for a public health approach. Geneva: World Health Organization Copyright (c) World Health Organization 2016; 2016.
144. Gunthard HF, Saag MS, Benson CA, et al. Antiretroviral drugs for treatment and prevention of HIV infection in adults: 2016 recommendations of the international antiviral society-USA panel. JAMA. 2016;316(2):191–210.
145. HHS. Guidelines for the use of antiretroviral agents in adults and adolescents living with HIV. 2017. https://aidsinfo.nih.gov/guidelines/html/1/adult-and-adolescent-arv/11/what-to-start.
146. Radix A, Sevelius J, Deutsch MB. Transgender women, hormonal therapy and HIV treatment: a comprehensive review of the literature and recommendations for best practices. J Int AIDS Soc. 2016;19(3 Suppl 2):20810.
147. Sellers CJ, Wohl DA. Antiretroviral therapy: when to start. Infect Dis Clin North Am. 2014;28(3):403–20.
148. Pacifici GM, Gucci A, Giuliani L. Testosterone sulphation and glucuronidation in the human liver: interindividual variability. Eur J Drug Metab Pharmacokinet. 1997;22(3):253–8.
149. Crum NF, Furtek KJ, Olson PE, Amling CL, Wallace MR. A review of hypogonadism and erectile dysfunction among HIV-infected men during the pre- and post-HAART eras: diagnosis, pathogenesis, and management. AIDS Patient Care STDs. 2005;19(10):655–71.
150. Bhatia R, Murphy AB, Raper JL, et al. Testosterone replacement therapy among HIV-infected men in the CFAR network of integrated clinical systems. AIDS (London, England). 2015;29(1):77–81.
151. Blick G. Optimal diagnostic measures and thresholds for hypogonadism in men with HIV/AIDS: comparison between 2 transdermal testosterone replacement therapy gels. Postgrad Med. 2013;125(2):30–9.
152. Hembree WC, Cohen-Kettenis P, Delemarre-van de Waal HA, et al. Endocrine treatment of transsexual persons: an endocrine society clinical practice guideline. J Clin Endocrinol Metab. 2009;94(9):3132–54.
153. Wansom T, Guadamuz TE, Vasan S. Transgender populations and HIV: unique risks, challenges and opportunities. J Virus Eradication. 2016;2(2):87–93.
154. Cheng ZN, Shu Y, Liu ZQ, Wang LS, Ou-Yang DS, Zhou HH. Role of cytochrome P450 in estradiol metabolism in vitro. Acta Pharmacol Sin. 2001;22(2):148–54.
155. Aweeka FT, Rosenkranz SL, Segal Y, et al. The impact of sex and contraceptive therapy on the plasma and intracellular pharmacokinetics of zidovudine. AIDS (London, England). 2006;20(14):1833–41.
156. Zhang M, Huang Q, Huang Y, et al. Beta-estradiol attenuates the anti-HIV-1 efficacy of Stavudine (D4T) in primary PBL. Retrovirology. 2008;5(1):82.
157. Ho JY, Chen MJ, Sheu WH, et al. Differential effects of oral conjugated equine estrogen and transdermal estrogen on atherosclerotic vascular disease risk markers and endothelial

function in healthy postmenopausal women. Hum Reprod (Oxford, England). 2006;21(10):2715–20.
158. Bjornsson TD, Callaghan JT, Einolf HJ, et al. The conduct of in vitro and in vivo drug-drug interaction studies: a PhRMA perspective. J Clin Pharmacol. 2003;43(5):443–69.
159. Larder B. Mechanisms of HIV-1 drug resistance. AIDS (London, England). 2001;15: S27–34.
160. Sevelius JM, Carrico A, Johnson MO. Antiretroviral therapy adherence among transgender women living with HIV. J Assoc Nurses AIDS Care JANAC. 2010;21(3):256–64.
161. Baguso GN, Gay CL, Lee KA. Medication adherence among transgender women living with HIV. AIDS Care. 2016;28(8):976–81.
162. Wiewel EW, Torian LV, Merchant P, Braunstein SL, Shepard CW. HIV diagnoses and care among transgender persons and comparison with men who have sex with men: New York City, 2006–2011. Am J Public Health. 2016;106(3):497–502.

Chapter 14
Transgender Care and Medical Education

Tamar Reisman, Dennis Dacarett-Galeano and Zil Goldstein

Introduction

Although conversation surrounding transgender healthcare has notably increased in the public sphere over recent years, health equity for transgender and gender nonconforming individuals is far from realized. The lesbian, gay, bisexual, and transgender community as a whole has seen great progress and success in achieving increased visibility and acceptance toward equality since the mid-twentieth century; nevertheless, people of trans experience consistently report a lack of access to quality care across all geographic, infrastructural, and sociocultural contexts.

A commonly reported barrier to care is the paucity of sensitive and competent healthcare providers [1, 2]. Patients from certain subgroups, such as racial and ethnic minorities, the elderly, and rural populations, may have particular challenges securing adequate care [3, 4]. Although substantial research on gender and sexual minority health education for clinicians has been conducted in the past few decades, it has been weighted heavily toward studying the health needs of gay men and lesbians. Transgender health education has traditionally been absent from the medical schools curriculum [2]. Exposure to a clinical curriculum that places an emphasis on transgender health can help cultivate competent, respectful clinicians who are sensitive to the unique health needs of this patient group [2].

T. Reisman (✉)
Department of Internal Medicine, Division of Endocrinology, Diabetes and Bone Disease, Icahn School of Medicine at Mount Sinai, New York, NY, USA
e-mail: tamar.reisman@mssm.edu

D. Dacarett-Galeano
Icahn School of Medicine at Mount Sinai, New York, NY, USA

Z. Goldstein
Department of Medical Education, The Mount Sinai Health System, New York, NY, USA

L. Poretsky and W. C. Hembree (eds.), *Transgender Medicine*, Contemporary Endocrinology, https://doi.org/10.1007/978-3-030-05683-4_14

Gender Dysphoria and Historical Discrimination in Medicine

Historically, the transgender community has had a tenuous relationship with medicine as an institution. Gender-affirming therapies, from hormones to surgical procedures, were overwhelmingly restricted in the United States until the second half of the twentieth century. In 1952, the story of Christine Jorgensen, a transgender woman who traveled to Europe to undergo hormonal and surgical therapies to affirm her gender identity, was published in the New York Daily News and made a possible national public discussion and medical debate surrounding therapeutic and surgical interventions to affirm transgender identity. Throughout the 1950s and 1960s, hundreds of transgender individuals from the United States requested care from Dr. Christian Hamburger, the Danish endocrinologist who had seen Christine Jorgensen, however, the Danish Ministry of Justice officiated that they would prohibit nonnationals from entering the country to receive care. At that time, Dr. Hamburger referred his client requests to Dr. Harry Benjamin, an endocrinologist and sexologist in the United States, who would then quickly become the American leader in treating the condition known today as gender dysphoria [5]. Joanne Meyerowitz, the author of the first book to use primary sources to trace the cultural and historical origins of the efforts to affirm a patient's gender identity through medical and surgical therapies in the United States [6], describes that transgender individuals have pushed the boundaries of medicine to accommodate their unique needs by persistently advocating past reluctance and "gatekeeping" they encountered along the way. This historically unjust relationship between the transgender community and the institution of medicine as one of "gatekeeping," according to Meyerowitz, still manifests itself in lasting, pervasive effects on the access to care is for individuals of trans and gender-nonconforming experience [7].

As recently as in 2013, claiming gender identity or expression incongruent with the sex assigned at birth was seen as a disorder in the Diagnostic and Statistical Manual of Mental Disorders. Today's DSM-V describes gender dysphoria as the psychological distress associated with gender nonconforming rather than an illness that should be cured or corrected: "a marked incongruence between one's experienced/expressed gender and assigned gender of at least 6 months' duration … [that] is associated with clinically significant distress or impairment in … important areas of functioning" [8–10]. Both during and after the reevaluation of gender identity disorder in the DSM, some advocated that the recent DSM classification of gender dysphoria remains stigmatizing. Others, including many LGBTQ organizations such as Lambda Legal and ultimately, the DSM-V Workgroup on Sexual and Gender Identity Disorders argued that, in large part because the medical payment models of medicine depend on a traditional diagnosis that is then accompanied by clinical indications for treatment, a classification such as gender dysphoria should stay in place [7, 10, 11]. Given the recent change in the medical approach to transgender health care and this historical shift in the transgender community's advocacy for equity, it is important to acknowledge and understand that gender identity disorder is no longer a diagnosis in use in addition to the fact that nonnormative gender expressions and identities have frequently been documented historically and observed cross-culturally and therefore, should not be seen through the traditionally clinical lens of pathology used in medical encounters [1, 12].

Data collection on gender identity and the prevalence of gender dysphoria has been limited by multiple factors [12]. Despite the challenges, The Williams Institute, using population-based data from 19 states, offers a conservative estimate that in the United States, 0.6% of adults, or roughly about 1.4 million people, identify as transgender [13]. Not all gender nonconforming individuals seek medical care with a desire to acquire transition-related services. Individuals who are studied and documented in epidemiological research are those that have sought transition-related care. Today, the treatment paradigm for those experiencing gender dysphoria is to alleviate patient's distress, if any, and not to guide patients to conform to a gender [12].

Present-Day Barriers to Care and Social Determinants of Health

In the spring of 2009, Lambda Legal, a national organization devoted to LGBT civil rights, administered the first survey to explore the healthcare barriers that gender and sexual minorities face in accessing care on a national level. The survey found that 70% of transgender and gender-nonconforming individuals faced some form of discrimination in the healthcare setting [14]. The National Center for Transgender Equality found that 19% of people of trans experience reported being refused medical care, 50% endorsed that they had to teach their medical providers about transgender care, and that 28% delayed seeking medical attention when needed due to historical discrimination [15].

In addition to challenges within the clinical encounter, people of trans experience suffer from significant stigma and oppression at individual, interpersonal, sociopolitical, and institutional levels that manifest in significant health disparities [7, 16]. In 2015, The National Center for Transgender Equality found that people of trans experience reported higher incidence of family violence, job insecurity, economic hardship, and home instability than the general population of the United States. Almost one-third of those surveyed who were employed endorsed that they had at one point experienced being fired, denied a promotion, or another form of mistreatment due to their gender identity or expression. Compared to the general population, the report highlighted that transgender people were more likely to be unemployed (15% vs. 5%) and impoverished (29% vs. 12%) and that 30% of transgender and gender-nonconforming individuals had experienced homelessness at some point in their lifetime. Moreover, transgender people of color were found to face increased burden. When data were stratified by race and ethnicity, unemployment among transgender people of color was found to be four times greater than the general population and the poverty rate over three times higher. Stemming from this pervasive discrimination, the report found that people of trans experience suffer from staggering rates of psychological distress. 39% of those surveyed experienced serious psychological distress in the month prior and 40% at one point had attempted suicide. Because of the level of prejudice, stigma, and oppression that the transgender community continues to face in and out of the healthcare setting in addition to the community's dependency on the medical system for personal affirmation and safety, it is particularly important for healthcare providers to deliver competent, sensitive, appropriate, and gender-affirming care [10, 16, 17].

Unique Health Needs and Lack of Comfort Among Clinicians

When seeking care, patients of trans experience will have unique health needs that a clinician must thoroughly consider, regardless of whether gender-affirming therapies such as hormones or surgical procedures are sought [4]. In particular, clinicians must be sensitive and affirming of their patient's identity and pronouns, demonstrate competence, and take an attentive, individualized approach particularly in managing gender dysphoria and transition-related care, a patient's self-determined mental health needs, and/or considering an individual's risk factors for preventative health screenings [12, 18].

Many patients will want to access hormonal or surgical therapies to treat their gender dysphoria and/or to affirm their gender identity; numerous studies to date have shown that medical intervention improves gender dysphoria, mental health and functioning, sexual health, and overall quality of life [19]. Providers should be familiar with common hormone regimens, and gender-affirming surgeries, as well as other potentially useful interventions such as voice and communication therapy, image consultation, and counseling or psychotherapy. When working with a patient to delineate a treatment plan, the provider must understand the patient's reproductive goals, and understand the ways that hormone and surgical therapy can impact fertility. In certain cases, patients may benefit from a referral for egg retrieval and cryopreservation or sperm banking prior to initiation of hormone therapy. Such services should be known to the provider and appropriate referrals provided [4].

For a variety of reasons—discomfort on the part of the patients or providers, lack of awareness among healthcare providers, and discrimination in the healthcare system—transgender patients are less likely to undergo regular preventive screening [18]. Breast, cervical, ovarian, uterine, and prostate cancer risk and screening should be considered in patients who have the corresponding anatomy, and in general, patients should follow age-appropriate cancer screening guidelines.

For example, transgender women with risk factors for breast cancer, including those who have received hormone treatment for more than five years, should undergo mammography screening in accordance to general population standards according to age [20]. Providers should be aware of frequently encountered adverse effects of masculinizing and feminizing hormone regimens, and monitor patients for potential complications on a regular basis. General health risks involving feminizing hormones include venous thromboembolic disease, gallstones, weight gain, and hypertriglyceridemia while polycythemia, sleep apnea, and acne can occur in patients undergoing treatment with masculinizing hormones. Because much research to inform guidelines is underway and more is still needed, the World Professional Association for Transgender Health recommends consulting the literature and updated national guidelines frequently. Many individualized and updated guidelines for screening patients who undergo transition-related hormone therapy and/or surgical procedures in the United States are available such as the *Guidelines for the Primary and Gender-Affirming Care of Transgender and Gender Nonbinary People* developed by the University of California, San Francisco's Center of Excellence for Transgender Health, and the Endocrine Society's 2017 clinical guideline, *Endocrine Treatment of Gender-Dysphoric/Gender-Incongruent Persons* [12].

Clinicians should be aware and up to date on options that can be offered for surgically managing gender dysphoria. Transgender men can achieve facial and body hair growth, vocal deepening, increased musculature, and cessation of their menstrual cycle with hormone therapy alone, however, some may want surgical procedures such as mastectomy to manage their chest appearance as well as hysterectomy, oophorectomy, vaginectomy, scrotoplasty, and/or metoidioplasty/phalloplasty for genital reconstruction. The general outline of surgical procedures offered to transgender women includes breast reconstruction, orchiectomy, penectomy, vaginoplasty, labiaplasty, clitoroplasty, urethral meatus reconstruction, and facial feminization surgery. Similar to the approach to hormonal therapy, the clinician must be adept at offering all options and attending to what a patient has in mind for their care [1].

A clinician's approach to gender nonconformity and/or gender dysphoria should also be individualized. Although most young children who exhibit gender-nonconforming behaviors or dysphoria will not exhibit this behavior by the time of puberty, some may develop more intense emotions and distress as puberty begins and adolescence progresses. Although exhibiting gender-nonconforming behaviors and/or dysphoria in childhood is neither required nor correlated with experiencing dysphoria in adolescence and adulthood, patients who had intense gender dysphoria in childhood are known to exhibit persistence of their symptoms into adolescence and adulthood. Although social transitioning in early childhood is controversial among professionals, an adolescent's reaction to their pubertal changes is considered diagnostic. Suppressing puberty starting at Tanner Stage 2 using reversible therapies such as GnRH agonists has been shown to improve wellbeing in transgender youths. According to professional guidelines, treatment with feminizing/masculinizing hormone therapy should begin at age 16 or with parental consent.

Treatment should always include the patient's goals in mind with inclusion of the family, ideally; however, the most significant risk of withholding medical treatment from adolescents is long-term damaging psychological consequences.

Despite increased awareness of the transgender community's unique healthcare needs, medical providers have yet to be adequately trained in attending to these needs. In a study evaluating knowledge of transgender healthcare among practicing endocrinologists, over 80% of clinicians reported having never received training on the care of transgender patients [21]. In a survey of gynecologists' current attitudes, knowledge, and practice, 80% had not received training in residency on caring for transgender patients. 35.3 and 29% of providers felt comfortable providing care to transgender women and men, respectively; additionally, 59.4% were unaware of the breast cancer screening recommendations for transgender women [22]. The lack of specialized care demonstrated by surveys such as these is concerning at face-value and reveals the underlying lack of education provided throughout the medical education continuum. Transgender health education is lacking throughout textbooks and insufficiently integrated into educational curricula from the start of medical school through residency and fellowship training [23].

Medical Education—History and Present

General sexual health competency training among medical providers transformed in the late twentieth century as needs, from contraception to sexually transmitted infection counseling, became more defined. Prior to this expansion, which saw its crest during the sexual revolution of the 1970s, undergraduate medical education on sexuality existed in only three medical schools in the United States. By the mid-1970s, 95% of the medical schools in the United States offered some form of training in sexual health competency. In part owing to reconsidering the bounds of medical education in this period, formal training surrounding the unique healthcare needs of gender and sexual minorities emerged and continued amplifying as social movements paved the way toward increased recognition. Nevertheless, equity is far from achieved and interestingly, overall time devoted to sexuality education has seen a decrease since its peak in the 1970s [24].

With particular regards to lesbian, gay, bisexual, and transgender-related content in undergraduate medical education, a 2011 study featured in the Journal of the American Medical Association found that out of 176 medical schools in the United States and Canada, the median time devoted to teaching LGBT-related content throughout the four years was 5 h. Additionally, 33% reported no time dedicated during clinical training [25]. 67.3% of medical students evaluated their LGBT-related curriculum as fair or worse, describing that they felt most comfortable addressing HIV (78.5%) and sexually transmitted infections (68.9%) and least on transition-related care of transgender individuals (28.0%) [26]. A 2014 article in the American Journal of Public Health suggested that students who were given just 2 h of instruction on transgender health during their family medicine clerkship had more favorable attitudes and improved competency in transgender health [27]. Nevertheless, the study also reaffirmed prior understanding that, across the board, medical education continues to lack focused educational time toward addressing transgender health content.

It is critical that educators consider and measure the specific content of these courses, the methodology by which these courses are taught, and the impact on educational outcomes. All educational content should be current and evidence based. At present, there is a small but impactful body of literature examining the impact of transgender health curricula in medical schools.

Dr. Joshua Safer and colleagues have drawn more attention to teaching evidence-based transgender content. According to Safer, content should focus on the biologic evidence for a durable gender identity as an effective means of educating students about the etiology of gender identity and the appropriateness of cross-sex hormones as a treatment for transgender patients. In his 2016 Endocrine Practice article, he describes his study where first year medical students at Boston University were exposed to content regarding the biologic evidence for the durability of gender identity and the use of cross-sex hormone therapy as a legitimate treatment option for transgender patients. Responses to a questionnaire were assessed prior to and following exposure of this content. The addition of this content to the medical school curriculum was found to increase the students understanding of these topics [28]. In a similar study by Safer and colleagues, second year students at Boston University were given a pathophysiology course regarding the rigidity of gender identity, treatment regimens, and monitoring requirements. All medical students received an online, anonymous questionnaire one month prior and one month after receiving this course. The questionnaire asked about predicted comfort using hormones to treat transgender individuals. The views of second year students were compared to views of students not exposed to this new curriculum. Exposure of students to this content was associated with a significant increase in the students' self-reported willingness to care for transgender patients [29]. The successful results toward improving knowledge, skills, and attitude in medical students have also been replicated for resident physicians [30]. Park and Safer at the Boston University School of Medicine have shown that clinical exposure to transgender medicine improves student confidence and competency in transgender health more than instructional teaching on its own [31]. Ultimately, gaps in medical school curricula and opportunities for intervention have not been studied and reported systematically or sufficiently, much less knowledge gaps and opportunities to intervene among practicing physicians [32].

Due to the increased awareness that no standardized curricula existed to guide medical schools in adequately administering vital training, the Association of American Medical Colleges convened an advisory committee, comprised of students and faculty, on sexual orientation, gender identity, and sex development in 2012 and, shortly after in 2014, published *Implementing Curricular and Institutional Climate Changes to Improve Health Care Individuals Who are LGBT, Gender Nonconforming, or Born with DSD: A Resource for Medical Educators*. In efforts to empower institutions to take charge of curricular content, the document builds recommendations for institutions to assess and create their own programming on top of eight professional competency domains: patient care, knowledge for practice, practice-based learning and improvement, interpersonal and communication skills, professionalism, systems-based practice, inter-professional collaboration, and personal and professional development [15]. They also propose the idea of "structural competency," which emphasizes the recognition of upstream forces beyond individual and interpersonal interactions, like stigma and inequality, in achieving and sustaining health [33]. Current and future providers must cultivate both professional and structural competency in order to alleviate health disparities and provide quality care.

In recent years, many educational initiatives at medical institutions, including the AAMC's advisory committee, have arisen out of student-led curricular reform and student-faculty partnerships. In 2009, student leaders at the University of California, San Francisco came together under the guidance of Dr. Madeline B. Deutsch to develop a pioneering 10-session course and formally assess the impact of the curriculum. Because of the course, knowledge surrounding topics such as medication management related to gender affirmation, practices for collecting data on gender identity, and federal policies that impact transgender health significantly increased. In addition, scores related to transphobic attitudes significantly decreased using a validated nine-item scale [34]. Today, this elective, which can serve as a model for other institutions looking to expand their programming in a substantial and meaningful way, attracts over 250 participants at the institution [35]. At Case Western Reserve University School of Medicine in Cleveland, OH, four student leaders designed a mandatory session for first years at Case Western Reserve University School of Medicine, which included a student presentation, a patient panel, and a small-group session that together totaled 2 h. Student knowledge and confidence in providing care were assessed pre- and post-session using anonymous student-generated identifiers. The course assessment showed improvement in both, demonstrating that the introduction of transgender medicine content early into a medical school curriculum can significantly impact medical student clinical development [36]. More recently, the Icahn School at Mount Sinai became first academic institution to offer advanced fellowships in transgender health in the divisions of psychiatry and plastic surgery. Mount Sinai also offers a structured transgender health elective for medical students, allowing them to rotate with internists, surgeons and mental health providers engaged in transgender care.

The AAMC's *Implementing Curricular and Institutional Climate Changes to Improve Health Care Individuals Who are LGBT, Gender Nonconforming, or Born with DSD: A Resource for Medical Educators* provides supportive guidelines and role description for more effective trainee–faculty–administrative partnership and collaboration. Trainees can and should support curriculum change by taking on advocacy and research projects with a reasonable, narrow, and specific question; faculty can structurally identify barriers for inclusion, think thoroughly about implementation, and support students in their own medical education projects; and finally, administrators can enforce an inclusive climate by supporting internal and external partnerships [15].

Successful curricular change only comes alongside an inclusive climate. Unfortunately, a recent study from the Stanford Lesbian, Gay, Bisexual, and Transgender Medical Education Research Group found that among 5812 respondents at 176 medical schools in the United States and Canada, 29.5% of sexual minorities conceal their sexual identity in medical school and a staggering 60% concealed their gender identity; moreover, up to 43.5% of respondents cited fear of discrimination in medical school as their reason for concealing [37]. According to the AAMC's guidelines, institutional climate should be evaluated across five major categories: efforts to educate, protections against mistreatment, promotion of equality, leadership and commitment, and having a welcoming patient care environment. With efforts in improving institutional climate, efforts at equity are more fully realized.

References

1. Wiley K, Knudson G, Khan SI, et al. Serving transgender people: clinical care considerations and service delivery models in transgender health. Lancet. 2016;388:401–11.
2. Safer JD, Coleman E, Feldman J, et al. Barriers to healthcare for transgender individuals. Curr Opin Endocrinol Diabetes Obes. 2016;23:168–71.
3. Institute of Medicine Committee on Lesbian, Gay, Bisexual, and Transgender Health Issues and Research Gaps and Opportunities. The health of lesbian, gay, bisexual, and transgender people: building a foundation for better understanding. Washington, DC: National Academic Press; 2011.
4. Winter S, Diamond M, Green J, et al. Transgender people: health at the margins of society. Lancet. 2016;388:390–400.
5. Meyerowitz JJ. How sex changed: a history of transsexuality in the United States. Cambridge, MA: Harvard University Press; 2002.
6. Susan S, Stephen W. The transgender studies reader. New York: Routledge; 2006.
7. White Hughto JM, Reisner SL, Pachankis JE. Transgender stigma and health: a critical review of stigma determinants, mechanisms, and interventions. Soc Sci Med. 2015;147:222–31.
8. APA. Diagnostic and statistical manual of mental disorders: DSM V. Washington, DC: American Psychiatric Publishing; 2013.
9. APA. Diagnostic and statistical manual of mental disorders: DSM II. Washington, DC: American Psychiatric Publishing; 1968.
10. Stroumsa D. The state of transgender health care: policy, law, and medical frameworks. Am J Public Health. 2014;104:31–8.
11. Drescher J. Queer diagnoses revisited: the past and future of homosexuality and gender diagnoses in DSM and ICD. Int Rev Psychiatry. 2015;27:386–95.
12. World Professional Association for Transgender Health. Standards of care for the health of transsexual, transgender, and gender nonconforming people. 7th version. World Professional Association for Transgender Health; 2012.
13. Flores AR, Herman JL, Gates GJ, et al. How many adults identify as transgender in the United States? Los Angeles. CA: The Williams Institute; 2016.
14. Lambda Legal. When health care isn't caring: Lambda Legal's survey on discrimination against LGBT peopled people living with HIV; 2009.
15. Hollenbach AD, Eckstrand KL, Dreger AD. Implementing curricular and institutional climate changes to improve health care for individuals who are LGBT, gender nonconforming, or born with DSD: a resource for medical educators. Washington DC: Association of American Medical Colleges; 2014.

16. James SE, Herman JL, Rankin S, et al. The report of the 2015 US transgender survey. Washington, DC: National Center for Transgender Equality; 2016.
17. Grant JM, Tanis J, Herman JL, et al. National transgender discrimination survey report on health and health care. Washington, DC: National Center for Transgender Equality and the National Gay and Lesbian Task Force; 2010.
18. Vogel L. Screening programs may overlook transgender people. CMAJ. 2014;186.
19. Murad MH, Elamin MB, Garcia M, et al. Hormonal therapy and sex reassignment: a systematic review and meta-analysis of quality of life and psychosocial outcomes. Clin Endocrinol. 2010;72:214–31.
20. Sonnenblick EB, Shah AD, Goldstein Z, Reisman T. Breast imaging of transgender individuals: a review. Curr Radiol Rep. 2018;6:1.
21. Davidge-Pitts C, Nippoldt TB, Danoff A, et al. Transgender health in endocrinology: current status of endocrinology fellowship programs and practicing clinicians. J Clin Endocrinol Metab. 2017;102(4):1286–90.
22. Unger CA. Care of the transgender patient: a survey of gynecologists' current knowledge and practice. J Women's Health. 2015;24:114–8.
23. Radix AE, Lelutiu-Weinberger C, Gamarel KE. Satisfaction and healthcare utilization of transgender and gender non-conforming individuals in NYC: a community-based participatory study. LGBT Health. 2014;1:302–8.
24. Shindel A, Baazeeem A, Eardley I, et al. Sexual health in undergraduate medical education: existing and future needs and platforms. J Sex Med. 2016;13:1013–26.
25. Obedin-Maliver J, Goldsmith ES, Steward L, et al. Lesbian, gay, bisexual, and transgender-related content in undergraduate medical education. JAMA. 2011;306:971–7.
26. White W, Brenman S, Paradis E, et al. Lesbian, gay, bisexual, and transgender patient care: medical students' preparedness and comfort. Teach Learn Med. 2015;27:254–63.
27. Dowshen N, Nguyen GT, Gilber K, et al. Improving transgender health education for future doctors. Am J Public Health. 2014;104:e5–6.
28. Eriksson SE, Safer JD. Evidence-based curricular content improves student knowledge and changes attitudes towards transgender medicine. Endocr Pract. 2016;22:837–41.
29. Safer JD, Pearce EN. A simple curriculum content change increased medical student comfort with transgender medicine. Endocr Pract. 2013;19:633–7.
30. Thomas DD, Safer JD. A simple intervention raised resident-physician willingness to assist transgender patients seeking hormone therapy. Endocr Pract. 2015;21:1134–42.
31. Park JA, Safer JD. Clinical exposure to transgender medicine improves students' preparedness above levels seen with didactic teaching alone: a key addition to the Boston University Model for teaching transgender healthcare. Transgender Health. 2018;3(1):10–6.
32. Safer JD. The large gaps in transgender medical knowledge among providers must be measured and addressed. Endocr Pract. 2016;22:902–3.
33. Donald C, DasGupta S, Metzl J, et al. Queer frontiers in medicine: a structural competency approach. Acad Med. 2017;92:345–50.
34. Braun HM, Garcia-Grossman IR, Quiñones-Rivera A, et al. Outcome and impact evaluation of a transgender health course of health profession students. LGBT Health. 2017;4:55–61.
35. Braun HM, Ramirez D, Zahner GJ, et al. The LGBTQI health forum: an innovative inter professional initiative to support curricular reform. Med Educ Online. 2017;22(1):1306419.
36. Grosz AM, Gutierrez D, Lui AA, et al. A student-led introduction to lesbian, gay, bisexual, and transgender health for first-year medical students. Fam Med. 2017;49:52–6.
37. Mansh M, White W, Gee-Tong L, et al. Sexual and gender minority identity disclosure during undergraduate medical education: "in the closet" in medical school. Acad Med. 2015;90: 634–44.

Chapter 15
The Social Elements of TGNC's Individual's Journey to Living Authentically

Donna B. Riley

Introduction

The range of transgender experience is evolving in response to increased knowledge and understanding of what it means to be transgender or gender nonconforming (TGNC) in contemporary society. These shifts are related to the breakdown of the concept of gender as a binary consisting only of "male" or "female" gender designations. Now, many leading scholars and activists acknowledge the concept of gender as a continuum of experiences that may be fluid over time [1–3] as well as an emerging positive shift in social and cultural attitudes and support for TGNC individuals. The purpose of this chapter is to discuss the social process of TGNC individuals' journey to living authentically in their self-identified gender. It would be negligent of me to omit the excessive risk of stigmatization and oppression experienced by TGNC community members. In addition to other scholars, I will include quotes and data from my study entitled *Lost and Found: Transgender Elders' Journey Toward Authenticity* [4].

Disparate Risk

For many years, social psychological research has examined the social dynamics of intergroup relations, stigmatizing beliefs and discriminatory behavior. Just as the definition of "stigma" has been increasingly attributed to social processes, models of the adverse effects of stigma have emphasized its social origins. A number of models have been proposed based on the analysis of stigma toward minority groups across a wide variety of settings, e.g., the mentally ill [5–7], transgender people

D. B. Riley (✉)
School of Social Welfare, Stony Brook University, Stony Brook, NY, USA
e-mail: donna.riley@stonybrook.edu

L. Poretsky and W. C. Hembree (eds.), *Transgender Medicine*, Contemporary Endocrinology, https://doi.org/10.1007/978-3-030-05683-4_15

[8, 9], and people who identify as homosexual [10–12]. It is beyond the scope of this analysis to review the effect of stigma on all marginalized people. It is essential, however, to highlight that studies reveal the significant impact of stigma on mental health and quality of life of each affected party [13–15].

One of the primary models of stigma focuses on the "justification of the status quo", which concentrates on psychological processes that contribute to the preservation of existing personal and social arrangements that result in stigma [16]. As asserted by Watson et al. [17] "psychological justification offers a motivational model of the processes that comprise stigma; namely, that stereotypes, prejudice, and discrimination serve the individual, group, or social goals" [17].

Focusing on the psychological justification of stigma, three models have emerged from the literature: ego-justification, group-justification, and system-justification [16]. Ego-justification occurs when "…individuals stereotype because it justifies their personal status or conduct in relation to others. This assumption that stereotypes serve to justify the behavior of individuals figured prominently in the early social psychological literature" [18]. Tajfel [19] expanded the initial ego-justification hypothesis to the level of intergroup relations, which emphasize the degree to which the in-group consolidates itself in order to distinguish itself from other groups. Lastly, system-justification "…designates any motivational tendency to defend, bolster, or rationalize existing social, economic, and political arrangements…System justification is an inherently conservative inclination to preserve "the way things are"" [20].

Given the large number of stigmatized corporations that exist in any given society, some tries have been made to supply classifications or taxonomies of stigmatization of these groups. Goffman [21] categorized the stigmatized into three major groups, along with "abominations of the body" (e.g., the bodily disabled), "tribal identities" (e.g., race, gender, religion, or nationality), and "blemishes of person character" (e.g., alcoholism, intellectual illness, unemployment, or homosexuality).

Taking Goffman's work a step further, Jones et al. [22] proposed six interdependent dimensions that individuals use to describe stigmas. As outlined by Dovidio et al. [23], these include the first dimension, "conceivability," or the extent to which the stigmatizing characteristic is necessarily visible (e.g., facial disfigurement vs. transsexuality). The second dimension, "course of the mark," relates to whether the mark may become more salient or progressively debilitating over time (e.g., HIV/AIDS vs. blindness). The third dimension, "disruptiveness," is the degree to which the stigmatizing characteristic (e.g., stuttering) interferes with the flow of interpersonal interactions. The fourth dimension, "aesthetics," is subjective reactions to the unattractiveness of the stigma. The fifth dimension is the "origin" of the stigmatizing mark (such as congenital, accidental, or intentional), which can also involve the person's responsibility for creating the mark. The final dimension is identified as "peril," which involves the perceived danger of the stigmatizing conditions by others (e.g., having a highly contagious, lethal disease vs. being overweight). These dimensions have potential consequences for how we react to and differentiate among various stigmas [24].

Crocker, Major, and Steele focused on "visibility" and "controllability" as the most important dimensions of stigma, because they are apparent and readily obvious to the observer, and to the individuals themselves: "the stigma can provide the primary schema through which everything about them is understood by others" [25]. About the experience of transgender persons, "visibility" is understood as the ability of the MTF transgender person to "pass" as female versus members of heteronormative society's ability to clock[1] MTF transgender people as inauthentic females. Visibility may determine the extent to which transgender people are denigrated, discredited, and construed as invalid relative to heteronormative individuals.

The concept of "controllability" related to stigma involves the person's responsibility for being stigmatized in the first place [23]. This component of stigma is vital in this discussion because it centers around the causation debate; people whose stigmas are perceived to be controllable (i.e., to be a choice) face higher levels of delegitimization and prejudice than those whose stigmas are perceived to be uncontrollable [24]. For example, lay theories about the etiology of transsexualism may significantly affect an individual's stigmatizing attitude toward transgender people. Those who hold psychological theories that transgender identity is a pathology or a mental illness may treat transgender people with higher levels of stigmatization and delegitimization. Conversely, those who hold biological, theories, where sexual differentiation is seen as biologically based might not perceive transgender people as mentally ill or as aberrations of fundamental human nature.

Internalized Stigma/Transphobia

The adverse effects of stigma and labeling have been discussed in the psychological and sociological literature [21, 22]. For example, stigmatization is related to adverse effects on self-esteem, employment, and social acceptance [24]. Goffman [21] discusses the anxiety with which the stigmatized individual approaches interactions in society. Such an individual "may perceive, usually quite correctly, that whatever others profess, they do not really 'accept' him and are not ready to make contact with him on equal grounds" [21]. Sullivan explains that "the fear that others can disrespect a person because of something he shows means that he is always insecure in his contact with other people; and this insecurity arises…from something which he knows he cannot fix" [26].

Similarly, Allport [27] describes "vigilance" as one of the traits used by oppressed individuals to develop defensive strategies to manage their minority status. This concept helps explain the stressful effects of stigma. A high level of socially accepted stigma by the dominant culture leads minority group members to maintain a high degree of vigilance (expectations of rejection, discrimination,

[1]Clock: to be recognized as transgender, defined by research respondents (Riley, 2015).

and violence) about the minority component of their identity in interactions with dominant group members. By definition, such cautiousness is perpetual in that it is over and over again and constantly evoked in the regular daily existence of the minority individual. This cautiousness is upsetting as it requires the effort of extensive vitality and assets in adjusting to this treatment [27]. Hetrick and Martin [28] describe "wanting to hide" as the most common coping strategy for lesbian adolescents and note that individuals in such a position must consistently monitor their behaviors in all circumstances; how they dress, speak, walk, and talk becomes a constant source of possible discovery. Hiding behaviors are employed to cloak the minority identity, and the result is internalized stress.

Minority Stress Theory

Like members of other stigmatized minority groups, transgender individuals must contend with negative societal attitudes and stigma. This stigma as a psychosocial stress is derived from minority status [29–31]. Consistent with social stress discourse [31] and the evidence of social causality of distress [32], researchers propose that such stress leads to adverse mental health outcomes.

The concept of minority stress is not based on one theory but is gleaned from several social and psychological theoretical frameworks. In general, minority stress can be described as related to the juxtaposition of minority and dominant values and the resulting conflict of the social environment experienced by minority group members [31]. Lazarus and Folkman [33] describe such a conflict between individuals and their experience of society as the essence of all social stress. Several theories describe alienation and incongruence between individual needs and social structures [34, 35]. Indeed, when a minority individual exists in a stigmatizing and discriminating society, the conflict between that person and the dominant culture can be onerous and the stress significant.

Social comparison theory provides a different additional perspective on the origin of stress. These theories view the social environment as endowing people with meaning to their world and organization to their experiences [36]. Negative regard from others, therefore, leads to negative self-regard [37] and adverse mental health outcomes [38].

Societal reaction theory directly addresses the effects of stigma and negative social attitudes on stigmatized individuals. According to societal reaction theory, deviance may lead to labeling and adverse societal reaction. Bettcher states, "If a person is subjected to discrimination or violence because this person is taken to violate gender norms, perhaps because the person is wearing a dress, this is no doubt because the person is being transphobically viewed as a man" [39]. As a consequence of negative societal reactions, stigmatized individuals develop adaptive responses that may include mental health symptoms.

Transphobia/Transprejudice

It is crucial for our discussion to present the conceptual model of transgender discrimination, described by King et al. [40] as "transprejudice." I propose that transprejudice is the most appropriate approach for conceptualizing the culturally influenced belief structures surrounding gender nonconformity in the United States for TGNC individuals. The respondents in Riley [4] consisted of individuals from the baby boomer generation. Respondents' life narratives exhibited vast social change toward the trans community during their lifetime. Further, Riley [4] included a definition of transprejudice that describes not only the evolving social climate for the participants' lives but also the effect of this prejudice on the TGNC individuals' self-perception or internalized transphobia.

Scholars agree on the destructiveness of homophobia, genderism, and sexism [41–45]. Sexual stigma, sexual prejudice, heterosexism, and their attitudinal and behavioral corollaries (stigma, prejudice, intolerance, and discrimination) are perennial experiences of some subgroups of society. The previous section has provided a conceptual framework for analyzing anti-transgender attitudes and beliefs.

In American society, transgender people encounter medical pathologization, social stigmatization, and legal delegitimization of their identities, behaviors, and indeed, their lives. As a consequence of their cross-gender identification or behavior, they suffer prejudice and discrimination on both personal and institutional levels. In the United States, transgender people are excluded from specific legal and civil protections that are readily available to non-transgender persons and even other protected classes. Currah and Minter make the observation that "[f]or the most part, transgender people have not been excluded from civil rights protections because of conceptual or philosophical failures in legal reasoning, but rather because they have not been viewed as worthy of protection or, in some cases, even as human" [46]. Now, through the growing understanding of the prejudice and oppression that TGNC individuals face, the increasing visibility of the TGNC community has consequentially affected the social concept of gender and the social representation of trans people.

Day-to-Day Needs, Barriers, and Resources

Housing, Employment, and Income Instability

Scheim and Bauer [47] conducted a study which revealed an alarming economic disparity between TGNC respondents and the U.S. population. At the time of the study, 29% of TGNC respondents were living below the national poverty level, compared to the national average of 12%. Upon further examination, they found that TGNC respondents were unemployed by three times the national unemployment rate at the time, which was 5%, presenting at a staggering 15%. The same study cited only 16% of the respondents owning a home, while the national average was 63%. Lastly, the study found that 30% of the respondents were homeless at some point in their lifetime.

Mandated Healthcare Inclusion

As of 2018, there have been some definitive advances in how individual states address the issue of insurance discrimination against TGNC people. Colorado, Hawaii, Illinois, and Pennsylvania ban insurance exclusions for transgender health care. California, Connecticut, Delaware, the District of Columbia, Maryland, Massachusetts, Minnesota, Nevada, New Jersey, New York, Oregon, Rhode Island, and Vermont ban insurance exclusions for transgender health care and provide health benefits for state employees that include transgender care [48].

Over 25% of Fortune 500 companies have also followed suit, as well as cities such as Berkeley and San Francisco. States such as California also outline an appeals process for individuals whose claims are denied. The following is from a bulletin California recently issued:

> [California law] prohibits health plans from discriminating against individuals because of the individual's gender, including gender identity or gender expression. [...] If a health plan denies an individual's request for services on the basis that the services are not medically necessary or that the services do not meet the health plan's utilization management criteria, the health plan's decision is subject to review through the Department's Independent Medical Review (IMR) process. [...] The Department directs health plans to revise all current health plan documents to remove benefit and coverage exclusions and limitations related to gender transition services. [49]

At present, the majority of private insurance plans include coverage exclusions aimed explicitly at denying TGNC people the ability to access treatment or procedures associated with transitioning—also known as sexual reassignment [50]. Additionally, insurance plans often exclude coverage of healthcare services for TGNC individuals that would have otherwise been covered, had the person in question not been TGNC. These services can include behavioral health, medical, and surgical procedures. Often, insurance providers' exclusionary clause is justified on the basis that the treatment is not medically necessary, but rather viewed as a cosmetic procedure. Therefore, the TGNC person's claim is consequently denied when it may otherwise have been covered for treatment not related to gender identity [50]. This exclusion ignores all existing research on TGNC people that demonstrates the profound challenges faced by individuals whose natal sex is incompatible with their gender identity including depression, elevated risk of suicide, divorce, and difficulties at work [51].

Furthermore, TGNC-inclusive health care is sometimes provided more exclusively on a city-by-city basis. This was the case in San Francisco when its innovative healthcare program for city residents removed the exclusion for TGNC care within the last few years. Most recently, the city of Philadelphia passed an

LGBT-inclusive healthcare bill that provides incentives to businesses that offer or expand this type of insurance coverage for their employees. The bill includes two credits, one of which focuses exclusively on offering coverage to employees for TGNC care [52].

According to the Corporate Equality Index 2018 reported by the Human Rights Campaign (HRC) [53], 58% of Fortune 500 companies offer their employees health insurance that is inclusive of TGNC-related medical costs [48]. TGNC advocates are concerned that insurance companies in states where bulletins have recently been mandated may continue to deny medical procedures, requiring individuals to endure a potentially lengthy appeals process to have their claims approved. As more and more states and cities clarify their laws concerning TGNC care, the chances of this happening will likely be reduced. Approaches to TGNC health care and health insurance coverage have certainly improved over the past few years, but there is still a long road ahead to ensuring that all 50 states provide adequate nondiscrimination coverage to trans and gender nonconforming residents.

Perception of Medical and Mental Health Providers

Austin and Goodman [54] conducted a study of the TGNC community's perception of medical and mental health providers. The findings were consistent with Riley's [4] respondents in that they reported difficulty in locating knowledgeable and supportive medical and mental health providers. In Austin and Goodman's [55], the study included 65 TGNC respondents; 24% reported that finding a supportive endocrinologist did not apply to them. Of the remaining 49 respondents, 42% had difficulty finding a knowledgeable and experienced TGNC endocrinologist. For 44 of the TGNC respondents seeking surgeons for TGNC-specific care, 33% had trouble accessing surgeons with TGNC-specific knowledge. Austin and Goodman also discovered that:

> [w]hile finding a knowledgeable primary care physician was less problematic for participants, with more than half (53%) reporting that it was easy to access a knowledgeable primary care physician ... 53% struggled to access a primary care provider perceived to be supportive of transgender people. [55], p. 24

Policy Implications

Scholars agree that the barriers to healthy living among TGNC people have significant policy implications [4, 56]. These studies illuminate prejudice and discrimination against the TGNC community at individual and institutional levels. Individual discrimination may be directed and interpersonal or indirect and impersonal. Institutional discrimination occurs when the practices, rules, benefits, and policies that apply to heteronormative men and women do not exist for TGNC people.

Anti-discrimination Laws

The findings in Riley [4] demonstrate the need for the enactment of anti-discrimination legislation in the United States inclusive of transgender individuals; they will provide support for the implementation of protective legislation for sexual orientation and the gender identity minority population. One must be keenly aware of the criticism that legislation will not change societal attitudes or indeed be considered a solution to reducing or eliminating discrimination based on sexual orientation or gender identity. However, legislative protection of equal rights is a potentially useful instrument for social change, specifically regarding the threat of legal action taken against those who commit discriminatory acts.

The Employment Non-Discrimination Act (ENDA) would provide basic protections against workplace discrimination on the basis of sexual orientation or gender identity (Case, 2014). ENDA affords essential employment protection to all Americans from discrimination based on irrational prejudice. This bill would accompany the existing civil rights laws, including Title VII of the Civil Rights Act of 1964 and the Americans with Disabilities Act. "The bill explicitly prohibits preferential treatment and quotas and does not permit disparate impact suits…[I]t exempts small businesses, religious organizations, and the military and does not require that domestic partner benefits be provided to the same-sex partners of employees" [57]. Nonetheless, the Employment Non-Discrimination Act (ENDA) should be enacted in concert with both school-based and educational interventions aimed at providing the appropriate information related to human diversity and civil rights, both of which are currently lacking in the United States.

Social Representation Theory

Social Representation Theory (SRT) addresses both social products and processes. As a product, social representation is defined as a widely shared set of beliefs—a systematic framework for evaluating events. As a process, social representation is the entirety of the activity (including communications, exchange, and argumentation) in which individuals and groups engage to make sense of their changing physical selves and their environment [58]. SRT addresses the social construct of meaning, and how society explains phenomena in the sociocultural environment. It theorizes the way in which society creates models, narratives, rhetoric, and arguments that interpret or make sense of new information. Social representations are ever evolving [39].

Connell [59] explains that the social interactions of multiple individuals generate social representations, creating an evolution of a widely shared set of beliefs. For this reason, as transgender visibility increases, societal understanding begins to adopt diversity and inclusiveness of the trans community. With this visibility, the social representation of "transgender" allows other trans people that are passing as their natal sex to begin to see new options for personal identity development.

In terms of the trans experience, the individual's perception of themselves and society plays heavily into the identities of marginalized minorities. Riley [4] demonstrates that within invisible minorities, as the transgender community has often been described by scholars [60–62], the digital age has given rise to multiple new options and opportunities for trans people to recognize, explore, and validate their identities. Through increased exposure to diverse people, ideologies, and experiences, advancements in technology have facilitated a change in the social representation of trans people at an exponential rate.

As an example, in Riley [4], Bridget described transitioning from presenting as her natal sex to her core identity twice, first in 1990 and the second time in 2012. She illustrated the difference between her expectations in 1990 versus 2012; the positive sociocultural changes within the transgender community shifted her expectations of transitioning. She recalled that in her 2012 transition, the visibility of the trans-identified community validated her identity as a transwoman. This experience was in contrast to her first transition, when she expected to ultimately transition to female, erasing her previous identity.

Social Identity Integration Theory

To examine how social identities develop and become integrated, it is essential to explain how they are organized cognitively within the self. Researchers view the self as a multifaceted cognitive structure [63, 64] that can be defined as "a collection of at least semi-related and highly domain-specific knowledge structures" [65]. The concept of "self" corresponds with the answer to the question "Who am I?" Although social identities deal specifically with group memberships, they can also be perceived as one specific type of self-component comprising the global self (Deaux, 1991). Social identity can be defined as "that part of the individual's self-concept which derives from his or her knowledge of membership to a social group (or groups) together with the value and the emotional significance attached to it" [19].

Amiot et al. [66] developed a four-stage model of social identity development and integration of the self. In the following pages, I adapt their theory to apply to the TGNC community (see Fig. 15.1). The first stage represents an anticipatory phase that initiates the process of identity integration. This stage takes place before one encounters a change in life and before any actual contact with a new social group. The second stage of their model is categorization. In this stage, group members are confronted with an actual change in their lives and with the existence of a new social group. The third stage, compartmentalization, accounts for the development of social identities. At this stage, the multiplicity of an individual's old and new social identities becomes recognized more explicitly as he or she identifies with different social groups and realizes that he or she belongs to these various groups. This stage occurs as group members have increased contact with members of other groups and as different social identities are activated simultaneously.

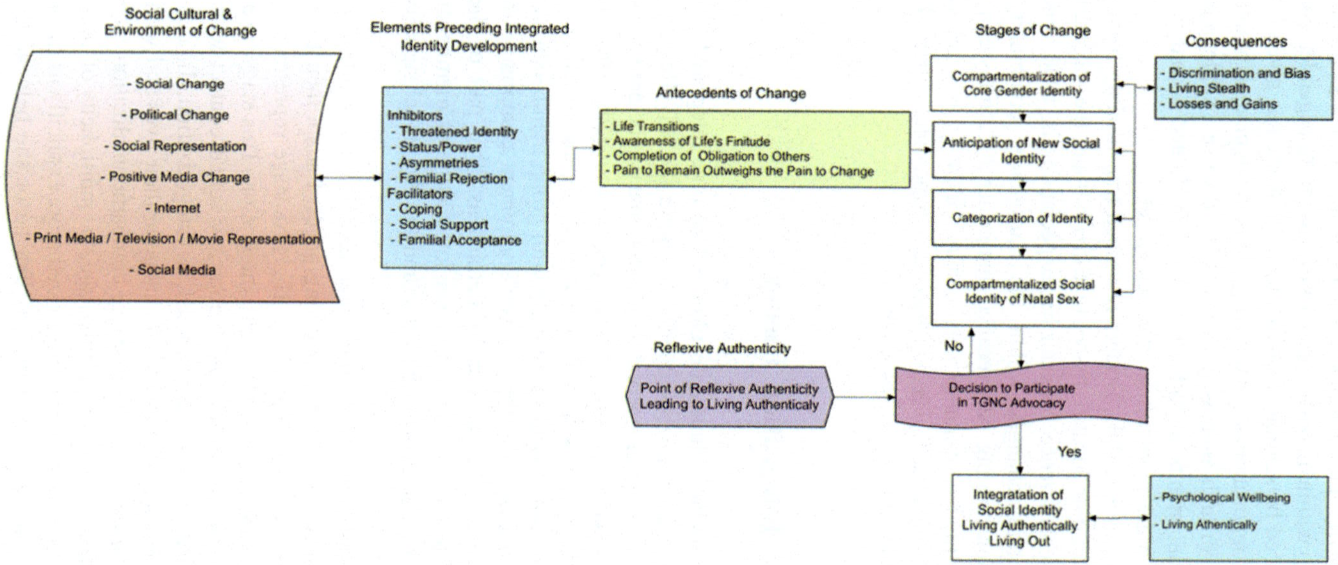

Fig. 15.1 Conceptual framework of reflexive authenticity

The fourth stage is integration. At this stage, individuals come to recognize that multiple and distinct social identities are simultaneously crucial to their self.

Adapting this model to the TGNC community, I identified a second compartmentalized social identity stage before the final stage: integration of social identity. This second compartmentalized social identity generally occurs in social transition. In this stage, the TGNC member is often concerned that if others are aware of their pronounced birth gender, it would spoil their new gender identity.

The Social Transition of TGNC Individuals

The following conceptual model will serve as a representation of the process. Each stage will then be explained further.

Conceptual Framework

Stages of Initial Awareness

Early Awareness

It is common for TGNC individuals to describe the dominant theme of early awareness as "feeling different" or that "something was wrong"; but, at these early ages, they lacked the verbal capacity to articulate their feelings of discomfort. A vast majority indicate that these feelings emerged between the ages of 4 and 7 years. Many elder members of the TGNC community recall reading the story of Christine Jorgenson which put words and concepts into their abstract feelings. Suddenly, they could describe their internal conflict. Gagne et al. [67] identify this conflict as *emergence*. This awareness gives rise to the exploration of internal gender identity through events such as cross-dressing or revealing gender identity to others. These behaviors often lead to extreme negative feedback from family members or authority figures.

Negative Feedback

The majority of TGNC individuals describe experiencing negative feedback from parents or authority figures in reaction to their attempts at authentic gender expression, which they perceived as a threat to their core gender identity [4]. Early awareness of gender identity and expression leads to compartmentalization of the core identity to protect the threatened identity.

Stage 1: Compartmentalization of Core Gender Identity

A "threat" cannot be adequately characterized by its form or type alone. The definition of a threat in this case must be derived from its effect on a person's identity. Breakwell defines the threat to identity as follows: "A threat to identity occurs when the process of identity, assimilation-accommodation, and evaluation are, for some reason, unable to comply with the principles of continuity, distinctiveness, and self-esteem, which habitually guide their operation" [68]. In other words, when a person's core identity is threatened, TGNC members will monitor their verbal, nonverbal, and visual cues to protect the yet emerged authentic identity.

Coping with Threatened Identity

Breakwell [68] states that on an interpersonal level, there are some identifiable interpersonal action strategies used when faced with threats to identity. She describes the four interpersonal coping mechanisms as (1) isolation "The individual occupying the threatening position seeks to minimize its impact by isolating himself or herself from other people" [68], (2) negativism: "…entails the opposite tactic [to isolation]: it involves the outright conflict with anyone who would challenge the identity structure" [68], (3) passing: "… totally convert, and normally occurs where the characteristics which identify the threatening position are easily hidden or erased" [68], and (4) compliance: "… accepting the behavioral prescriptions associated with the threatening position; living up to expectations [of the threatened identity]" [68].

Passing as One's Natal Sex. Many TGNC community members initially use *passing as one's natal sex*, as a coping mechanism to protect their threatened internal transgender identity. This coping mechanism is used, for example, when a male-to-female transgender person (MTF) individual endeavors to pass as male out of fear that their TGNC identity will be discovered. Moreover, the vast majority also employ *isolation* during different periods in their lives to cope with their threatened TGNC identity.

Interpersonal strategies are those that rely on "changing relationships with others to cope with the threat" such as self-isolation and passing. Passing as one's natal sex necessitates building personas and lives that others expect of them, including marital relationships [68]. Also, TGNC individuals often purposely self-isolate before transitioning and report intentionally having few friends out of fear that others might see through their constructed and false natal sex personas [4].

Making the Decision to Transition

In recent studies of transgender elders, three themes emerged from the data from the respondents: (1) feeling ready to transition after fulfilling the obligation to others, (2) the pain to remain outweighing the pain to change, and (3) awareness of life's finitude [4].

Feeling Ready to Transition After Fulfilling Obligation to Others

The majority of middle-age TGNC individuals speak of waiting to transition out of obligation to others, such as nuclear families and families of origin. In this way, they could also keep their careers intact for financial security. Scholars discuss the coping processes for emotional experiences at different stages of the gender transitioning process [4, 69]. In a recent study, Riley [4] reported that "responsibility to others" was significant in the respondents waiting to transition. Similarly, the respondents in the present study specifically used "obligation to others," as a standard phrase.

Many TGNC elders explain that having fulfilled their obligations to others, they then felt able to care for themselves. When the respondents relayed events such as retiring from a long-time career, being widowed, or launching their adult children, their experience was coded as "obligation to others fulfilled."

Pain to Remain Outweighs the Pain to Change

Often TGNC individuals report that their increasing emotional pain, depression, and hopelessness drove them to realize that life without transitioning was not worth the pain. Beyond the sense of fulfillment of obligations, many of the respondents also spoke of the psychological pain of passing as their natal sex [4]. This pain led to increased depression and in four cases, suicide attempts. Breakwell [68] discusses the double-edged sword of passing, while it may help individuals gain the social status of the persona presented, "… [T]he consequence of the enactment of fraud cannot be underestimated. The person who passes must live a lie. This has psychological implications. Further, the passer lives with the continual fear of discovery and exposure" [68]. Respondents spoke of the increasing sense of urgency to transition as they age. They reported it was too painful to continue living a lie.

Awareness of Life's Finitude

> Human activities are essentially oriented toward the future; when we select a particular goal or course of action, we assume that our future self will experience the expected or anticipated outcomes. When our future becomes uncertain, it makes naturally less sense to defer gratifications and forgo an immediate advantage for some future benefit. [70]

Personal goals are described as future-oriented representations of what individuals strive for in possible life achievements [71]. TGNC elder individuals often speak of their awareness of their fading life reserve; they felt an urgency to work toward the lifetime goal of living as their authentic selves and subsequently transitioned. In my clinical practice working with TGNC patients, these same issues arise, regardless of age. However, the late age of transition for some of these individuals underscores the importance of emotional pain that TGNC people endure: hiding and delaying their transition for, on average, four decades. These patients explain that continuing to live their remaining years presenting as their natal sex was unimaginable; thinking about it would only exacerbate their depression. TGNC individuals transitioning later in life often relay that before deciding to transition, they did not care for their physical body. After transitioning, their mind and body matched. They then felt renewed to care for themselves. In Riley [4] Natalie, a 62-year-old transwoman used the phrase, "rebirth at 62." She went on to detail how this complete self-acceptance gave her hope and energy to live authentically into her elder years. She was among nineteen transgender elders who defined successful aging as "living authentically." Many of the respondents spoke about making up for lost time and living life to the fullest. For example, some spoke of a "bucket list," and others spoke of finding meaning in their lives [4].

As this awareness set in, respondents moved into the anticipation stage, by seeking information about what transitioning might be like. Further, information-seeking now included professional resources to begin a physical and emotional transition. Deciding to transition leads to anticipatory identity. Whether TGNC individuals are dealing with their gender dysphoria in their teens or later in life, in coping with their threatened core identity, they decide to transition to their core identity.

Stage 2: Anticipation Phase

The internal awareness of gender identity and a new motive to create change led respondents to seek information. They wanted answers to a variety of questions: specifically, about how to go about transitioning from their natal sex to their core gender identity.

Amiot et al. [66] identify the anticipation stage of identity integration as a preparation stage. Indeed, all of the respondents spoke about seeking out transgender information early in their lives to confirm that they were not alone in their feelings of gender incongruity. Respondents sought venues where they could explore their authentic gender identity and gather the resources to transition, socially and medically. In discussing their developing awareness of possibilities, many respondents spoke of the historical timeline of the technological revolution.

Seeking Information Respondents' experience of personal "sense-making" changed over time. According to Dervin, personal sense-making is defined as "behavior, both internal (i.e., cognitive) and external (i.e., procedural), which allows the individual to construct and design his/her movements through time-space" [72]. TGNC persons express how they sought to meet their own informational needs. Before the Internet, it was challenging to identify available resources when they initially sought information to make sense of their internal gender feelings.

Through print media, television, and the Internet, respondents spoke of finding information and resources to aid in the process of self-acceptance. Further, changing media perspectives provided them with insights and mechanisms for reaching out to others—for testing the waters as they expressed (at first, tentatively and then, more boldly) their TGNC identity and their authentic selves. The TGNC community speaks of the impact of progressively changing social representation of the transgender community that rode on the coattails of the gay civil rights movement.

Transgender Support Groups
Forsman et al. [73] found that informal social contacts, such as family members and lifelong relationships between friends, affect the mental well-being of older adults. Well-being is enhanced due to shared life events, social support, mutual appreciation, trust, and a sense of belonging through everyday social activities.

All of the respondents in Riley [4] spoke of the importance of transgender support groups and how participation evoked a sense of belonging to the transgender community. All of the respondents in the integrated social identity (ISI) category spoke of the sense of belonging they had in their participation in transgender support groups/community activities. Participation in these groups gave rise to their future participation in trans advocacy. Respondents reported that transgender advocacy gave them a great sense of life meaning. As the respondents gained knowledge, support, and friendships through transgender support groups, they began to feel a "duty" to give back and "carry the torch." When participants felt they gained enough information from the support groups, they spoke of continuing to participate so they could help others find their way. Others recognized that their trans voice could help change policies and laws for trans people who remained closeted and fearful of coming out.

Lambert et al. [73] conducted four studies to explore the connection between belonging and meaning. All four of their studies elucidate the importance of relationships. They found that "social relationships promote the perception that life is meaningful and that relationships that promote a sense of belonging are especially likely to promote a belief that one's life is meaningful" [74]. Humans seem to have a biological need for social relationships [75]. Baumeister [76] contends that human beings have an inherent need to understand themselves as social beings in a larger society. One might expect, then, that a sense of meaning in life depends, at least in part, on a feeling of belonging. Numerous studies have indicated that individuals who report having found meaning in life also report more desirable perspectives and more positive perceptions of the world [77–79].

While respondents in Riley spoke about "personal meaning," they recognized that meaning itself is not solely personal, but rather culturally inclusive. When speaking of personal meaning, TGNC respondents understood the importance of cooperation to achieve a more substantial future cultural change for TGNC community human rights in America. Integrated social identity (ISI) respondents spoke of their fight for transgender rights and the possibilities for future trans equality [4]. They were all, currently or formerly, politically active and committed to building social and political acceptance of the transgender community.

Social Representation: An Identity-Shaping Social Context
Studies have supported the concept that societal change can have a significant impact on different aspects of one's social identity [74]. Furthermore, a growing

number of studies have provided evidence for the variations based on the societal change that occur in group members' social identities over time [80].

The respondents in Riley [4] detailed historical events that drove a cultural shift during their lives and how this shift impacted their self-perceptions. The following table is a historical representation of the TGNC cultural evolution that the respondents recognized as essential for the growth of the TGNC community (see Table 1).

Table 1 Historical timeline as related by the participants

Average birth year of participants: 1949	
1952—Christine Jorgenson news article	1950–1959
1965—Johns Hopkins: The first hospital in the nation to formally establish a sex change program 1966—Harry Benjamin's "Transsexual Phenomenon"—scientific proof 1967—*Christine Jorgenson: A Personal Autobiography* 1968—Hellfire Club 1968—Rachel Harlow article in *Philadelphia Magazine* 1969—Stonewall—Sylvia Rivera 1969—Lee Brewster opens Lee's Mardi Gras Boutique	1960–1969
1970s—Phil Donahue & Dinah Shore TV—FTM & MTF 1970—STAR: Transvestite Action Revolutionaries 1970—First NYC Pride Parade held: Trans people excluded 1971—Movie *Dr. Jekyll & Mrs. Hyde* 1971—Ed Sullivan Show: Jim Baily 1973—The *XX* (Twenty) Club established, supporting pre- and post-operative transsexuals 1973—Gigi's Gay Bar—Detroit 1975—Renee Richards 1977—Confide Group NJ 1978—Transgender Tapestry Magazine—Porn & Gay bookstores 1978—"Transgenderist" term—The "Transcendents" or "Trans" People, Virginia Prince	
Mid 1980s—Dial-up bulletin boards, magazine articles 1980s—CompuServe: the first online service provider in the United States. Precursor of AOL 1980—Version of Nancy Drew book, *The Clue in the Old Stagecoach*—a female character named George 1985—Stryker identifies 1985 as the beginning of the trans movement 1985—AOL Founded: May 24, 1985 1986—Night of A Thousand Gowns 1988—*The "Empire" Strikes Back: A Posttranssexual Manifesto*, by Sandy Stone 1988—Tri-Ess on the *Phil Donahue Show* 1989—NYC Gender Identity Project and Survivors of Transsexuality Anonymous founded	1980–1989
1991—Gazebo: AOL Chatroom 1992–2001—The Vault, S & M club 1992—*Crying Game* movie normalizes trans people	1990–1999

(continued)

Table 1 (continued)

Average birth year of participants: 1949	
1993—Mustang Sally's Saloon 1994—First NYC Gay Pride parade inclusive of trans people 1994—Melanie Philips Website 1994—Transsexual Menace activism group, founded in 1994 by Riki Wilchins 1994—Transy House Opens—a home for homeless transgender individuals Mid-1990s—David Valentine, *Imagining Transgender: An Ethnography of a Category* 1996—Transsexual Road Map: a consumer website for transgender people 1996—2002: VITALE LETTER a weekly online newsletter about gender 1997—FemmeFever founded 1998—The Colorado Gold Rush Conference 1998—Gwendolyn Ann Smith founded Transgender Day of Remembrance 1998—Metropolitan Gender Network 1999—Janet's Closet—Detroit 1999—*Boys Don't Cry* film 1999—LITE—Long Island Transgender Experience	1990–1999
2000—Average year of transition for participants in the study 2001—IFGE—International Foundation for Gender Education 2002—NYC Human Rights Law passed 2002—The Philadelphia Trans-Health Conference (PTHC) founded by transgender activists 2003—National Center for Transgender Equality (NCTE) founded 2006—Facebook opens registration to everyone 2004—Southern Comfort Conference—Donna Rose on aging 2005—Transgender Legal Defense & Education Fund founded 2008—*The Oprah Show* aired several shows regarding transgender people	2000–2009
2010—The Community Kinship (CK Life) 2011—Chaz Bono—on *Dancing with the Stars*	2010–2012

Respondents in Riley [4] explained that the positive evolution of the social representation of the trans community afforded them identities beyond the strict dichotomous binary gender. For discussion, the historical events were broken down into decade-specific events. Regarding the 1950 and 60s, all of the respondents spoke of becoming aware of Christine Jorgensen. They recalled how her story provided language to their internal feelings. While Ms. Jorgensen's story gave verbiage to their internal gender feelings, it also left some respondents in a quandary. Benjamin's [81] book *The Transsexual Phenomenon* was a set of guidelines that connected sexual orientation to gender identity; therefore, post-transition, a trans person would appear and present in society as a heterosexual person. Those who did not fit these criteria moved to the club scene where alternate lifestyles were welcomed. In these clubs, individuals used words like a female mimic, drag queen, or transgenderist. Respondents spoke of the vibrant underground world in the 1960s, in clubs such as Hell Fire, Mustang Sally's, and The Vault.

The 1970s brought television shows that broadcast interviews of transgender people in the media spotlight. Shows such as the *Phil Donahue Show* and *Dinah's Place* (with Dinah Shore) introduced transgender individuals, with whom the respondents in Riley [4] could identify. For example, transmen respondents spoke of becoming aware that transition was not only for transwomen, thus confirming feelings that transmen also existed and that this was a valid identity. Although these interviewees' stories resonated with the respondents, they reported that the public perception of transgender individuals was that of an "othered" identity. Respondents explained that by the mid-70s, there was a trans acceptance within gay nightclubs, where they could present their core identity in relative safety. Respondents also related that some early transgender support groups were forming, allowing them to meet other transgender people and share their stories.

Mikayla, a respondent in Riley [4], spoke of her perception of the climate in the 1970s for trans people and the fear that kept her closeted: "If in '75 and '76 I had come out and said, I wanted to be a woman, I wouldn't have had a job" [Mikayla, MTF, age 78, 17 years post-transition].

The 1980s brought about the beginning of the computer age with dial-up bulletin boards. For the first time, trans people could connect to other trans individuals anonymously from the privacy of their homes. Magazine articles with positive stories of transwomen became more prevalent, including the first publication of *Tapestry Quarterly Magazine*. This publication included information written for, about, and by transgender individuals. This magazine was the beginning of print media that presented transgender articles without the sensationalism of earlier newspaper articles, such as the media coverage about Christine Jorgensen and Renee Richards.

The majority of respondents in Riley [4] spoke of the impact of the commercial Internet. CompuServe broke new ground in 1980 as the first online service to offer a real-time chat function online. In this medium, individuals could speak anonymously in real time about their feelings and thoughts about being trans. Respondents noted that this was a safe place to express their core identity and receive validation of their core gender. One of the respondents, Molly, a 70-year-old transwoman, recalled that Susan Stryker identified 1985 as the beginning of the transgender civil rights movement. Stryker [82] expanded her declaration by highlighting the public scuffle between Janice Raymond, a transphobic lesbian separatist, and Sandy Stone, a lesbian, transgender woman. Respondents spoke of how the Internet increased the visibility of transgender people and their diverse expressions under the umbrella term "trans." Respondents explained that within this decade particularly, they felt a sense of belonging to the trans community. They spoke about how these social connections increased the possibilities of how they could self-actuate and self-define their identities. As an example, one of the respondents, Renee, a 69-year-old transwoman, self-identified as a "transbian.[2]"

[2]Renee defined transbian as a transwoman who is attracted to transwomen.

The 1990s ushered in a significant political movement. Suddenly, the acronym LGBT became prominent. With this symbolic gesture, transgender individuals were now included in pride parades nationwide. Further, the respondents in Riley [4] discussed the increased emergence of websites with information and social connections in the trans community. Additionally, respondents described the positive image shift in the media portrayal of transgender people. As an example, they spoke of the movie *The Crying Game*. In this film, they saw the portrayal of a transgender woman's emotional struggle, rather than the previously depicted psychotic killer of the 1980 film *Dressed to Kill.* All of the respondents acknowledged the dramatic change of the category "trans" in society over the past 20 years. Respondents also spoke about the importance of transgender conferences where trans individuals could meet and appreciate the diversity of other conference attendants.

Adrianna, a 55-year-old transwoman participant in Riley [4], told of the impact the changing representation of the trans community had on her own identity. Initially, as she was attracted to women, Adrianna had identified as a cross-dresser. However, as the transgender social representation changed, she recognized the importance of self-defining her gender. She did not have to fit the narrow confines of the socially constructed stereotypical woman:

> I identified more as a male when I was younger, with a cross-dressing aspect to me, and then as I got older the feminine side of me came out more and more, and more. And now I'm pretty much there and fully female, with a little bit of butch tendencies. [Adrianna, MTF, age 55, five years post-transition]

Natalie summed up the positive change in the social representation of transgender people: "Because of the publicity that's out there, because of the internet. It's not just Jerry Springer … it's not a just grotesque monster like people who I don't think are sincere, it's just sensationalism." [Natalie, MTF, one-year post-transition] [4].

She detailed the positive role models that were out over the last 10–20 years, as opposed to television shows that sensationalized the topic. Natalie specified: "So for me, I think the good news in the transgender world is that for most people, it's not the first time they've heard of it. It's not just Christine Jorgenson. It's teachers … it's doctors."

On February 13, 2014, Facebook initiated multiple gender options for their members, giving them 56 gender choices [83]. This change speaks volumes about the transformations in our society today. Facebook's change has opened the door to potential socially acceptable identities beyond a strict gender binary.

With growing self-acceptance and support, many TGNC people now categorized their social identity as "transgender" and gained a sense of community belonging.

Stage 3: Categorization of Social Identity

Categorization of identity/acceptance of transgender identity often leads to transition.

Emergence—Transition

> We must be willing to let go of the life we planned so as to have the life that is waiting for us".—Joseph Campbell[3]

Lev's [84] book, *Transgender Emergence*, describes the process of transition as the internal gender identity emerging from within where it has remained purposefully hidden from the world, out of fear of discrimination or violence. As indicated in the findings of Riley [4], the respondents often used the expression "leap of faith" to describe the moment where they began to present to the world as their core gender. The majority of respondents explained, in hindsight, that their initial presentations often very stereotypically depicted their aspirational gender identity. It was at this point that the theoretical construct of "passing," not as their natal gender, but as their authentic selves, became the goal, to manage the stigma of being transgender again. Social comparison theory, first established by Leon Festinger [85], postulates that people constantly evaluate themselves and compare themselves to others. There are two types of comparisons: downward and upward. Downward comparisons occur when people compare themselves to someone else and find the other person to be lacking. Upward comparisons, however, are when people compare themselves to others and find *themselves* to be lacking. In Riley [4] as the respondents first transitioned, they often used upward comparison—reaching for an unattainable gender presentation as portrayed in the media. The findings regarding the transwomen respondents were consistent with Festinger [85] who concluded that cultural norms for thinness and beauty play a large role in women's chronic dissatisfaction with their bodies. Respondents spoke about how initially they established their idealized self within the culturally determined stereotypes of what it means to be a "beautiful woman" or a "masculine man" [86].

In contrast to respondents' early upward comparisons with media icons, using the Internet, respondents were able to read stories and gain access to other transgender individuals—more positive role models—allowing for horizontal comparison which helped them build positive self-esteem. Social comparisons have become a relevant mechanism for learning about the appearance-related social expectations among peers and for evaluating the self [87]. As an example, many of the transwomen in Riley [4] spoke of the initial importance of makeup and outward female presentation; over time, living authentically, they recognized they did not need to go to such lengths to identify as women. Mikayla, a 78-year-old transwoman who transitioned 17 years ago, clarified how early in her transition, she would spend countless hours watching and observing women:

---

[3]Joseph Campbell was an American mythologist, writer, and lecturer, best known for his work in comparative mythology and comparative religion. This quote was sourced from a book of his unpublished works, *Reflections on the Art of Living: A Joseph Campbell Companion*, edited by Diane Osbon.

> I think a great deal of difference is how we view those insignificant things that a woman takes for granted that we think are so interesting that eventually become second nature. You think, all right, when I first transition; you will make sure your makeup is on right. That [you look] perfect … I don't even wear makeup anymore. After sixteen years, I'm just an old lady who goes from one place to another. Old ladies don't wear makeup. Our value of what a woman is when we want to transition is much more important when we begin the transition than later on. [Mikayla, MTF, age 78, 17 years post-transition]

Acceptance or Rejection of Trans Identity

Respondents detailed how "emergence" included disclosing their transgender identity and their plans to transition to family, friends, and co-workers. They received varying reactions, from acceptance to conditional acceptance, and sometimes, to outright rejection. Since the vast majority of the population is at least relatively comfortable with their gender identity, it becomes challenging for cis-gendered people (non-TGNC people) to relate or to understand the transgender experience; therefore, the outcome of disclosure is difficult to predict. Before disclosing their transgender identity, respondents in Riley [4] reported hoping for acceptance and support but feared loss and rejection.

The literature on TGNC family relationships is limited and mostly dated. Additionally, these qualitative studies used much more broadly defined transgender communities (e.g., cross-dressers) for their inclusion criteria [88]. Scholars suggest that family relationships, including intimate partner relationships, are essential to individual well-being [89], children [90, 91], parents [92], and siblings [93, 94]. This research also suggests that the coming out process affects the quality of family relationships. None of these studies examined the nature of the well-being of TGNC individuals regarding life satisfaction and self-esteem or specifically how these constructs related to the quality of family relationships.

Israel [95] states, "Individuals, who have at least one parent or a close family member often find just enough love and support to make it through unimaginable hardships associated with a harsh, transphobic society" [95]. For participants in Riley [4], support and acceptance were found to be significant in four primary domains: (1) nuclear families, (2) families of origin, (3) friendships, and (4) careers.

Respondents in Riley [4] whose parents were still alive hoped for acceptance and support. The majority of respondents whose parents were deceased before their transition regretted not having the opportunity to gain their parents' love and acceptance of their true selves. On the other hand, one transwoman was so fearful of rejection that she deliberately waited until her parents had passed to transition.

The majority of respondents spoke about isolating before transition and having few friendships, while in post-transition they began to build more friendships and social connections. "Social support is a key concept in social gerontology; there is empirical evidence of its relationships with health, well-being, and quality of life in old age" [96], p. 645. The respondents regarded social contacts as an essential element for well-being. Conversely, they felt that loneliness would lead to depression and age poorly.

> Well, obviously, health is always an issue, that's one thing. But, there's also a mental health issue that I think is important. I'm sure that there are probably some people that are very isolated, that don't have friends … that have no social life. [Lynn, Dual-Gendered, age 58, 11 years post-transition]

Lynn, as with all the respondents in the integrated social identity (ISI) category in Riley [4], spoke of an increasing number of friendships post-transition. Many respondents had come to a place where they valued friendships and were either rebuilding old relationships or building new friendships post-transition; they became more social.

As the average age of transition for the study cohort was 52 years old, many had already retired from their primary careers. Fourteen respondents reported that they were unable to retire or had to subsidize their social security income due to the financial cost of transitioning. The respondents who needed to continue working often faced discriminations on multiple levels. Many of the respondents used the phrase "triple whammy," when searching for employment; they reported experiencing trans-discrimination, ageism, and sexism. It was even common for the respondents with advanced academic degrees to experience difficulty securing meaningful employment.

Among those who experienced a positive reaction in the workplace, there was a consensus that such acceptance related to the importance of having achieved a successful reputation in their career before coming out. For the respondents who "came out" at work, many used humor to ease the tension and were surprised that they received acceptance and support.

Stage 4: Compartmentalized Natal Sex Identity Post-Transition

Initially, post-transition leads to the compartmentalization of the previous identity to protect the threatened new identity from being spoiled by others' knowledge of their natal sex. "Conflicting social identities may be managed through compartmentalizing and dealing with each in a context-dependent way" [97]. All of the respondents initially entered the compartmentalized social identity phase post-transition. At this stage of social identity development, compartmentalization does not have to imply a contextual presentation of either male or female. Some respondents described themselves as living "stealth": not allowing others to know their natal sex at birth, which differed from their core or authentic gender as they identified it. One of the respondents, who had transitioned and had been living stealth, described this state as "immigrating to a new gender land and living in constant fear of expulsion." The respondents in Riley [4] defined "stealth" as not allowing others to know their natal sex at birth which differs from their core or authentic gender they identified it.

At this stage, the respondent's natal sex identity and their post-transition social gender identity are kept compartmentalized and distinct; the possible intra-individual contradictions and similarities between the identities are not yet recognized [98]. In other words, at this point, they kept both their pre-transition and post-transition identities separate and could not recognize how both identities could exist as one person.

Stage 5: Integrated Social Identity Through Reflexive Authenticity

The distinction between compartmentalized social identity (CSI) and integrated social identity (ISI) respondents in Riley [4] related to their self-perception post-transition. Within the ISI group of respondents, they self-identified as "transgender," versus CSI respondents post-transition held firmly to categorizing themselves as "cisgendered." Therefore, the CSI group carefully hid their natal sex and felt people who knew of their transgender history would treat them as less than human.

Social identity can be defined as "that part of the individual's self-concept which derives from his or her knowledge of membership to a social group (or groups) together with the value and the emotional significance attached to it" [99].

In Riley [4], respondents were assigned into two categories, compartmentalized social identity (CSI) post-transition or integrated social identity (ISI) post-transition. Those who were assigned ISI had moved past the need to be stealth. They reported that by recognizing similarities in both their pre- and post-transition selves, they now felt comfortable in their skin and were living authentically. In doing so, they had ruptured the strict boundary of the compartmentalized social identity and melded their personas together into one integrated social identity.

According to Amiot and Jaspal [58], achieving an integrated social identity occurs by (1) recognition and resolution of conflict between different critical social identities; (2) establishment of interrelations between identities and recognizing the similarities between them; (3) creation of higher order categorizations to resolve the conflict; and (4) overlap between identities, such that total out-groups or partial in-groups become total in-groups. Amiot & Jaspal [58] reported that at this stage, the whole life experience comes together to form one identity. "This process allows the simultaneous identification as a whole authentic self" [58].

Transgender Advocacy

Several scholars agree that individual trans activism, not only on a personal level but in the social representation of the transgender community as well, increases self-esteem and social connectedness [4, 100, 102]. Self-esteem refers to a stable sense of personal worth [37] as well as the competence to cope with life stressors [102].

Those trans respondents whose characteristics placed them in the integrated social identity category spoke about committing to improving circumstances politically and socially for the transgender community. Specifically, they described working to pass anti-discrimination laws inclusive of gender identity and gender expression, as well as educating greater society about the transgender experience through both personal conversations and lectures. They spoke of the importance of visibility of transgender people in our society, thereby changing the social representation of transgender individuals and countering stereotypes. Riley [4] indicates the importance of expanding Raj's [100] theory of trans activism as a therapeutic tool. Raj recommends using trans activism in individual therapeutic counseling as a tool for self-empowerment and discusses the maximum ability of people to act autonomously and to settle on their own free decisions.

TGNC community members often express that transgender advocacy helped build their self-esteem [4]. Additionally, it encouraged respondents to form a healthy recognition between their pre- and post-transition identities as they discovered what they titled their "authentic self."

Authenticity

> Who can say why I heard its music the way I did? All I know is that from earliest memory I disliked being called 'he' and longed to be addressed as 'she.' I wanted to look like what I considered myself to be, and perceived that I was profoundly misplaced – all of which evoked in me the utter sadness of feeling irremediably lost and alone in a situation impossible to rectify… These feelings were real. I am agnostic as to their origin. I did not choose them. I chose only how I would inhabit the architecture of their affect. [82]

The theme of authenticity in Riley [4] emerged from respondents who described that through transitioning, they had become more authentic individuals. Maddy [103] defined authenticity as understanding and accepting one's personal traits. According to the respondents, the authentic self included the little boy or little girl that corresponded to their natal sex. Also, the authentic self included the person that the participants wanted to be. The authentic self did not manifest during the times of imitation of others or when the participants hid behind facades. According to Ryan and Deci [104], an authentic person engages in authentic behaviors that exist as "self-authored and endorsed" [104]. The participants in Riley [4] described the authentic self as the person whom they hid, guarded, protected, or defended. Moreover, this person was the one the participants wanted to set free, liberate, heal, develop, and mature. None of the respondents said they regretted their transition. They relayed how they were finally living as their "true selves." Further, all of the respondents noted that they felt younger than their chronological age and that their emotions had vastly improved. The vast majority reported they no longer suffered from depression. Additionally, respondents who identified as living authentically no longer purposefully self-isolated.

The respondents spoke of the process of becoming comfortable in their skin and being less concerned with what others thought of them. Acceptance of both pre-transition and post-transition identities and participation in transgender advocacy lead to an integrated social identity/living authentically.

Social Connectedness

Notwithstanding the difficulties persevered by TGNC people, numerous exhibit momentous versatility, accomplishment of progress, prosperity, and a constructive feeling of self and network despite lopsidedly large amounts of minority stress [4, 54, 62, 105, 106]. Recent research with TGNC individuals suggests the importance of social support and social or community connectedness and activism on positive mental health outcomes [4, 107, 108]. Specifically, mounting subjective research has featured a novel feeling of versatility among assorted examples of transgender people. In late grounded hypothesis investigations of TGNC youth and senior people, accounts featured trips toward legitimacy and self-acknowledgment that were frequently saturated with encounters of persecution; by the by, members described stories of prominent tolerance, tirelessness, quality, and rising certainty [4, 54, 62]. Scholars have highlighted sources of resilience that include the ability to exhibit self-worth in the face of oppression, hope for the future, social activism, and acting as a positive role model for others [4, 62, 101, 106].

Discussion

Advancements in technologies from television in the mid-1950s through the use of personal computers and the internet have facilitated social change at an exponential rate through increased exposure to diverse people, ideologies, and experiences. This has been especially significant in establishing and connecting the transgender community. Moreover, social connections to other transgender individuals, transgender support groups, and transgender social groups led respondents to participate in transgender advocacy groups where members' activities worked to achieve the three group goals. Breakwell [68] lists these goals as (1) change value of the group attributes, (2) change characteristics associated with the social category, and (3) change the social order and dominant ideologies.

In my study [4], TGNC individuals demonstrated that they had developed narratives of coping with their gender identity from early childhood until the present [4]. These respondents' narratives drew new insight into a process that Lev [84] says occurs in the final stage of the TGNC identity development model, and shed new light on the post-transition phase. This further illustrated the importance of connecting both social identities—the pre-transition and post-transition social identities. A common narrative that TGNC individuals use to describe the process of moving toward authenticity is that initially, their priority in post-transition was "passing" to protect their newly presented core identity. This finding is consistent with Amiot et al. [66] compartmentalized social identity stage on the journey toward identity integration.

Respondents expressed that advocating as a self-identifying transgender person helped build their self-esteem. Further, it allowed recognition of behaviors and similarities between their pre- and post-transition identities, into a healthy identity that they unanimously titled their "authentic self."

Final Thoughts

The goal of this chapter was to help medical and mental health professionals understand the journey toward authenticity that TGNC individuals go through to live authentically. Within this process, I emphasize the importance of the social context in which these individuals travel. It is not a solo journey, but one better served through support, connection to other TGNC people, and a society that accepts the obsolescence of the concept of a gender binary. Burdge [1] states that social workers "should reject a dichotomous understanding of gender in favor of more accurate and affirming conceptualizations of gender" [1]. Rejection of binary gender models is crucial for social workers and all health professions as the gender binary is the foundation on which transgender oppression depends.

References

1. Burdge BJ. Bending gender, ending gender: theoretical foundations for social work practice with the transgender community. Soc Work. 2007;52(3):243–50. https://doi.org/10.1093/sw/52.3.243.
2. Monro S. Beyond male and female: poststructuralism and the spectrum of gender. Int J Transgenderism. 2005;8(1):3–22. https://doi.org/10.1300/j485v08n01_02.
3. Saltzburg S, Davis TS. Co-authoring gender-queer youth identities: discursive tellings and retellings. J Ethn Cult Divers Soc Work. 2010;19(2):87–108. https://doi.org/10.1080/15313200903124028.
4. Riley DB. Lost and found: transgender elders' journey toward authenticity (Doctoral dissertation). 2015. Retrieved from ProQuest Dissertations Publishing. https://search.proquest.com/openview/b7db4f6ced1037cbd337ffb18f9fd007/1?pq-origsite=gscholar&cbl=18750&diss=y.
5. Corrigan PW. On the stigma of mental illness: practical strategies for research and social change. Washington, DC: American Psychological Association; 2005.
6. Corrigan PW, Green A, Lundin R, Kubiak MA, Penn DL. Familiarity with and social distance from people who have serious mental illness. Psychiatr Serv. 2001;52(7):953–8. https://doi.org/10.1176/appi.ps.52.7.953.
7. King D. Respect and equality: transsexual and transgender rights. Soc Leg Stud. 2003;12(4):559–60.
8. Weiss JT. The gender caste system: identity, privacy, and heteronormativity. Law Sex Rev Lesbian Gay Bisexual Transgender Leg Issues. 2001;10(123):128–97.
9. Austin T, Eyler A. Hate crimes and violence against the transgendered. Peace Rev. 1999;11(3):461–8. https://doi.org/10.1080/10402659908426291.
10. Burn SM. Heterosexuals' use of 'fag' and 'queer' to deride one another: a contributor to heterosexism and stigma. J Homosex. 2000;40(2):1–11. https://doi.org/10.1300/J082v40n02_01.
11. Herek GM. Beyond "homophobia": thinking about sexual prejudice and stigma in the twenty-first century. Sex Res Soc Policy J NSRC. 2004;1(2):6–24. https://doi.org/10.1525/srsp.2004.1.2.6.
12. Herek GM, Capitanio JP. AIDS stigma and sexual prejudice. Am Behav Sci. 1999;42(7):1130. https://doi.org/10.1177/00027649921954804.
13. Hinshaw SP. The stigmatization of mental illness in children and parents: developmental issues, family concerns, and research needs. J Child Psychol Psychiatry. 2005;46(7):714–34. https://doi.org/10.1111/j.1469-7610.2005.01456.x.

14. Major B, McCoy SK, Kaiser CR, Quinton WJ. Prejudice and self-esteem: a transactional model. In: Stroebe W, Hewstone M, editors. European review of social psychology. London: Psychological Press; 2003. p. 77–104.
15. Schmitt MT, Branscome NR. The meaning and consequences of perceived discrimination in disadvantaged and privileged social groups. In: Stroebe W, Hewstone M, editors. European journal of social psychology. London: Psychological Press; 2002. p. 167–99.
16. Jost JT, Banaji MR. The role of stereotyping in system-justification and the production of false consciousness. Br J Soc Psychol. 1994;33(1):1–27. https://doi.org/10.1111/j.2044-8309.1994.tb01008.x.
17. Watson AC, Ottati V, Corrigan P. From whence comes mental illness stigma? Int J Soc Psychiatry. 2003;49(2):142–57. https://doi.org/10.1177/0020764003049002007.
18. Jost JT, Sidanius J. Political psychology. New York, NY: Psychology Press; 2004.
19. Tajfel H. Differentiation between social groups: studies in the social psychology of intergroup relations. London: Academic Press; 1978.
20. Jost JT, Andrews R. System justification theory. In: Christie DJ, editor. The encyclopedia of peace psychology. Malden, MA: Wiley-Blackwell; 2012. p. 1092.
21. Goffman E. Stigma: notes on the management of spoiled identity. Englewood Cliffs, NJ: Prentice-Hall; 1963.
22. Jones EE, Farina A, Hastorf A, Marks H, Miller D, Scott R, French R. Social stigma: the psychology of marked relationships. New York, NY: W.H. Freeman and Co; 1984.
23. Dovidio JF, Major B, Crocker J. Stigma: introduction and overview. In: Heatherton TF, Kleck RE, Hebl MR, Hull JG, editors. The social psychology of stigma. Fort Worth, TX: Harcourt Brace Jovanovich; 2000.
24. Weiner B, Perry RP, Magnusson J. An attributional analysis of reactions to stigmas. J Pers Soc Psychol. 1988;55(5):738–48. https://doi.org/10.1037//0022-3514.55.5.738.
25. Crocker J, Major B, Steele C. Social stigma. In: Gilbert D, Fiske S, Lindzey G, editors. The handbook of social psychology. 4th ed. Boston, MA: McGraw-Hill; 1998. p. 504–53.
26. Sullivan HS. Clinical studies in psychiatry. New York, NY: W. W. Norton & Company; 1956.
27. Allport GW. The nature of prejudice. Cambridge, MA: Addison-Wesley; 1954.
28. Hetrick ES, Martin AD. Ego-dystonic homosexuality: a developmental view. In: Hetrick ES, Stein TS, editors. Innovations in psychotherapy with homosexuals. Washington, DC: American Psychiatric Association Press; 1984. p. 2–21.
29. Brooks VR. Minority stress and lesbian women. Lexington, MA: Lexington Books; 1981.
30. Meyer IH. Prejudice, social stress, and mental health in lesbian, gay, and bisexual populations: conceptual issues and research evidence. Psychol Bull. 2003;129(5):674–97. https://doi.org/10.1037/0033-2909.129.5.674.
31. Mirowsky J II, Ross CE. Minority status, ethnic culture, and distress: a comparison of blacks, whites, Mexicans, and Mexican Americans. Am J Sociol. 1980;86(3):479–95.
32. Dohrenwend BP. Socioeconomic status and psychiatric disorders: An update on the social causation—social selection issue. Epidemiol Psichiatr Soc. 1993;2(02):71–4. https://doi.org/10.1017/s1121189x00006825.
33. Lazarus RS, Folkman S. Coping and adaptation. In: Gentry WD, editor. Handbook of behavioral medicine. New York, NY: Guilford Press; 1984. p. 11–21.
34. Durkheim E. Suicide: a study in sociology. New York, NY: The Free Press; 1952.
35. Merton RK. Social theory and social structure. New York, NY: The Free Press; 1968.
36. Stryker S, Statham A. Symbolic interaction and role theory. In: Lindsey G, Aronsen L, editors. Handbook of social psychology. New York, NY: McGraw-Hill; 1985. p. 311–78.
37. Rosenberg M. Conceiving the self. New York, NY: Basic Books; 1979.
38. Crocker J, Major B. Social stigma and self-esteem: the self-protective properties of stigma. Psychol Rev. 1989;96(4):608–30. https://doi.org/10.1037//0033-295x.96.4.608.
39. Bettcher TM. Trapped in the wrong theory: rethinking trans oppression and resistance. Signs J Women Cult Soc. 2014;39(2):383–406. https://doi.org/10.1086/673088.

40. King ME, Winter S, Webster B. Contact reduces transprejudice: a study on attitudes towards transgenderism and transgender civil rights in Hong Kong. Int J Sex Health. 2009;21(1): 17–34. https://doi.org/10.1080/19317610802434609.
41. Guindon MH, Green AG, Hanna FJ. Intolerance and psychopathology: toward a general diagnosis for racism, sexicism, and homophobia. Am J Orthopsychiatry. 2003;73(2):167–76. https://doi.org/10.1037/0002-9432.73.2.167.
42. Hanna FJ, Talley WB, Guindon MH. The power of perception: toward a model of cultural oppression and liberation. J Couns Dev. 2000;78(4):430–41. https://doi.org/10.1002/j.1556-6676.2000.tb01926.x.
43. Herek GM. Sexual prejudice and gender: do heterosexuals attitudes toward lesbians and gay men differ? J Soc Issues. 2000;56(2):251–66. https://doi.org/10.1111/0022-4537.00164.
44. Liang CTH, Alimo C. The impact of white heterosexual students' interactions on attitudes toward lesbian, gay and bisexual people: a longitudinal study. J Coll Stud Dev. 2005;46(3): 237–50. https://doi.org/10.1353/csd.2005.0028.
45. Masser B, Phillips L. "What do other people think?"—the role of prejudice and social norms in the expression of opinions against gay men. Aust J Psychol. 2003;55(3):184–90. https://doi.org/10.1080/0004953042000298652.
46. Currah P, Minter S. Unprincipled exclusions: the struggle to achieve judicial and legislative equality for transgender people. In: Schaffner EBL, editor. Regulating sex: the politics of intimacy and identity. New York, NY: Routledge; 2005. p. 35–48.
47. Scheim AI, Bauer GR. Sex and gender diversity among transgender persons in Ontario, Canada: results from a respondent-driven sampling survey. J Sex Res. 2015;52(1):1–14. https://doi.org/10.1080/00224499.2014.893553.
48. Human Rights Campaign Foundation. State maps of laws & policies. 2018a. Retrieved June 23, 2018, from https://www.hrc.org/state-maps/transgender-healthcare.
49. Brown EG Jr, Barnhart BA. Gender nondiscrimination requirements. California Health and Human Services Agency, Department of Managed Health Care. (Health and Safety Code section 1365.5). 2013. Retrieved December 2, 2015 from https://www.dmhc.ca.gov/Portals/0/LawsAndRegulations/DirectorsLettersAndOpinions/dl12k.pdf.
50. Stroumsa D. The state of transgender health care: policy, law, and medical frameworks. Am J Public Health. 2014;104(3):31–8. https://doi.org/10.2105/AJPH.2013.301789.
51. Haas AP, Rodgers PL, Herman JL. Suicide attempts among transgender and gender non-conforming adults: findings of the national transgender discrimination survey. 2014, January. Retrieved November 10, 2015, from https://williamsinstitute.law.ucla.edu/wp-content/uploads/AFSP-Williams-Suicide-Report-Final.pdf.
52. Cahill S, Makadon H. Sexual orientation and gender identity data collection in clinical settings and in electronic health records: a key to ending LGBT health disparities. LGBT Health. 2014;1(1):34–41. https://doi.org/10.1089/lgbt.2013.0001.
53. Human Rights Campaign Foundation. Corporate equality index 2018: rating workplaces on lesbian, gay, bisexual, transgender, and queer equality. 2018b. Retrieved June 12. 2018, from https://assets2.hrc.org/files/assets/resources/CEI-2018-FullReport.pdf?_ga=2.212880852.1367531959.1529887025-1768334379.1529779793.
54. Austin A. "There I am": a grounded theory study of young adults navigating a transgender or gender nonconforming identity within a context of oppression and invisibility. Sex Roles. 2016;75(5–6):215–30. https://doi.org/10.1007/s11199-016-0600-7.
55. Austin A, Goodman R. Perceptions of transition-related health and mental health services among transgender adults. J Gay Lesbian Soc Serv. 2018;30(1):17–32. https://doi.org/10.1080/10538720.2017.1408515.
56. James SE, Herman JL, Rankin S, Keisling M, Mottet L, Anafi M. The report of the 2015 U.S. transgender survey. 2016. Washington, DC: National Center for Transgender Equality.
57. Kirsten Gillibrand, United States Senator for New York. *Schumer, Gillibrand co-sponsoring legislation to end workplace discrimination based on sexual orientation and gender identity* [press release]. (2009, August 06). Retrieved June 2, 2018, from https://www.gillibrand.

senate.gov/news/press/release/ schumer-gillibrand-co-sponsoring-legislation-to-end-workplace-discrimination-based-on-sexual-orientation-and-gender-identity.
58. Amiot CE, Jaspal R. Identity integration, psychological coherence and identity threat: linking identity process theory and the notion of integration. In: Jaspal R, Breakwell GM, editors. Identity process theory: identity, social action and social change. Cambridge: Cambridge Press; 2014. p. 155–76.
59. Connell RW. Gender and power: society, the person and sexual politics. Stanford, CA: Stanford University Press; 1987.
60. de Vries B. LGBT aging: research and policy directions. Public Policy Aging Rep. 2011; 21(3):34. https://doi.org/10.1093/ppar/21.3.34.
61. Kreps GL. Foreward. In Peterkin AD, Willes K, Allen M, Manning J, Ross K, Scholl JC, … Moltz R, editors. Health care disparities and the LGBT population. New York, NY: Lexington Books; 2014.
62. Witten TM. It's not all darkness: robustness, resilience, and successful transgender aging. LGBT Health. 2013;1(1):24–33. https://doi.org/10.1089/lgbt.2013.0017.
63. Markus H. Self-schemata and processing information about the self. J Pers Soc Psychol. 1977;35(2):63–78. https://doi.org/10.1037//0022-3514.35.2.63.
64. Markus H, Wurf E. The dynamic self-concept: a social psychological perspective. Annu Rev Psychol. 1987;38(1):299–337. https://doi.org/10.1146/annurev.ps.38.020187.001503.
65. Fiske ST, Taylor SE. Social cognition. 2nd ed. New York, NY: Random House; 1991.
66. Amiot CE, de la Sablonnière R, Terry DJ, Smith JR. Integration of social identities in the self: toward a cognitive-developmental model. Personal Soc Psychol Rev. 2007;11(4):364–88. https://doi.org/10.1177/1088868307304091.
67. Gagne P, Tewksbury R, McGaughey D. Coming out and crossing over: identity formation and proclamation in a transgender community. Gend and Soc. 1997;11(4):478–508. https://doi.org/10.1177/089124397011004006.
68. Breakwell GM. Coping with threatened identities, vol. 904. London: Methuen; 1986.
69. Budge SL, Katz-Wise SL, Tebbe EN, Howard KA, Schneider CL, Rodriguez A. Transgender emotional and coping processes. Couns Psychol. 2012;41(4):601–47. https://doi.org/10.1177/0011000011432753.
70. Witten TM. Graceful exits: intersection of aging, transgender identities, and the family/community. J GLBT Fam Stud. 2009;5(1–2):35–61. https://doi.org/10.1080/15504280802595378.
71. Brandtstädter J, Rothermund K, Kranz D, Kühn W. Final decentrations: personal goals, rationality perspectives, and the awareness of life's finitude. Eur Psychol. 2010;15(2):152. https://doi.org/10.1027/1016-9040/a000019.
72. Dervin B. Information as a user construct: the relevance of perceived information needs to synthesis and interpretation. In: Ward SA, Reed LJ, editors. Knowledge structure and use: implication for synthesis and interpretation. Philadelphia, PA: Temple University Press; 1983. p. 155–83.
73. Forsman AK, Herberts C, Nyqvist F, Wahlbeck K, Schierenbeck I. Understanding the role of social capital for mental wellbeing among older adults. Ageing Soc. 2012;33(05):804–25. https://doi.org/10.1017/s0144686x12000256.
74. Lambert NM, Stillman TF, Hicks JA, Kamble S, Baumeister RF, Fincham FD. To belong is to matter. Pers Soc Psychol Bull. 2013;39(11):1418–27. https://doi.org/10.1177/0146167213499186.
75. Baumeister RF, Leary MR. The need to belong: desire for interpersonal attachments as a fundamental human motivation. Psychol Bull. 1995;117(3):497–529. https://doi.org/10.1037//0033-2909.117.3.497.
76. Baumeister RF. The cultural animal: human nature, meaning, and social life. Oxford: Oxford University Press; 2005.
77. Lewis AM. Terror management theory applied clinically: implications for existential-integrative psychotherapy. Death Stud. 2013;38(6):412–7. https://doi.org/10.1080/07481187.2012.753557.

78. Sharpe D, Viney LL. Weltanschauung and the purpose-in-life test. J Clin Psychol. 1973; 29(4):489–91. https://doi.org/10.1002/1097-4679(197310)29:4%3c489:AID-JCLP2270290429%3e3.0.CO;2-D.
79. Simon L, Arndt J, Greenberg J, Pyszczynski T, Solomon S. Terror management and meaning: evidence that the opportunity to defend the worldview in response to mortality salience increases the meaningfulness of life in the mildly depressed. J Pers. 1998;66(3): 359–82. https://doi.org/10.1111/1467-6494.00016.
80. Jaspal R, Breakwell GM. Identity process theory: identity, social action and social change. UK: Cambridge University Press; 2014.
81. Benjamin H. The transsexual phenomenon. New York: Julian Press; 1966.
82. Stryker S. Transgender history. Berkeley, CA: Seal Press; 2008.
83. Weber P. Facebook offers users 56 new gender options: here's what they mean. The Week. 2014, February 14. Retrieved June 14, 2015, from http://theweek.com/article/index/256474/facebook-offers-users-56-new-gender-options-heres-what-they-mean.
84. Lev AI. Transgender emergence: therapeutic guidelines for working with gender-variant people and their families. Binghamton, NY: Routledge; 2004.
85. Festinger L. A theory of social comparison processes. Hum Relat. 1954;7(2):117–40. https://doi.org/10.4135/9781412972017.n235.
86. Strahan EJ, Wilson AE, Cressman KE, Buote VM. Comparing to perfection: how cultural norms for appearance affect social comparisons and self-image. Body Image. 2006;3(3): 211–27. https://doi.org/10.1016/j.bodyim.2006.07.004.
87. Kilbourne, J. (1994). Still killing us softly: advertising and the obsession with thinness. Fem Perspect Eat Disord, 395–418. https://doi.org/10.1037/e549522004-001.
88. Jones D. Social comparison and body image: attractiveness comparisons to models and peers among adolescent girls and boys. Sex Roles. 2001;45(9–10):645–64. https://doi.org/10.1023/A:1014815725852.
89. Nuttbrock L, Rosenblum A, Blumenstein R. Transgender identity affirmation and mental health. Int J Transgenderism. 2002;6(4):1–15.
90. Brown GR, Denny D. Women in the closet: relationships with transgendered men. In: Denny D, editor. Current concepts in transgender identity. New York, NY: Garland Press; 1998. p. 353–71.
91. Prince VC. Understanding cross dressing. Los Angeles, CA: Chevalier; 1976.
92. Boszormenyi-Nagy I. Invisible loyalties. New York, NY: Routledge; 2014.
93. Bolin A. In search of eve: transsexual rites of passage. Westport, CT: Bergin & Garvey; 1988.
94. Parker G, Barr R. Parental representations of transsexuals. Arch Sex Behav. 1982;11(3): 221–30. https://doi.org/10.1007/bf01544990.
95. Israel GE. Translove: transgender persons and their families. In: Bigner JJ, editor. An introduction to GLBT family studies. New York, NY: Routledge; 2013. p. 51–65.
96. Fernández-Ballesteros R. Social support and quality of life among older people in Spain. J Soc Issues. 2002;58(4):645–59. https://doi.org/10.1111/1540-4560.00282.
97. Kohut H, Goldberg A, Stepansky PE. How does analysis cure?. Chicago, IL: University of Chicago Press; 1984.
98. Crisp RJ. The psychology of social and cultural diversity. Malden, MA: Wiley-Blackwell; 2010.
99. Levitt HM, Hiestand KR. A quest for authenticity: contemporary butch gender. Sex Roles. 2004;50(9/10):605–21. https://doi.org/10.1023/b:sers.0000027565.59109.80.
100. Raj R. Transactivism as therapy: a client self-empowerment model linking personal and social agency. J Gay Lesbian Ment Health. 2007;11(3):77–98. https://doi.org/10.1080/19359705.2007.9962484.
101. Singh AA, Hays DG, Watson LS. Strength in the face of adversity: resilience strategies of transgender individuals. J Couns Dev. 2011;89(1):20–7. https://doi.org/10.1002/j.1556-6678.2011.tb00057.x.

102. Brand FS, Jax K. Focusing the meaning (s) of resilience: resilience as a descriptive concept and a boundary object. Ecol Soc. 2007;12(1):12. https://doi.org/10.3410/f.1159209.619531.
103. Maddy MD. Maximizing potential: a grounded theory study. (Doctoral dissertation). 2007. Retrieved June 6, 2015, from ProQuest Dissertations and Theses http://search.proquest.com/docview/304705069?accountid=14172.
104. Ryan RM, Deci EL. Self-determination theory and the facilitation of intrinsic motivation, social development, and well-being. Am Psychol. 2000;55(1):68–78. https://doi.org/10.1037//0003-066x.55.1.68.
105. Beemyn BG, Rankin S. The lives of transgender people. New York, NY: Columbia University Press; 2011.
106. McFadden SH, Frankowski S, Flick H, Witten TM. Resilience and multiple stigmatized identities: lessons from transgender persons' reflections on aging. In: Sinnott JD, editor. Positive psychology: advances in understanding adult motivation. New York, NY: Springer; 2013. p. 247–67.
107. Bariola E, Lyons A, Leonard W, Pitts M, Badcock P, Couch M. Demographic and psychosocial factors associated with psychological distress and resilience among transgender individuals. Am J Public Health. 2015;105(10):2108–16. https://doi.org/10.2105/ajph.2015.302763.
108. Testa RJ, Jimenez CL, Rankin S. Risk and resilience during transgender identity development: the effects of awareness and engagement with other transgender people on affect. J Gay Lesbian Ment Health. 2014;18(1):31–46. https://doi.org/10.1080/19359705.2013.805177.

Chapter 16
Legal Issues for Transgender Individuals

Noah E. Lewis

Introduction

Healthcare providers play an important role not only in delivering health care to transgender individuals but also in assisting patients with nonmedical aspects of their treatment for gender dysphoria. Providers must routinely provide documentation for legal gender changes, insurance appeals, medical leave, disability benefits, and more. Providers are also called upon to advocate with schools, employers, insurance companies, and unsupportive family members. Finally, patients may tell providers of legal problems they are experiencing such as discrimination, family law issues, or housing barriers. Providers with a basic understanding of transgender legal rights are in a better position to engage in effective advocacy as well as encourage people to seek out legal assistance and assert their rights.

Preparing Your Practice for Trans Clients

All healthcare practices can expect to see a transgender patient—either a new patient or an existing patient who begins to transition. Being proactive about adopting best practices for transgender patients is the best way to create a respectful and welcoming environment as well as avoid discrimination. A useful resource for any health care practice is *Creating Equal Access to Quality Health Care for Transgender Patients: Transgender-Affirming Hospital Policies*, a comprehensive resource that covers nondiscrimination policies, patient bills of rights, access to

N. E. Lewis (✉)
Transcend Legal, 3553 82nd St. #6D, Jackson Heights, NY 11372, USA
e-mail: nlewis@transcendlegal.org

L. Poretsky and W. C. Hembree (eds.), *Transgender Medicine*, Contemporary Endocrinology, https://doi.org/10.1007/978-3-030-05683-4_16

transgender-related care, protocol for interaction with trans patients, room assignments, restrooms, and access to personal items that assist gender presentation [1]. Adhering to those best practices will help to ensure that a hospital or provider is meeting their obligations under nondiscrimination laws.

Legal Duties to Trans Patients

Virtually all healthcare providers in the U.S. have a legal obligation to provide respectful, culturally competent care to transgender patients. Protections for transgender patients arise from nondiscrimination laws, professional licensing standards, and professional standards of conduct.

Federal law prohibits transgender discrimination in health care. Section 1557 of the Patient Protection and Affordable Care Act prohibits discrimination on the basis of sex, disability, age, race, color, and national origin in health programs or activities that receive federal funding. Courts have repeatedly found that Section 1557 protects transgender people under the category of sex. The category of disability would also apply. The law applies to entities receiving federal financial assistance through their participation in Medicare (excluding Medicare Part B) or Medicaid. This includes a broad range of providers beyond hospitals and doctors' offices, such as home health agencies, physical therapy practices, speech pathology programs, and drug treatment facilities.

Courts have also found that people with gender dysphoria are protected under the Americans With Disabilities Act, and, for government-run programs, Section 504 of the Rehabilitation Act of 1973, both of which prohibit disability discrimination in places of public accommodation [2].

State and local public accommodations laws similarly apply to provider offices, and trans people may be protected under the category of gender identity or transgender status [3], or in many more states, under the categories of sex and disability. Obligations of fair treatment can also arise from licensing boards and hospital accreditors, such as The Joint Commission, which prohibits discrimination based on gender identity or expression [4].

If a patient reports experiencing discrimination from another provider, it is helpful to advise them of the many places to file a complaint such as a patient advocate, state or local human rights commission, provider licensing boards, or the Office of Civil Rights of the federal Department of Health and Human Services [5]. Advise them that there are deadlines to take legal action and that they should promptly contact an attorney or legal organization. Encouraging individuals to file complaints is important because even if it does not resolve their individual situation, a record is established that could demonstrate a pattern of discrimination in the future. Local transgender organizations can be a source for locating local trans-friendly legal resources; Lambda Legal has compiled a list of such organizations [6].

Inclusive Client Intake Forms

Client intake forms can help set the tone for a respectful and inclusive practice. Review patient intake forms to ensure that they are collecting accurate information when it comes to transgender patients. An intake form that simply has a box for "sex" with the options "male or female," is ambiguous—does this refer to legal sex, physical sex, or self-identified sex? Is the question being asked for insurance purposes or does it relate to medical history? Similarly, asking simply for "name" will not capture important information if someone uses a name other than their legal name, as do many cisgender patients as well.

When clarifying the intake form, collecting the following data will ensure that transgender people's information is adequately and appropriately captured [7].

- Legal name
- Name used
- Pronouns (Note: not "preferred" pronouns.)
- Sex on insurance records: ❒ female ❒ male
- Gender: ❒ female ❒ male ❒ nonbinary
- Sex labeled at birth: ❒ female ❒ male ❒ intersex
- Are you transgender? ❒ no ❒ yes ❒ don't know

Name and Pronouns

Transgender people commonly report being misgendered—particularly in hospitals—since many different staff members come into contact with the patient and not all of them have familiarity with the patient's trans status. Transgender people in such situations can feel vulnerable due to the power imbalance of needing to challenge those responsible for providing essential care. All staff must be educated to use the name and pronoun the patient uses and that, if they make a mistake, to simply correct themselves and move on. While accidental slip-ups may not rise to the level of discrimination, deliberate misgendering can, as could fail to adequately educate and discipline staff.

Another problem area is with electronic medical records. Trans people who have previously been admitted to a hospital report the hospital using their old name and gender when being admitted even if that does not match their current ID document. If a person has not had a legal name change, there should be a provision to have their preferred name appear on their records as common law name changes are valid.

When announcing names in the waiting room, using only the patient's last name avoids using a gendered honorific or gendered first name. People may not want to be unnecessarily gendered or outed with their pronoun and preferred name in front of others.

Sex-Specific Facilities

Sex-specific restrooms, room assignments, residential treatment programs are another common source of transgender discrimination. The general legal rule is that transgender people must be treated according to their affirmed sex regardless of whether or not they have had any specific medical treatments such as hormones or surgery. For sex-specific screening centers or programs, all individuals with a specific body part evaluated by the screening program must be included, i.e., both transgender women and transgender men who have breasts must be allowed to participate in a mammography clinic.

Consent to Care

Obtaining Informed Consent

Transgender-related health care is still subject to higher societal scrutiny than other forms of medical treatment. Robust informed-consent procedures can help to alleviate provider concerns about delivering this care, particularly to minors. As many transgender health centers provide hormones on an informed consent basis, there are many sample informed-consent protocols and documents available for initiating treatment from centers such as Callen-Lorde Community Health Center, Fenway Health, or Howard Brown Health Center.

Consent When Treating a Minor

In situations where puberty suppression treatment is warranted, treatment cannot be delayed without the minor facing lifelong, irreversible changes to their body. Hormone and surgery access can also be equally pressing, especially where the minor is experiencing anxiety, depression, social isolation, or suicidal ideation. Being proactive about ensuring the necessary legal consent is in place early on will help to avoid negative health consequences for the minor.

The age of majority to consent to medical treatment is generally 18 years in most states. If the minor cannot legally consent directly, consent must be obtained from the parent or legal guardian. Youth in out-of-home care will generally still need to obtain parental consent for treatment even if they are not living with a parent. Youth in state custody, including child welfare systems and juvenile justice systems, must be provided with all medically necessary transgender-related care.

When Neither Parent Is Supportive

If a parent or guardian is not supportive, options include trying to educate the caregiver, such as by connecting them with culturally appropriate resources, or exploring options for treatment without parental consent. If both of a patient's parents are blocking treatment for a minor, there may be legal options available to the minor. The safest course of action when parental consent cannot be obtained is to have the minor consult with an attorney to explore all of their options.

In some states, people under 18 are legally able to consent to their own treatment [8]. Some states have clear statutory authority for people under 18, e.g., minors in Alabama can consent at age 14 and in Oregon at 15. There are also exceptions in most states conferring the ability to consent for people who are married, pregnant, parents, or serving in the military. A number of states provide that if a minor is able to meet informed consent standards, they can consent to their own treatment. If a minor lives apart from their parents and is financially self-sufficient, some states allow for emancipation either through a court order to establish such a status at the outset or at the time a controversy arises, such as a disagreement over medical treatment between the patient and their parents. Some states also recognize a "mature minor" doctrine where a sufficiently mature minor is able to consent to their own treatment.

Using contraception to eliminate the risk of pregnancy as well as stop the menstrual cycle is an important treatment option for many trans adolescents. Many states have laws that allow minors to access contraception without parental consent or notification, and in all states, adolescents of any age can access contraception at federally funded Title X clinics without parental notice or consent.

In some extreme instances, trans minors with unsupportive parents desire that child protective services get involved because they are being denied medically necessary treatment, which can be considered neglect. In such situations, providers can document the minor's medical needs and help to educate the agency staff.

Courts are increasingly more willing to order that a child receive transgender-related treatment over the objections of parents. For example, an Ohio court applied a "best interests of the child" standard and granted custody to the grandparents of a 17-year-old trans man when his parents would not allow him to access testosterone therapy [9].

Parental Consent When Parents Disagree

When parents disagree about whether their minor child should socially transition or have access to puberty suppression treatment, hormones, or surgery, providers can play a role in educating the nonsupportive parent. Supportive parents in such a situation are advised to proceed with caution and providers must be aware of the precariousness of the situation.

If the parents are married, the supportive parent or the provider should continue to inform the other parent of all doctor's appointments; the other parent should be encouraged to attend, meet other supportive parents, and see a therapist themselves if they are willing. Providers can recommend a second opinion as well as books and documentaries that other parents have found to be helpful.

If the parents are divorced, most often both parents retain control over medical decision-making. It is therefore important to ensure that both parents are aware of the child's treatment. If one parent allows the child to socially or medically transition without the other parent's consent, the unsupportive parent may use this to go to court to seek a modification of the child custody order that either requires their involvement in medical decisions or awards them sole custody. If a parent who has been supportive of a child's transition has lost custody of their children in court, the child can be forced by the other parent to live as their sex assigned at birth until they turn 18.

Providers can assist minors by being proactive in documenting all efforts to educate and involve both parents in the minor's treatment. Keeping contemporaneous notes about the provider's own opinion regarding the best treatment for the child will be helpful in the event of a legal dispute about care [10]. A provider may be called upon to testify about the best interests of the child. The provider has the opportunity to educate the court about transgender youth and ally any concerns that the supportive parent is pushing the child to be transgender.

Insurance Coverage for Trans-Related Health Care

Many transgender people and providers still assume that paying out of pocket is the only way to obtain hormones, surgery, or puberty suppression treatment. This is particularly true if the surgery needed is facial gender reassignment surgery or breast augmentation. But in general, if a person has health insurance, they should be able to get coverage for trans-related care, though sometimes it requires going through the appeals process or contacting an attorney.

Advocacy, increased transgender visibility, and legal changes have all led to unprecedented levels of transgender people having insurance coverage at all and furthermore having insurance coverage that does not exclude trans-related care. The enactment of the Patient Protection and Affordable Care Act (ACA) in March 2010 was instrumental in expanding access to coverage by prohibiting insurers from refusing to issue plans to transgender people due to having the preexisting condition of gender dysphoria. Medicaid expansion, the establishment of the Marketplace, and tax subsidies for premiums all led to increased coverage for transgender people.

Transgender exclusions have also increasingly been removed from health insurance plans. In the Human Rights Campaign Foundation's *Corporate Equality Index 2018*, over three quarters (79%) of the businesses ranked—and over half of Fortune 500 businesses—offer transgender-inclusive healthcare coverage. That is up from 0 in 2002 [11]. Medicare removed its blanket exclusion in 2014 as did the Federal Employee Health Benefits program in 2016. At least 19 states and the

District of Columbia have prohibitions on transgender discrimination in health insurance, and the same number have explicit transgender coverage in state Medicaid plans [12].

Assessing Whether a Plan Will Cover Trans Care

If a patient asks if their plan will cover transgender-related care, there are two documents that will help them answer that question: (1) their specific insurance plan document and (2) the insurance company's general clinical policy on gender dysphoria treatments.

The individual's plan document is specific to their insurance policy. The document has many different names—it might be called a Certificate of Coverage, a Summary Plan Description, a Member Handbook, a Benefits Certificate, or a Certificate of Insurance. A person can obtain the plan booklet by calling the number on the back of their card, logging into the insurance company's website, or if it is an employer-based plan, looking on the company's benefits website or asking Human Resources for a copy of the plan.

The full plan booklet will contain a list of exclusions. The exclusions or limitations section might list an exclusion for "transsexual surgery," "sex transformations," "gender reassignment surgery" or "sex change." If there is an exclusion for trans-related care, the person should immediately consult with an attorney as such exclusions can be challenged as unlawful discrimination.

If there is no exclusion, then the next step is to get a copy of the insurance company's clinical medical policy on treatments for gender dysphoria. Transcend Legal's website contains links to over 120 such policies [13]. Those policies are generic and apply to all plans that insurance company offers or administers. These policies list what evidence the insurance company wants to see before it will approve a surgery as medically necessary. Providers should review these requirements and make sure the therapist letters and supporting medical documentation meet all of the criteria.

If the patient does not meet all of the criteria, providers should include an explanation as to why any particular criterion or criteria should not apply to this patient. For example, some policies state that a person must be 18 before undergoing surgery, so in that case, the providers should document why surgery is important for the individual at this time even though they are not yet 18. Some policies also classify certain procedures, such as breast augmentation, as cosmetic. In that case, the person knows that they will receive a denial letter and will have to go through the appeals process. In situations where not all of the criteria are met or the treatment is listed as not covered, encourage the person to promptly seek legal assistance.

The best way to know if an insurance plan will cover that patient's trans-related care is to apply for preauthorization. Especially when there is a question about coverage or the individual knows they will be denied, applying for preauthorization as quickly as possible will allow the person sufficient time to challenge the denial.

Preauthorization requests submitted even 90 days prior to surgery may not allow sufficient time to challenge a denial depending on the nature of the denial and the plan. Accordingly, submitting the preauthorization request immediately after the consultation—using a placeholder date of service if necessary—affords the person the best chance of being able to successfully appeal and maintain their surgery date.

Common Types of Denials

There are three main types of insurance denials trans people face: sex-specific care, categorical exclusions, and medical necessity denials. There are also barriers to coverage that come from a lack of qualified in-network providers and low reimbursement rates.

Denials of Sex-Specific Care

The easiest type of denial to resolve is a denial of a sex-specific service that does not match the sex on the person's insurance records. A transgender man who is listed as male on his insurance may receive a denial for gynecological care or contraception. A transgender woman may face denials for prostate testing. These denials are computer-generated based on a perceived coding mismatch.

It is unlawful for an insurer to refuse to pay a claim simply because of a gender coding mismatch. First, make sure that the claim was submitted with the member's sex as they have it recorded with their insurance. If the claim was submitted correctly, the provider or member can simply call the insurance company and explain that the service was correct. Do not hesitate to ask to speak with a supervisor if the first representative is not helpful. A phone call should be sufficient to resolve the issue, but also be mindful of deadlines to file an appeal and file a written appeal if necessary. Another option is to file a complaint with the insurance company's civil rights coordinator, which is separate from the internal appeals process. Because a civil rights complaint does not count as filing an appeal, be aware of any imminent deadlines to file the internal appeal.

If an insurance company asserts that the person must change their gender marker back in order to access the service, explain that that is not accurate and it is also a privacy concern. Gender markers appear, for example, when an individual goes to a pharmacy, and transgender people should not be forced to have a gender marker that would publicize their transgender status.

To prevent the issue going forward, asking the insurer to put a note in the file can be helpful. And when submitting Medicare claims, institutions may use condition code 45 (ambiguous gender category) and physicians can use the KX modifier (requirements specified in the medical policy have been met) to flag that the service is correct despite the gender mismatch.

A related question patients often have is if they should change the sex designation on their insurance when they change their name. Some fear they will be denied not only sex-specific services but also transgender-related care if their sex designation is already changed. The standard for whether transition-related care is provided is a diagnosis of gender dysphoria and medical necessity, not someone's administrative sex. Changing the sex designation at the time of the name change is thus recommended.

Categorical Exclusions

Some plans still explicitly exclude all transgender-related health care. And increasingly, some plan documents have explicit coverage for some types of gender dysphoria treatment, such as genital reassignment surgeries, but explicitly exclude other services such as facial reassignment surgery or voice therapy. All of these categorical exclusions—whether total or partial—are likely unlawful and unenforceable for a variety of reasons.

First, the plan booklet might simply be out of date, so the person should ask if there have been any subsequent modifications that removed the exclusion.

Second, if it is an insurance plan regulated by one of the many states whose insurance departments have issued guidelines or regulations saying that there cannot be categorical exclusions for some or all trans-related care, then the exclusion is invalid and the person can contact an attorney or the state insurance department for assistance. If it is an employer-based plan, the state where the insurance plan was issued might be different from the state where the person lives, and it is the state where the plan was issued that governs, not the state where they live.

Third, the exclusion is almost certainly unlawful. If the denial letter cites a transgender-specific exclusion in the plan document itself—as opposed to an insurance company's clinical criteria on gender dysphoria treatments—this is a red flag that an attorney should be contacted immediately. In these situations, even if a provider can demonstrate medical necessity, the plan can still deny care under the exclusion. Prompt legal assistance is required because there are deadlines to file an appeal or bring discrimination claims.

Medical Necessity Denials

Denials based on lack of medical necessity require assistance from medical and mental health providers to write letters in support of the appeal. Insurance companies usually deny care as not medically necessary based on their clinical policies on gender dysphoria treatments. Common medical necessity denials include denying surgery for people under 18 and categorizing surgeries such as breast augmentation and facial gender reassignment surgery as "cosmetic." Sometimes only part of a surgery is deemed "cosmetic," such as nipple reconstruction in conjunction with mastectomy, or scrotoplasty as part of phalloplasty.

These denials generally have several levels of appeal available: peer-to-peer, one or two levels of internal appeal with the insurance company, and often an external appeal to an independent medical review agency. Engaging in a peer-to-peer review can resolve some types of issues but is less successful where the insurance company has a written policy of not covering the treatment.

Whether the patient is working with an attorney or the provider is handling the appeal, providers will need to write letters in support of the appeal. A provider letter submitted for an insurance appeal will likely contain much more detail than a typical surgery referral letter. Helpful elements include the following:

- Qualifications and experience of the provider, including experience with trans patients;
- The patient has been diagnosed with gender dysphoria and a description of their history and symptoms;
- Length of time on hormones and social transition;
- Current treatments have been insufficient to alleviate gender dysphoria;
- Tell the patient's story, including a discussion of specific examples of problems and limitations the person is having because of the incongruent body parts;
- Reasons for any exceptions to the insurance company's criteria that are being requested;
- Harms associated with delaying the treatment;
- Treatment is provided in accordance with the WPATH Standards of Care;
- The surgery changes sex characteristics for the purpose of treating gender dysphoria, not to improve appearance;
- In the provider's opinion, the surgery is medically necessary and will help to alleviate the patient's gender dysphoria.

Note: If the appeals process does not work, the person may have the ability to file a lawsuit seeking care under the terms of the plan. But a court can generally look only at the information that the insurance company had in front of it at the time it made its decision. Assume that the person will not have the ability to introduce new evidence later on. So, if the appeal is not comprehensive, i.e., including peer-reviewed medical literature and other documents about the accepted standard of care, they may be forfeiting their rights. For this reason, it is best to consult with an attorney prior to exhausting the internal appeals process.

Legal Protections to Challenge Insurance Denials

No transgender person should be denied medically necessary care under insurance, and those who are have many legal avenues to challenge such denials. Section 1557 of ACA created nondiscrimination protections in health care. Since Section 1557 applies to any health program or activity that receives federal funding, it includes virtually all providers, hospitals, and insurance companies. The Office of Civil Rights (OCR) of the federal Department of Health and Human Services is tasked with enforcing Section 1557. In 2016 OCR issued regulations to clarify the nondiscrimination protections under Section 1557. The regulations clarified that "sex" included gender identity. The regulations also contained three explicit protections regarding transgender individuals: (1) that they must be treated according to their gender identity, (2) that covered health plans cannot contain categorical exclusions for gender transition treatments, and (3) that plans cannot make discriminatory denials of coverage for gender transition-related care.

The implementing regulations were called into question in a lawsuit brought by Catholic healthcare providers and five states, *Franciscan Alliance v. Burwell*, 227 F. Supp. 3d 660 (N.D. Tex. 2016), but Section 1557 is a statute passed by Congress and remains in force. Courts have entertained claims under Section 1557 and found that transgender exclusions are discrimination under Section 1557.

For government-run plans, in addition to Section 1557, constitutional protections such as Equal Protection also apply. For Medicare and Medicaid, federal protections under those statutes apply as well.

For employer-based plans, Title VII of the Civil Rights Act of 1964 applies to all states. Title VII prohibits sex discrimination in employment. The Americans with Disabilities Act also applies to employer-based plans and prohibits discrimination based on the disability of gender dysphoria. Companies that are federal contractors are also specifically prohibited from discriminating on the basis of gender identity, including having transgender exclusions in health plans. For state and local government plans, state and local nondiscrimination laws are another source of protection. Finally, the Employee Retirement Income Security Act (ERISA) governs private employer-based health plans. If medically necessary care is denied absent a specific transgender exclusion, a lawsuit under ERISA can be brought to enforce the terms of the plan.

Medical Leave and Short-Term Disability

Transgender people who are unable to work due to their gender dysphoria or while recovering from surgery will need documentation from a provider. Patients should be aware that if they have a short-term disability policy, they can use it for their post-surgery recovery to receive part of their income during that time. Such plans may not deny coverage for disability benefits simply because the procedure is trans-related. If someone has been denied because the insurance company says their surgery is elective or cosmetic, they should seek legal assistance or file a complaint with the state insurance agency. Similarly, an employee eligible for unpaid leave under the Family and Medical Leave Act cannot be denied leave simply because the surgery is trans-related or the employer has deemed it "cosmetic."

Name and Gender Changes

Some transgender people may be intimidated about applying for a legal name and gender change, feel overwhelmed by the process, or be unable to afford it. According to the 2015 U.S. Transgender Survey of nearly 28,000 transgender people, only roughly 1 in 10 respondents (11%) had all of their IDs and records accurately listing both their current name and sex [14]. More than two-thirds (68%) reported that *none* of their IDs or records had both their current name and sex [14].

Encouraging transgender people to apply for a legal name and gender change is an important way to help them improve their wellbeing. Having inaccurate identity documents subjects trans people to increased risk of harassment and discrimination in everyday situations such as renting an apartment, being called by name in a doctor's office, interacting with law enforcement, or any situation where one must show proof of identity. A lack of appropriate identity documents can also deter people from applying for jobs, school, benefits, or even a library card. Having to present an ID that does not match one's appearance can, at best, cause embarrassment or confusion, or worse—subject the person to discrimination, accusations of fraud, or violence. Nearly one-third (32%) of individuals who have shown ID with a name or gender that did not match their appearance have experienced negative experiences such as being harassed, denied services, or attacked [14].

Legal Name Changes

Transgender people nearly universally require a court-ordered name change to bring their identity documents in accord with their current name. While all people are free to adopt and use any name they wish as long as it is not for fraudulent purposes, such a common law name change cannot, post-9/11, be used to update identity documents.

The process for obtaining a legal name change depends on the state in which the individual lives and varies by county. Required documents, associated fees, and hearing before a judge, for example, are all ways in which jurisdictions differ. There are many pro bono name change projects throughout the country, and many court clerks also have sample name change petitions. The National Center for Transgender Equality's (NCTE) ID Documents Center is a good starting place to search for name change assistance and resources in a particular state [15].

Most states require some form of publication of the name change such as in a newspaper or at the courthouse. There are usually exceptions to this in the case where it would threaten someone's safety. If a person is concerned about their safety or wants to seal the records of their name change, they should seek out legal assistance.

In the case of a name change for a minor, one parent must file the petition and the other parent must consent. If the other parent is not supportive, the judge still has the ability to grant the name change. And if it would be a safety risk to notify the other parent of the name change, such a requirement can usually be waived.

Medical documentation of transgender status should not be required for a legal name change. One possible exception is if the name change is for a minor, and a judge has some discretion to determine if it is in the best interests of the child. If both parents are supportive, there is no real basis to require medical evidence.

If the petitioner is unable to afford the costs associated with obtaining a name change, they may be eligible to file a fee waiver request. Court clerks have sample forms for requesting a fee waiver, which may be known as filing *in forma pauperis* or requesting poor person status.

Legal Sex

"Legal sex" is not monolithic. Each identity document has its own procedure for changing a sex designation and must be updated separately. In the event of a dispute about recognizing an individual's sex, a judge can issue a decision that may or may not accord with a person's identity documents.

Updating Documents to Reflect a New Name and Gender

If a person is updating both their name and gender, it is easiest to correct both at the same time. A certified copy of a court-ordered name change is used to update the name. For name changes with private entities, a photocopy or scan of the name change order is sufficient. Gender updates will generally require a provider letter or court order as detailed below.

Federal Identity Documents

The sex designation on all federal documents including Social Security, passports, and immigration documents can be updated with a letter from an M.D. or D.O. stating that the individual has undergone "appropriate clinical treatment." There is no particular medical requirement for what that treatment must be. It can simply mean therapy or even social transition; it is up to the provider whether they feel comfortable making that statement. It is best to use verbatim the template provided by the State Department, which will work for all federal documents [15]. Provide the patient with two original copies, ideally signed in blue ink so that anyone examining the letter will readily be able to see that it is an original signature, not a photocopy.

Passports

Aside from being necessary for international travel, a corrected passport can be used in many situations in lieu of a corrected birth certificate for people who are unable to correct the sex on their birth certificate.

An “X” gender marker is recognized by the United Nations’ International Civil Aviation Organisation (ICAO), which sets forth international travel document standards. Many countries issue passports with sex designations other than “M” or “F.” A federal court in the case of *Zzyym v. Pompeo* ordered U.S. State Department to revisit its sex designation policy, but the Department has not issued a nonbinary passport to an intersex person as of this writing.

For transgender people who travel regularly and can afford it, applying for a Global Entry card or TSA Pre✓ status allows people to bypass body scanners for all flights. Because the body scanners are gendered, transgender people’s bodies or prosthetics can trigger an anomalous reading and require the person to undergo intrusive questioning and a pat down.

Social Security

Changing the name and gender with Social Security does not change an individual’s Social Security number. Updating the name with Social Security is what will allow someone to receive a paycheck and file taxes in their new name.

Selective Service

Changing one’s sex with Social Security will have Selective Service implications for transgender men. People who were assigned female at birth are not required to register for the draft. However, all men are required to register in order to access federal student loans or government jobs. Accordingly, people listed as male with Social Security will need to register, which they can do online if they are under 26. Alternatively, if they are too old to register or do not want to, they can apply for a Status Information Letter, which says the person was not required to register but does not state the reason.

People who were assigned male at birth are required to register with Selective Service. This is true even if someone corrects her birth certificate and Social Security records to female prior to turning 18. Trans women under 26 can register online; they will just have to select “male” to register as it will not let females register.

State Identity Documents

NCTE maintains a list of the requirements to update the name and gender on each state’s driver’s licenses and non-driver ID cards [15]. Most states no longer require surgery to update these documents. Some states have forms that providers are to use and others will accept the same letter that was used to update federal documents.

For a minor who does not have a state ID yet, it is preferable to correct their birth certificate or get a passport in the new name and gender and use that to apply for a state ID for the first time.

Several states are issuing nonbinary IDs, but the logistical implications of these documents have not yet been fully determined. For example, a gender must be listed when booking a flight, and the options are limited to male or female. People choosing a nonbinary designation should be aware that their ID may not always result in recognition of their nonbinary status, particularly where federal rules are involved.

Birth Certificates

The procedure for correcting the sex on a birth certificate depends on where the person was born. The requirements for each state can be found on NCTE's ID document center [15]. Most states will seal the old record in the case of a gender change. About half of the states require a court order to update the sex on the birth certificate. In that case, it is mostly up to the judge to determine what proof is necessary and most states do not require proof of surgery. The other half of states use an administrative process of submitting the correction application the vital records agency. Most states require a letter from a provider, with about half requiring surgery and half not. An increasing number of states have eliminated the requirement of a provider letter altogether and have moved to a self-attestation model where the individual can correct their sex via an affidavit from themselves. Nonbinary designations are also increasingly permitted. A few states still prohibit birth certificate corrections even if the person has had surgery.

Name and Gender Changes with Private Entities

In addition to changing the name and gender on one's government ID documents, transgender people must individually contact every other entity or account with their name on it. This includes schools, banks, insurance companies, loans, utilities, retirement accounts, etc. Most schools will reissue a diploma with the new name for a fee. If the person is listed as a beneficiary in a will, IRA, college fund, life insurance policy or the like, it is best to update the name.

Conclusion

Providers can greatly assist transgender people by providing supportive documentation when requested. Moreover, providers have an important role to play in helping patients to identify legal issues and connecting them to legal services when necessary. Finally, providers have always played an influential role in advocating for transgender people in settings such as schools, employment, and insurance coverage, and such work is essential in eliminating discrimination and creating a healthy environment for trans people.

References

1. Lambda L et al. Creating equal access to quality health care for transgender patients: transgender-affirming hospital policies. https://www.lambdalegal.org/publications/fs_transgender-affirming-hospital-policies (2016).
2. Barry K, Levi J. Blatt v. Cabela's Retail, Inc. and a new path for transgender rights. Yale LJF. 2017;127:373–394.
3. Movement Advancement Project. Equality maps: non-discrimination laws. http://www.lgbtmap.org/equality-maps/non_discrimination_laws (2018). Accessed 16 Aug 2018.
4. The Joint Commission. Advancing effective communication, cultural competence, and patient- and family-centered care for the lesbian, gay, bisexual, and transgender (LGBT) community; 2011.
5. Transcend Legal. Medical discrimination fact sheets. https://transcendlegal.org/medical-discrimination-fact-sheets (2018). Accessed 16 Aug 2018.
6. Lambda L. Nationwide trans resources. https://www.lambdalegal.org/know-your-rights/trans-nationwide-resources (2018). Accessed 16 Aug 2018.
7. Health F. Client registration. http://fenwayhealth.org/documents/patient-services/FenwayClient_Registration_v11.pdf (2016).
8. Coleman DL, Rosoff PM. The legal authority of mature minors to consent to general medical treatment. Pediatrics. 2013;131:786–93. https://doi.org/10.1542/peds.2012-2470.
9. In re: JNS. No. F17-334 X Hamilton County Juvenile Ct; 2018, Feb 16.
10. Levi JL, Connors C. Transgender youth, medical professionals, and the law: what you should know. Adolesc Med. 2018;29:131–51.
11. Human Rights Campaign Foundation. Corporate equality index 2018. https://www.hrc.org/campaigns/corporate-equality-index (2018). Accessed 16 Aug 2018.
12. National Center for Transgender Equality. Health care action center. https://transequality.org/health-care-action-center (2018). Accessed 16 Aug 2018.
13. Transcend Legal. Transgender insurance medical policies. https://transcendlegal.org/health-insurance-medical-policies (2018). Accessed 16 Aug 2018.
14. James SE et al. The report of the 2015 U.S. transgender survey. http://www.transequality.org/sites/default/files/docs/usts/USTS%20Full%20Report%20-%20FINAL%201.6.17.pdf (2016).
15. National Center for Transgender Equality. ID documents center. https://transequality.org/documents (2018). Accessed 16 Aug 2018.

Chapter 17
Ethics of Gender-Affirming Care

Warren M. Seigel, Kelly McBride Folkers and Nancy Neveloff Dubler

Introduction

The ethical practice of medicine requires identifying the interests and rights of patients and creating a corresponding set of obligations and duties to fulfill those interests and rights. Throughout the last century, medical ethicists have struggled to recognize the requirements of patients within their social, ethnic, and class divides, and to encourage and force accommodation of their needs and wants in medical practice. That said, data reveal that medical providers are disinclined to recognize their own professional, social, and class biases about listening and responding to patients' voices, wants, needs, and desires. For example, we know that poor people of color are less likely to have their rights and interests identified and responded to than those not burdened by these socioeconomic characteristics. To create a responsive ethics of medical practice one must recognize the provider's perception of the "otherness" of some patients and confront those biases, as they may prevent the practitioner from meeting the patient where they are situated.

Since the inception of the LGBTQ+ rights movement, starting with the Stonewall riots in 1969, hospitals and healthcare institutions have made tremendous efforts to meet the needs of LGBTQ+ patients and to decrease homophobia and heteronormativity in healthcare. During the AIDS epidemic from 1981 forward, patients with HIV/AIDS, many of whom were gay men, advocated for the medical

W. M. Seigel
Department of Pediatrics/Division of Adolescent Medicine/Bioethics Consultation Service, NYC Health + Hospitals/Coney Island, Brooklyn, NY, USA

K. M. Folkers · N. N. Dubler
Division of Medical Ethics, Department of Population Health, NYU School of Medicine, New York, NY, USA

N. N. Dubler (✉)
NYC Health + Hospitals, New York, USA
e-mail: nancyadubler@gmail.com

L. Poretsky and W. C. Hembree (eds.), *Transgender Medicine*, Contemporary Endocrinology, https://doi.org/10.1007/978-3-030-05683-4_17

and research communities to address the specific needs and behaviors of their community. They demanded that medical practitioners create more inclusive practices. Accommodations were ultimately reached that made it possible for HIV/AIDS patients to receive excellent preventive care and effective interventions. Nonetheless, discrimination continues against LGBTQ+ patients, including the increasing numbers of patients who identify as transgender and gender nonconforming (TGNC). There remains a substantial need to design ethical and medical systems that address the evolving and complex needs of this population.

It is an axiom that nothing in medical ethics is permanent. In recent years, health professionals caring for children, adolescents, and young adults report an increase in the incidence of patients who self-identify as transgender. This increase in the population who publicly identify as TGNC has been quantified and examined through survey data [1]. Youth who do not unambiguously conform to societal gender norms often experience depression due to harassment, bullying, discrimination, and ostracism beyond that of their cisgender peers [2]. They are at significantly higher risk for substance abuse, physical, sexual and emotional abuse, coercion, suicidal ideation, and death by suicide [3].

Caring for children whose behavior and discourse suggest the presence of gender dysphoria or that they may be TGNC is ethically complex for pediatricians and parents. As humans have been predominantly classified into binary categories of "male" and "female," it may be even more complex for children who identify with a nonbinary gender as they navigate puberty and adolescence.

Transgender children can present a challenge to the caregiver. Their medical needs are constantly changing. Their sophistication as moral agents is emerging. Underlying their rapid evolution is the biological timer that will prohibit or permit an easier transition to their gender expression. Anxiety and uncertainty permeate this developing field of practice despite increasing expertise and developed guidelines for the standard of care. The reality presented by any particular child at any specific age may become uncertain and may change as they mature. The field of gender affirmation care is hampered by this continuously evolving background and the lack of long-term outcomes data to guide the selection of optimal treatments for these patients.

Bioethical processes and principles are best understood as part of an analysis of the life stories of patients. TGNC patients, by their nature and development, present conflicts about values and demand a range of options to best serve their interests. Ethical analyses gone awry might lead to treatment that is not in the best interests of a patient at a particular moment in their life.

The range of decision-making in medical care spans from deciding for others, which carries the heaviest ethical burden, to honoring and respecting the decision of a capable, legally authorized adult, which is the least weighty burden. Adult decision-making reflects the reasoning and rationale of an individual capable of assessing personal values, medical needs, risks and benefits, and the risks of foregoing treatment. In contrast, medical care decisions for children with gender dysphoria or TGNC children must be made in the best interest of the patient in advance of or during their development of adult decision-making capacity. The patient, family members, and increasingly, healthcare practitioners from whom families seek guidance feel such shifting burdens and perspectives. The uncertainties regarding best interest color the progress and process of ethical decision-making when caring for patients who experience dysphoria and may develop into TGNC adults.

Medical professionals can play a major role in supporting and improving the healthy development of TGNC youth and adults. In this chapter, we will focus attention on treating the TGNC population across the life cycle. We will intersperse the analysis with case descriptions of real patients who, while de-identified to retain anonymity, provide a context for the discussion of bioethical issues in their medical care.

Terminology and Description

Sexual orientation refers to a person's emotional and/or sexual attraction to other people. Sexual orientations can include sexual and/or romantic attraction to the opposite gender (heterosexual), same gender (homosexual), male and female (bisexual) genders, all genders (pansexual), or no genders (asexual). This list of sexual orientations is not exhaustive. A person's sexual orientation consists of three components which may or may not be congruent: desire, behavior, and identity.

Sexual identity refers to the experience of one's sexual desires. Homosexual, gay, lesbian, or bisexual identities (to name a few) involve a measure of one's self-acceptance as well as one's identification within a community. Sexual identity reflects how one thinks and feels about their sexual attraction and is not necessarily synonymous with sexual orientation, which is to whom one is emotionally and/or sexually attracted.

Gender identity refers to an individual's perception of and experience with belonging to a particular gender. This may or may not correspond to the gender one is assigned at birth. Gender identities include male, female, neither, both, or somewhere on the spectrum between what is traditionally considered male or female.

Gender roles refer to qualities that our society identifies as masculine or feminine and are an outward expression of our sense of ourselves and our gender.

Transgender is an umbrella term that refers to people whose self-identity is outside the boundaries of their biological sex and/or culturally determined gender expression. The term "transgender" originally was coined in the early 1970s at the beginnings of the LGBTQ+ rights movement in the US to refer to people who live full-time in a manner not associated with the gender that they were assigned at birth. Gender nonconforming and transgender youth often face enormous obstacles at home, at school, in foster care, and in the juvenile justice system. Historically, they have experienced a chronic state of conflict between the gender identity and role they were assigned at birth and the gender identity that most aligns with their lived experience. There is often an ongoing incongruence between who they feel they are and the perception others have of them. Some adults are able to integrate these tensions within well-formed personalities, but these internal struggles can be devastating to children and adolescents who do not experience social support aimed at affirming their gender identity.

Media coverage, increased interest in clinical practice, and increased public awareness have improved the visibility of TGNC people and their healthcare needs. Healthcare organizations with programs that aim to serve TGNC youth have reported a steady increase in the number of youth seeking services over the past 20 years. Current data suggest that approximately 1.4 million adults and 150,000 children identify as TGNC in the US [1]. Transgender people are known to be at a higher risk for mental health challenges as well as negative and often dangerous maladaptive behaviors because of stigma and discrimination. Transgender women, particularly those of color, are at the highest risk of violence and poor mental health.

Cisgender is a term used to describe individuals whose gender identities align with their assigned sex at birth.

All of these distinctions are further complicated because gender identity and sexual orientation may be independent variables.

A note about pronouns: the patients in each of the cases in this chapter will be addressed by the pronoun that aligns with their expressed gender identity preference. Though we note that the experience of gender dysphoria does not necessarily lead one to seek irreversible changes to one's secondary sexual characteristics, we believe it is important to respect each person's expressed gender identity by using pronouns consistent with their experiences. Indeed, new research has shown that the use of TGNC patients' chosen names in the clinic reduces poor mental health outcomes specific to this population [4]. Therefore, in the case discussions, we will refer to natal males who assert that they are female as "she" or "her" and to natal females who assert that they are male as "he" or "him." It is important to note that some TGNC people use neither "she" nor "he" and instead prefer "they" or "ze." For clarity and to respect the lived experiences of these children, we will use appropriate pronouns and use "they" to refer to the collective group of TGNC patients or a theoretical individual patient when discussing this population's needs as a whole.

Pediatrics and TGNC Patients

Case 1: The Case of the Furious 4-Year-Old

JP is a 4-year-old natal male who was born without complications to a 21-year-old mother and a 23-year-old father. JP's health and development were completely normal. Around 3 years of age, however, JP's parents noted that JP insisted that she was a girl, refused to wear pants or any articles of clothing that would usually be associated with boys, and consistently preferred items that were "sparkly" and "pretty." Today, while shopping for clothes for school, JP announced "I'm a girl and I'm going to dress like a girl. If I can't wear a dress to school, then I'm not going anymore!"

How can we assess the moral authority, wisdom, and insight of a 4-year-old? In this case, JP's authority equates to determination/power to disrupt family life, disregard rules and plans, and dictate the dress code that will permit the school-going enterprise to go forward. Parenting books alert parents to the "Terrible Twos": those irrational, explosive, and determined little emerging persons who demand what they want when they want it. But, 2-year-old little people can indeed be snatched up and physically moved. They can contribute much noise but have little effective ability to prevent the intervention that the parents felt would address the dismay of the moment. Many parenting books, however, fail to warn about the "'F'ing Fours": larger, but still little, people facing the same struggles for control and separation but with many more inches in height and length who can no longer easily be moved to a secure space and isolated from possibly disapproving onlookers.

A 4-year-old is a power into herself and has both the physical force and the emotional determination to insist on her will. Does this child have moral authority, wisdom, and insight? We can assume not. Does she have gender dysphoria? We don't know. Research seems to indicate that it is most likely that this child will "desist." But she has the power to bring the familial ship of state to an abrupt halt.

"Desistance," in this context, means the tendency for gender dysphoria to resolve itself over time as a child gets older. All else being equal, this research suggests that the most likely outcome for a very small child with gender dysphoria is that they will grow up to be cisgender [5]. However, there are major methodological and interpretative limitations and criticisms of this body of research, so much is not yet understood about the etiology of gender dysphoria [6]. So, it might be that this child will "desist" from her 4-year-old position. But, it might equally be so that this 4-year-old will seek medically irreversible change as she progresses in her physical, mental, and emotional development. Furthermore, it may be that this child will grow up with a gender expression that is nonbinary. Thus, it is important for parents and practitioners to note the child's discomfort with her gender and approach further mental health or medical care respecting the child's gender expression, although not necessarily her full autonomy, in relation to her ability to appreciate and understand her evolving gender identity.

Awareness of being a boy or a girl begins during the first year of a child's life when babies discover their genitals. Between the ages of 1 and 2, children become conscious of physical differences between genders. By the age of 3, children are easily able to label themselves as they acquire a strong concept of self [7].

During this same time of life, children learn gender role behavior—that is, doing things "that boys do" or "that girls do." Before the age of 3, children can differentiate gender-stereotyped toys. By 3 years of age, they have also become more aware of "boy" and "girl" activities, interests, and occupations. Many begin to play with youngsters of their own gender in activities identified with that gender. By the ages of 3–4 years old, most children can identify themselves as either a boy or a girl. By the time they enter kindergarten, children are able to articulate their gender identity [7].

What can we reliably say about the perception/reliability or moral agency of a 4-year-old? This is the same child who will, most certainly, have a tantrum if her sibling receives what she considers more than the fair share of meringue pie. Yet the choices for the parent and pediatrician are stark: break her will or follow her lead? It is difficult to conceive of the benefit of leaving a child battered, bruised, and hopeless in the face of her identification as a girl. This child is leading, however, and she knows that the importance of stipulating the terms and conditions of her participation in her family and in her educational community. How can we justify this leadership given that a 4-year-old has no notion of moral authority or agency or best interest? The answer lies in selecting the "least worst alternative" when the choices are respecting the "spoken choice" of the child, or leaving her defeated, battered, and hopeless in the face of the greater physical power of the parents and pediatrician [8, 9].

A European ethics group consensus on the management of intersex children suggested that there are three ethical principles that can be used to undergird decisions about care and guidance for intersex children. These can be applied to the TGNC population: (1) to foster the well-being of the child and the future adult, (2) to uphold the rights of children and adolescents to participate in and/or self-determine decisions that affect them now or later, and (3) to respect the family and parent–child relationships [10].

Could these principles help in resolving the case of this determined four-year-old? If they are to help, the parents and pediatrician/healthcare practitioner must accept that something serious is in the mind of this child. We are told in the case vignette that this has been a gradual evolution, within her 4 years of existence during which the child increasingly identifies herself as a girl. So, there is some relevant social history. Referring to the above principles, the child's well-being likely will not be furthered by total denial and rejection of her self-articulated positions. Certainly, offering her support now keeps open options for the future. The World Professional Association for Transgender Health (WPATH) recommends that mental health professionals work with the gender dysphoric child and their family to lessen the distress the child experiences with their gender, making sure not to impose a binary view of gender in this process. In some cases, in which there is an agreement between the pediatrician, mental health practitioner, and the parents, social transition to a new gender role may be appropriate [11]. Support for the family and child early on may help them to face the future with optimism.

Case 2: Adolescent Depressed Over Beginning Puberty

CJ is a 9-year-old natal female whose birth, health, and development have been normal. Recently, he announced to his family that he "feels deep down that I'm a boy" and has become increasingly depressed and despondent about beginning puberty. He was recently seen by his pediatrician who noted that he had breast buds, which indicated that puberty has started. Although the pediatrician seemed very happy and excited about CJ "turning into a young woman," CJ reports increasing anxiety and depression since this visit.

Having one's body change involuntarily is often disturbing to children, regardless of gender identity or expression. If the change foretells a process of becoming an adult in a gendered body that feels unwelcome and uncomfortable, it can be even more deeply upsetting. Unbeknownst to his family as well as his pediatrician, this child's response to the onset of puberty is at odds with what many of us would expect. He is, in fact, not happy about "turning into a young woman" and is now experiencing increased anxiety and depression due to the physical changes that he anticipates in the coming months.

Here we would like to reiterate the guidelines cited above: "(1) To foster the well-being of the child and the future adult, (2) to uphold the rights of children and adolescents to participate in and/or self-determine decisions that affect them now or later, and (3) to respect the family and parent–child relationships." These principles lead to an intervention by engaging the child and parents in a discussion with a sympathetic care practitioner, as well as exploring the child's feelings, preferences, interests, history, fears, anxieties, and notions of the future. All stakeholders in this discussion need to be cognizant of the need to respect the feelings and position of the child. They should avoid imposing more structure or supposing that more desire and determination exists than the situation might justify. This child may be uncomfortable with the pubertal changes associated with becoming a woman for reasons that have to do with highly sexualized images of women in modern society and the societal subjugation of women, rather than with gender dysphoria.

We do not know how long this child has felt that he is not a girl but is, in fact, a boy. This feeling may be longstanding but has never been openly discussed with his family and medical practitioners. Additionally, puberty either may have brought the issue to the forefront or confronted him with feelings that he had previously ignored or set aside. We cannot tell from this short vignette. What we do know is that:

The child's statement needs to be addressed carefully and thoughtfully to respect him as a person and offer him justice; he and his parents need to be supported by a pediatric professional who is open to and respectful about the issues that the patient is raising; an exploration of the child's gender identity at this moment in time should begin with an attempt to determine the proper course and conduct for his medical care; and all efforts should be made neither to push the child forward to a position that he might not really want nor to deny him an action that is really in his best interest and reflects his genuine interest and preferences.

According to the WPATH standard of care guidelines, hormone treatment that suppresses puberty may be administered to children and adolescents under the following minimum conditions: (1) the patient has demonstrated a long-lasting and intense pattern of gender nonconformity or dysphoria, (2) gender dysphoria emerged or worsened with puberty, (3) any co-existing medical, psychological, or social problems that could interfere with treatment have been addressed, and (4) the child or adolescent, to the extent they have capacity, has given informed consent along with parents or other caretakers or guardians who will support the patient through the treatment. Treatment with hormones that suppress puberty allows the adolescent to explore their gender nonconformity with "bought time" and to delay the development of secondary sex characteristics that the adolescent may find upsetting. In this case, the child is clearly uncomfortable with the development of breast buds, which indicates that this child has entered Tanner Stage 2 of puberty for natal females [11, 12].

While existing research has not evaluated the use of puberty suppressing hormones in children under the age of 12, such treatment is currently recommended for adolescents as young as 9 that have entered this stage of puberty, otherwise meet the WPATH criteria, and have been appropriately screened by a trained mental health professional. However, such a recommendation primarily is based upon professional consensus rather than validated outcomes. Thus, any decision to treat CJ with puberty suppressing hormones must be considered alongside the risks of such treatment, which exist somewhere between the standard of care and an experimental intervention as the hormones prescribed to suppress puberty are still being validated for long-term safety and efficacy. Some concerns regarding the safety of puberty suppressing hormones are mitigated by the reversibility of puberty suppression.

This case leaves us asking more questions than it answers. For example, we do not know how long the adolescent has been experiencing discomfort with his gender, nor do we know if he has any underlying medical or psychological health conditions that may be contributing to his distress. A pediatrician should convene a multidisciplinary care team that will take this adolescent's discomfort with puberty seriously and work toward affirming his gender experience.

Ambivalence is the natural state of being for pre-adolescents and adolescents. We have no idea in this vignette what this adolescent is saying and what the most ethical medical decision is at this time. What we can say with some certainty is that a sympathetic pediatrician/healthcare practitioner, with whom both the parents and the patient are at ease, should be involved in discussions and decisions going forward.

Currently, there are three unofficial views on treating the transgender adolescent. The first view states that it is best to wait until the adolescent is 18 when he can consent to treatment without a parent and has fully experienced puberty. Proponents of this view argue that individuals should experience all their adult characteristics, and only then can they decide on physical treatment.

Other experts support allowing the young person to experience puberty until Tanner stage 4 or 5, and then start GnRH analogues to halt further physical changes and perhaps initiate hormones to follow shortly thereafter at around age 15 or 16. Studies on this approach show good results with resolution of gender dysphoria and no regret by the adolescent relating to their gender affirmation. Their psychological well-being often improves as well [13].

Finally, another group of experts contends that if the diagnostic criteria for gender dysphoria are fulfilled, it makes sense to start puberty suppression, in the form of gonadotropin-releasing hormone (GnRH) analogues, at Tanner stage 2—around age 12 or 13 or even as young as 9—and initiate gender-affirming (commonly known as "cross sex") hormone treatment several years later. The advantages of administering GnRH analogues are that the changes are fully reversible; they provide extra time for psychotherapy and a relief of dysphoria as well as reactive depression, and they prevent the development of secondary sex characteristics that would require more invasive intervention later should the child's gender dysphoria persists [11].

Case 3: Suicidal Adolescent

LB is a 17-year-old natal male with no significant past medical history. A senior in high school this year, LB has always been noted to dress and act more feminine than his peers and has refused to go to gym class for the past 2 years. LB likes music, acting, theater, and dance, and has friends that are mainly girls. The family has always been very accepting of LB's behavior and thought that "this was just a phase that he will outgrow." LB had been an "A" student until sophomore year, when LB began cutting classes, became more withdrawn, and began spending more time alone and less time with friends or family. Today, LB is brought into the pediatric emergency room after having ingested multiple unknown medications that were found in the family's medicine cabinet in an admitted suicide attempt.

After being stabilized and treated medically, the patient disclosed to a mental health social worker that she has never felt "like a real male" and in fact has always "felt deep down inside me that I am a woman just trapped in a man's body." The patient further states that she has been increasingly bullied at school, although no one knows that she had been struggling with her gender for many years. She had, in fact, never told anyone until the suicide attempt. She does state that she has many good friends who are girls and she believes that they accept her for who she is, but for the past 2 years, the bullying at school has gotten worse. She had been contemplating suicide for the past 6 months. She admits that this was an intentional act on her part and states that she would "rather die than live like a freak!"

TGNC youth experience a higher risk of suicide than their cisgender peers. Studies of mental health outcomes in transgender youth have demonstrated that between a third to 45% of those studied have reported having thought seriously about ending their lives; one survey reported that 26% of respondents had attempted suicide [14, 15]. Violence and bullying toward LGBTQ+ youth have been documented extensively.

This child presents a most difficult case as her deep preferences have been stored up inside forcing her to exist in silence. She has gone through puberty, felt alone, been bullied, sought no solace until her suffering overwhelmed her. Depression won over optimism in the tussle between her emotions and actions.

Untangling the educational, medical, and emotional mess is the first step in the process of understanding, adjustment, and recovery. First, a skilled mental health professional must determine whether the depression behind the suicide attempt was part of an ongoing suicidal ideation that presents an ongoing threat to this patient's life or an initial cry for help that once responded to is contained. That is the initial determination that will indicate whether this child needs placement and supervision or understanding and therapy.

Second, the need of the child for openness and support must be addressed. It seems unusual that her drop in academic standing, refusal to go to gym class, and increasing isolation did not trigger more active intervention by her parents. What is the role that they have played in her increasing isolation? Each of the separate behaviors cried out for attention; the combination demonstrated a clear and present danger for this child. Are the parents transphobic, unaware emotionally and intellectually, hostile, or disengaged? How did this happen?

We are long beyond the stage of the "schizophrenigenic" mother. Parents, and mothers especially, are no longer considered the origin of homosexuality, bipolar disorder, or schizophrenia. However, total disregard for a growing pattern of dysfunction and isolation seems more pathological than accidental.

This is a case that needs intensive interventions by medical, mental health, and social service personnel and others to determine the level of danger, stabilize the situation, and begin to move forward. In the meantime, as this patient has stated that she has persistent and distressing feelings of gender dysphoria for many years, it would benefit her if her providers and family called her by the female pronoun and her chosen name. Recent research has shown that when providers call gender nonconforming patients by their chosen names, they experience better health outcomes and a more trustworthy doctor–patient relationship. Although she may not ultimately live as a transgender woman for the rest of her life, this teenager has the ability to express her preferences, which should be respected.

Caring for the Adult TGNC Patient

Discussing the rights of adult persons to make decisions about their own healthcare is generally a formulaic process that requires the initial determination that the patient is decisionally capable and can understand the options arrayed by the medical team to structure the choice of a course of care. The practitioners, led by the attending physician, must then present the diagnosis, prognosis, possible interventions, risks and benefits of each intervention, and the likely consequences of nonintervention. This is the standard schema for the process of informed consent.

What it is missing in this basic schema is the human interaction and the professional obligation of the physician to provide interpretation, support, and empathetic advice to this particular patient. In this expanded notion of sharing information and decision-making, the terms of informed consent—which has become more of a legal and risk-management label than an ethical aspiration—might more appropriately be changed to "advised consent" to encompass the doctor–patient relationship and its attendant obligations.

But even the change from "informed consent" to "advised consent" will not help in exploring and describing the status of ethical issues that apply to the decision of a person to enter the path and process of gender-affirming care. In the next brief discussion, we will address: the history of TGNC care and key persons in that history; the emergence of the more extended discussion of TGNC care in the last decade; and the factors of race, class, education, socioeconomic status, familial and community support, and strength of character, all of which play a role in shaping decisions to enter a gender-affirming pathway.

As a whole, LGBTQ+ people often experience worse health outcomes than their heterosexual and cisgender peers [16]. Experts call these differences "health disparities." On its website, the US Office of Disease Prevention and Health Promotion lists a number of alarming disparities identified by researchers thus far [17]. Lesbian women are less likely to get cancer screening with Pap tests and mammograms, and lesbian and bisexual women are more likely to be overweight or obese—both are risk factors for a host of health issues. Young gay and bisexual men—especially gay and bisexual men of color—disproportionately bear the burden of new HIV diagnoses. LGBTQ+ youth are two to three times more likely to attempt suicide. TGNC people of all ages experience higher rates of sexually transmitted infections, mental health issues, and suicide. Finally, LGBTQ+ populations have higher rates of alcohol abuse, smoking, and other drug abuse. These disparities exist for a number of reasons. There is ongoing stress caused by living in a society where LGBTQ+ people are stigmatized and subject to violence. There is a lower rate of insurance coverage in the LGBTQ+ community, which compounds the problem [18].

As the binary world of sexuality and gender disappears, the fluid and unconstrained world that emerges provides little guidance for physicians attempting to meet the medical needs of the queer community. Deciding to seek gender affirmation care is not solely about "health" care, even if it involves members of the medical profession in providing support, medical advice, hormones, and sometimes surgery. It is important to note that TGNC identities can be expressed and affirmed without medical intervention, and gender fluidity is becoming more acceptable within the queer community. The University of California, San Francisco, has published an approach to genderqueer, gender nonconforming, and gender nonbinary people in its guidelines for the care of TGNC people, which asserts the acceptance of varied gender expressions and how medicine should approach them [19]. However, gender affirmation care, in general, is still discussed in terms of a gender binary.

Most readers, newshounds, and ethically aware medical professionals encountered two transgender woman, Renee Richards and Jan Morris, as they first appeared in public life. Jennifer Boylan's book, *She's Not There: A Life in Two Genders*, began to examine and grapple with the feelings that might lead a person to act so aggressively to so change the basis of their being. Jennifer Boylan put to rest the notions that adolescent discontent, developmental issues, lack of peer identification, and the desire to mutilate oneself all played a part in this strange scenario. But, icons do not translate into patients, whose lives and dilemmas become part of the clinical material of medical ethics. Actual stories of real people became, as always, the basis for ethical examination.

Consider the Following Cases

Peter is a man who, as a female child, was always trailing off after his older brother and working to emulate everything about him. Peter insisted that he was a boy and that a mistake had been made assigning him to the female gender. He consistently acted, dressed, and posed as a male person. When he came to speak at the Annual Corser Symposium, the educational highlight of ethics discussion at the New York City Health + Hospitals Corporation, he narrated a long history of gender discontent, insistence on dressing as a boy as a young child and on beginning hormones as an adolescent to prevent puberty. That early intervention prevented the development of many of the secondary sex characteristics of female development and made the transition to a male gender relatively smooth and uncomplicated.

Maxine was designated female at birth but presented as a "tomboy" during much of their childhood. They stumbled through elementary school but were increasingly alienated in middle school as they began to experience female puberty. They suspected that they were gay but were not sufficiently comfortable with their parents to so state. The parents, both well educated, New York professionals, struggled with how to manage. Maxine suggested attending boarding school, to which they both agreed.

By sophomore year in high school, Maxine found other queer people at school, which allowed them to flourish and come out publicly as lesbian. Maxine was comfortable and happy and thought that they had accomplished "finding their place" in the world.

But, as a freshman in college, they discovered that there was a category called "transgender" of which they had not been aware. This category of understanding became increasingly appealing to Maxine. In their second year, they began using they/them pronouns, binding their breasts to great pain and discomfort, and receiving very intensive counseling, which lead to beginning hormone therapy a year later. At the end of their third year, it was clear the breast removal was a necessary next step. In their last year of college, they not only lived as an "out" nonbinary person (although not with necessarily fixed sexual preferences) but evolved legally with a name change to Max. They found their new identity "pleasing and pleasant." Would the future bring more surgery? Uncertain. Many trans persons who have had "top surgery" do not proceed further with surgery as bottom surgery is far less successful and less certain.

Joyce grew up as a tomboy. They came out to her parents as gay in high school, played soccer in college, and seemed to have a stable presence as a lesbian woman. As a very successful fifth-year associate in a major New York City law firm, they had successful relationships with other gay women. But they were increasingly uncomfortable with both their assigned gender and assumed identity. At age 33, they sought medical assistance to begin hormone treatment and made plans for top surgery.

Each of these stories demonstrates how the TGNC experience can evolve along with the individual. Some individuals seek a range of medical interventions, while some choose to seek none at all. Clinicians should be aware that TGNC individuals are not a "one-size-fits-all" population in terms of the choices and options they will seek to affirm their chosen gender identity. While Peter sought out gender affirmation care earlier in life, Joyce did not decide to seek medical intervention until into their 30s. Thus, gender-affirming care can be sought and received throughout the life cycle. Providers should approach adult patients individually, making no assumptions about each patient's experience as a TGNC person.

Another major issue that TGNC adults face in the clinic is discrimination. Many TGNC adults feel discouraged from seeking out routine clinical care unrelated to gender affirmation because they fear discrimination or intolerance in the healthcare setting, which may contribute to some of the health disparities that TGNC people face. Though 20 states and the District of Columbia provide insurance coverage mechanisms for transgender adults through anti-discrimination laws, Medicaid policy, or both, many TGNC people report delays or barriers to accessing gender-affirming and routine healthcare. Many procedures that are traditionally associated with one gender, like Pap tests or prostate exams, have been unfairly denied to TGNC adults because providers have been unable to bill for procedures that do not "match" a patient's gender marker. Moreover, the US Department of Health and Human Services, under the Trump administration, is increasing the enforcement of conscientious objection protections for healthcare providers, which may allow practitioners to discriminate against TGNC people on the basis of religious grounds. Thus, TGNC people seeking routine and gender-affirming care may be unable to obtain either; the landscape of practitioners offering such care may become more heterogeneous than it already is. Healthcare practitioners working with TGNC adults should be aware of the barriers they face in coming into the clinic and do their best to make the experience one that is affirming and positive.

One way to accomplish this goal is by referring to the patient by their chosen name and use their appropriate pronouns. Unfortunately, many healthcare professionals struggle with this, as a patient's legal name may not match their chosen name. Healthcare professionals should be sure to ask their TGNC patients what name they would like to be called and what their preferred pronouns are. These simple questions demonstrate to the patient that the healthcare professional is helping them to affirm their gender expression.

Conclusion

Social upheaval generates chaos at many levels. The expansion beyond binary gender categories has created new challenges in schools, state legislatures, federal regulatory process, and in the practice of medicine. Medical ethics cannot escape these challenges as the field mediates the tension that can arise between maintaining long-held ethical standards and new developments. This tension is especially true in pediatrics, in which the focus of medicine is on the evolving nature of the patient in the context of changing needs, wants, and desires. But it is also true in the care of adults and emerging adults. The search for clarity and comfort in adults or older adolescents is accompanied by chaos and confusion. It is these latter emotions that surround the care practitioner and challenge them to reach out and guide, rather than step back and retreat.

The characteristics of clinical ethics consultation (CEC) from the STADA model [20] can provide a framework for mediating tensions that arise in gender-affirming care for youth. This model is used by clinical ethics consultants in settings where an ethical issue arises in medical care for which mediation is needed to resolve the issue. In situations where CEC is employed, the consultant must reach a solution to the ethical issue by mediating the concerns of the patient, family members, and medical practitioners. The following steps can be employed when medical practitioners are assisting gender dysphoric patients and their family members with a clinical decision:

Sit with everyone to assess what is happening.

Tell me what is happening and how you feel about it.

Admire the ability of all to come together and talk.

Discuss the options.

Advise on what can or might or should happen to help the individual reach their goal.

There is no short answer for how all TGNC patients should be treated in the clinic. There is, however, process—quiet, open, and supportive listening and responding to the needs of this unique population.

References

1. Herman JL, Flores AR, Brown TN, Wilson BD, Conron KJ. Age of individuals who identify as transgender in the United States. The Williams Institute: UCLA School of Law; 2017.
2. Becerra-Culqui T, Liu Y, Nash R, Cromwell L, Flanders WD, Getahun D, Giammattei SV, Hunkeler EM, Lash TL, Millman A, Quinn VP, Robinson B, Roblin D, Sandberg DE, Silverberg MJ, Tangpricha V, Goodman M. Mental health of transgender and gender nonconforming youth compared with their peers. Pediatrics. 2018;141(5). https://doi.org/10.1542/peds.2017-3845.
3. de Vries AL, Doreleijers TA, Steensma TD, Cohen-Kettenis PT. Psychiatric comorbidity in gender dysphoric adolescents. J Child Psychol Psychiatry. 2011;52(11):1195–202.
4. Russell ST, Pollitt AM, Li G, Grossman AH. Chosen name use is linked to reduced depressive symptoms, suicidal ideation, and suicidal behavior among transgender youth. J Adolesc Health. 2018;S1054-139X(18):30085-5.
5. Wallien MS, Cohen-Kettenis PT. Psychosexual outcome of gender-dysphoric children. J Am Acad Child Adolesc Psychiatry. 2008;47:1413–23.
6. Newhook JT, Pyne J, Winters K, Feder S, Holmes C, Tosh J, Sinnott M, Jamieson A, Pickett S. A critical commentary on follow-up studies and "desistance" theories about transgender and gender-nonconforming children. Int J Transgenderism. 2018;19:212–24.
7. American Academy of Pediatrics. Caring for your school-age child: ages 5–12. New York: Bantam Books; 1995.
8. Collopy B, Dubler N, Zuckerman C. The ethics of home care: autonomy and accommodation. Hastings Cent Rep. 1990;20:1–16 suppl.

9. Dubler NN. Autonomy and accommodation: mediating individual choice in the home setting. Generations. 1990;14:29–31.
10. Wiesemann C, Ude-Koeller S, Sinnecker GH, Thyen U. Ethical principles and recommendations for the medical management of differences of sex development (DSD)/intersex in children and adolescents. Eur J Pediatr. 2010;169:671–9.
11. Coleman E, Bockting W, Botzer M, Cohen-Kettenis PT, Decuypere G, Feldman J, Fraser L, Green J, Knudson G, Meyer WJ, Monstrey S, Adler RK, Brown GR, Devor AH, Ehrbar R, Ettner R, Eyler E, Garofalo R, Karasic DH, Lev AI, Mayer G, Meyer-Bahlburg HF, Hall BP, Pfaefflin F, Rachlin K, Robinson B, Schechter LS, Tangpricha V, van Trotsenburg M, Vitale A, Winter S, Whittle S, Wylie K, Zucker KJ. Standards of care for the health of transsexual, transgender, and gender-nonconforming people, version 7. Int J Transgenderism. 2012;13:165–232.
12. Hembree WC, Cohen-Kettenis PT, Gooren L, Hannema SE, Meyer WJ, Murad MH, Rosenthal SM, Safer JD, Tangpricha V, T'Sjoen GG. Endocrine treatment of gender-dysphoric/gender-incongruent persons: an endocrine society clinical practice guideline. J Clin Endocrinol Metab. 2017;102:3869–903.
13. Smith YL, van Goozen SH, Cohen-Kettenis PT. Adolescents with gender identity disorder who were accepted or rejected for sex reassignment surgery: a prospective follow-up study. J Am Acad Child Adolesc Psychiatry. 2001;40:472–81.
14. Clements-Nolle K, Marx R, Katz M. Attempted suicide among transgender persons. J Homosex. 2006;51:53–69.
15. Grossman AH, D'Augelli AR. Transgender youth and life-threatening behaviors. Suicide Life Threat Behav. 2007;37:527–37.
16. PFLAG National Glossary of Terms [Online]. Parents, families and friends of lesbians and gays; 2018. Available: https://www.pflag.org/glossary. Accessed 26 July 2018.
17. Office of Disease Prevention and Health Promotion. Lesbian, gay, bisexual, and transgender health [Online]; 2018. Available: https://www.healthypeople.gov/2020/topics-objectives/topic/lesbian-gay-bisexual-and-transgender-health. Accessed 26 July 2018.
18. Padula WV, Baker K. Coverage for gender-affirming care: making health insurance work for transgender Americans. LGBT Health. 2017;4:244–7.
19. Deutsch MB (ed). Guidelines for the primary and gender-affirming care of transgender and gender nonbinary people. Center of Excellence for Transgender Health, University of California, San Francisco; 2016. Available: http://transhealth.ucsf.edu/protocols. Accessed 30 July 2018.
20. Dubler NN, Liebman CB. Bioethics mediation: a guide to shaping share solutions. Vanderbilt University Press, New York; 2011. p. 74–75.

Chapter 18
Spiritual Care of Transgender Persons

Jo Hirschmann, Emilee Walker-Cornetta and Susan Jelinek

Introduction

This chapter, which is intended to be used by chaplains as well as by clinicians, defines terms that are frequently used in the context of spiritual care and highlights research in the field of religiosity/spirituality (R/S) and health that has relevance for transgender populations. It also describes some features of chaplaincy care for transgender adults and adolescents through the presentation of cases. We proceed from the understanding that R/S beliefs and behaviors can be both supportive and harmful forces in people's lives. This is particularly true for transgender people, especially those who were raised in religious communities that do not embrace members who come out as transgender and/or transitioning. At the same time, the research literature shows, and our work as chaplains affirms, that religion and spirituality can be rich sources of support and meaning in transgender people's lives. This chapter invites all those who work with transgender people in healthcare settings to assess their patients' R/S needs and resources, whether this is in the context of transition-related healthcare, general medicine, or other clinical settings.

J. Hirschmann (✉)
Department of Spiritual Care and Education, Mount Sinai Beth Israel, New York, NY, USA
e-mail: jo.hirschmann@mountsinai.org

E. Walker-Cornetta
Department of Pastoral Care and Education, New York-Presbyterian Hospital, Columbia University Irving Medical Center, New York, NY, USA

S. Jelinek
Department of Pastoral Care, Cincinnati Children's Hospital Medical Center, Cincinnati, OH, USA

L. Poretsky and W. C. Hembree (eds.), *Transgender Medicine*, Contemporary Endocrinology, https://doi.org/10.1007/978-3-030-05683-4_18

Definitions

Although spirituality and religion are diffuse concepts with complex and overlapping usages, research about their interactions with health outcomes requires distinctive operational definitions [1]. In the current literature on R/S and health, religion is generally understood to designate participation in historic and established institutions, communities, and doctrinal systems that function to promote connection to the divine and guide one's living. The more inclusive of the two terms, spirituality typically refers to a person's "improvised and individual" experience of the sacred. It describes a range of human experiences related to ultimate beliefs and concerns that may or may not also be considered "religious" in nature [2]. The following definition of spirituality was developed for use in healthcare settings and is often cited in literature on R/S and health:

> [Spirituality is] the aspect of humanity that refers to the way individuals seek and express meaning and purpose and the way they experience their connectedness to the moment, to self, to others, to nature and to the significant or sacred. [3]

Significance of R/S in Clinical Settings

It is well known that many people look to R/S resources for strength and comfort in times of stress [4]. Pertinent to the healthcare context, a range of studies have demonstrated positive associations between R/S and quality of life in adult medical patients [1, 5–7]. Though many people find turning to R/S in difficult times to be rewarding, others may discover that R/S does not provide them with the support they need, or even compounds feelings of distress. This phenomenon is known as *spiritual struggle*, *spiritual distress*, or *negative religious coping*. It can include such experiences as feeling distant from or punished by God, questioning one's faith, or the loss of a sense of religious belonging [8–10]. Studies about the prevalence of spiritual struggle in healthcare settings have shown that up to half of patients may experience some spiritual struggle, with up to 15% of patients experiencing moderate or severe struggle [11, 12].

Despite these findings and the fact that a majority of patients would welcome the opportunity to discuss their spiritual needs with their physicians, only a small population of patients report having received spiritual care from their healthcare team [13–18]. Clinicians surveyed in these studies cited lack of training as the biggest barrier to routinely assessing patients' spiritual needs. Further development of spiritual screening tools and programs for clinician education would help ensure that patients in need of more comprehensive spiritual care—of the kind that may be provided by a trained, professional chaplain—receive access to it [12, 19, 20].

Spiritual Care and Chaplaincy

While all members of the clinical team ideally have some competence in identifying and meeting patients' R/S needs, chaplains may be called upon to assess and respond to needs that require greater expertise in the area of R/S coping. This distinction between *spiritual care generalists* (which refers to all members of the team other than chaplains) and *spiritual care specialists* (which refers to chaplains) will be explored in more detail below [21]. Chaplains acquire such expertise through graduate-level education in religion or theology, combined with minimum of four units of Clinical Pastoral Education (CPE). CPE is accredited by the Department of Education-recognized Association for Clinical Pastoral Education and is a case study method of training. Through clinical experience, individual supervision, and group reflection, CPE students learn how to provide tailored support to patients and families with diverse R/S and cultural backgrounds.

Critical elements of chaplaincy care include: (1) an assessment of patients' (and family members') spiritual beliefs and/or practices and how they impact coping, (2) interventions to support patients' access to their own spiritual resources and facilitate progress toward their spiritual goals, and (3) ongoing evaluation of the outcomes of those interventions. Research on chaplain activities in patient visits indicates that most interventions constitute what is called "empathetic" or "active" listening, the provision of emotional support, and religious activities such as prayer or other rituals [22–24]. Other possible goals of chaplaincy care include pursuing alignment between the plan of care and the patient's values, reducing a person's feelings of isolation, facilitating meaning-making, and promoting a sense of peace [25]. In a multisite survey of about 1500 hospital inpatients, of the nearly 70% who wanted to see a chaplain, 77% reported that an important reason to do so was "to be reminded of God's care and presence." Other reasons endorsed as important or very important were to provide support for their family and friends (71%), to be with them in times of anxiety (69%), to pray or read scripture with them (62%), and to counsel them regarding moral/ethical concerns or decisions (39%) [26].

While research on measurable outcomes of chaplaincy care is still relatively nascent, preliminary studies suggest that chaplains' interventions may be associated with increased levels of positive religious coping [27, 28]. In addition, several studies have shown that patients who consider their R/S needs to have been met by their healthcare team, including through visits with chaplains, report higher satisfaction with overall care [29–31].

Screening and Assessment Tools

Spiritual care generalists need tools for identifying R/S distress in patients, making referrals to chaplains, and identifying how patients' R/S lives may intersect with their healthcare needs. In settings where no chaplains are available, physicians,

Table 18.1 Tools used to identify and assess patients' R/S need

Tool	For spiritual care (SC) generalists or SC specialists?	Purpose
FICA© Spiritual History Tool	Developed for physicians and other SC generalists; to be used when taking a history in a medical setting	To understand how patients' R/S lives might affect their medical coping and decision-making
Rush Religious Struggle Screening Protocol	SC generalists	To identify patients who are experiencing R/S struggle and refer them to chaplains
Religious and Spiritual Struggles Scale	Developed for the purpose of conducting research but its categories could be used by chaplains as a spiritual assessment tool	To categorize and differentiate among six forms of R/S struggle

FICA© Spiritual History Tool

nurses, social workers, and other clinicians need tools to assess and then address patients' R/S concerns. Chaplains, meanwhile, need tools with which to conduct spiritual assessments, which then become the basis for choosing appropriate interventions.

Here, we offer examples of three such tools. In the case study section of this chapter, we will provide practical examples of how these tools might be employed with transgender patients. Table 18.1 offers an overview of these three tools, by whom they are intended to be used, and their purpose. Each tool is then described in more detail below.

The most widely-used spiritual history is the FICA, which was developed by Christina Puchalski for use by physicians. This screen is intended to be used by physicians as they take patients' histories. Utilizing the FICA tool helps physicians learn about how patients' R/S lives contribute to coping and decision-making in the context of illness. The FICA incorporates the following sections and questions:

F—Faith and Belief
"Do you consider yourself spiritual or religious?" or "Is spirituality something important to you?" or "Do you have spiritual beliefs that help you cope with stress/difficult times?"
If the patient responds "No," the healthcare provider might ask, "What gives your life meaning?" Sometimes patients respond with answers such as family, career, or nature. (The question about meaning should also be asked even if people answer yes to spirituality.)
I—Importance
"What importance does your spirituality have in your life? Has your spirituality influenced how you take care of yourself, your health? Does your spirituality influence you in your healthcare decision-making? (e.g. advance directives, treatment, etc.)"

C—Community
"Are you part of a spiritual community? Communities such as churches, temples, and mosques, or a group of like-minded friends, family, or yoga can serve as strong support systems for some patients. Can explore further: Is this of support to you and how? Is there a group of people you really love or who are important to you?"
A—Address in Care
"How would you like me, your healthcare provider, to address these issues in your healthcare?"

The Rush Religious Struggle Screening Protocol

This screening protocol was developed by chaplains at Rush University Medical Center and tested on a group of 96 medical rehabilitation patients (Fig 18.1). It was developed to be used by providers other than chaplains to assess whether hospitalized patients would benefit from a chaplain visit. It asks whether religion/spirituality plays a role in coping and enquires about how much strength and comfort a person is deriving right now from their religion or spirituality. In this study, the screening was administered by psychology and medical residents and, when chaplains made follow-up visits to patients and conducted spiritual assessments, the screening tool was found to have accurately identified R/S struggle in all but one case [32].

A 2016 QI project, led by Grossoehme and colleagues and described in more detail in the next section, tested the Rush Screening Protocol with adolescents and their caregivers in an outpatient transgender clinic [33]. In 2017, the screening protocol was tested in a study involving bone marrow transplant survivors and was found to have poor sensitivity and specificity [34]. While the protocol may need to be refined for maximum utility, we include it here because of its acceptability to patients, caregivers, and staff in Grossoehme et al.'s 2016 study [33]. The Rush Screening Protocol is reproduced here (Fig. 18.1) in the form it was used in Grossoehme et al.'s project. We provide an example of its use in the case study section of this chapter.

Religious and Spiritual Struggles Scale

This scale was introduced into the research literature in a 2014 article by Exline and colleagues [35], which describes the development and initial validation of a six-item self-report measure that categorizes different kinds of religious struggle. The paper builds upon Pargament's earlier work on positive and negative religious coping; Pargament is a coauthor of the paper.

The scale encompasses *transpersonal struggle* (in this case, struggle with the divine and/or with demonic entities), *interpersonal struggle* (i.e., struggle with other people), and *intrapersonal struggle* (i.e., struggle within oneself). Table 18.2

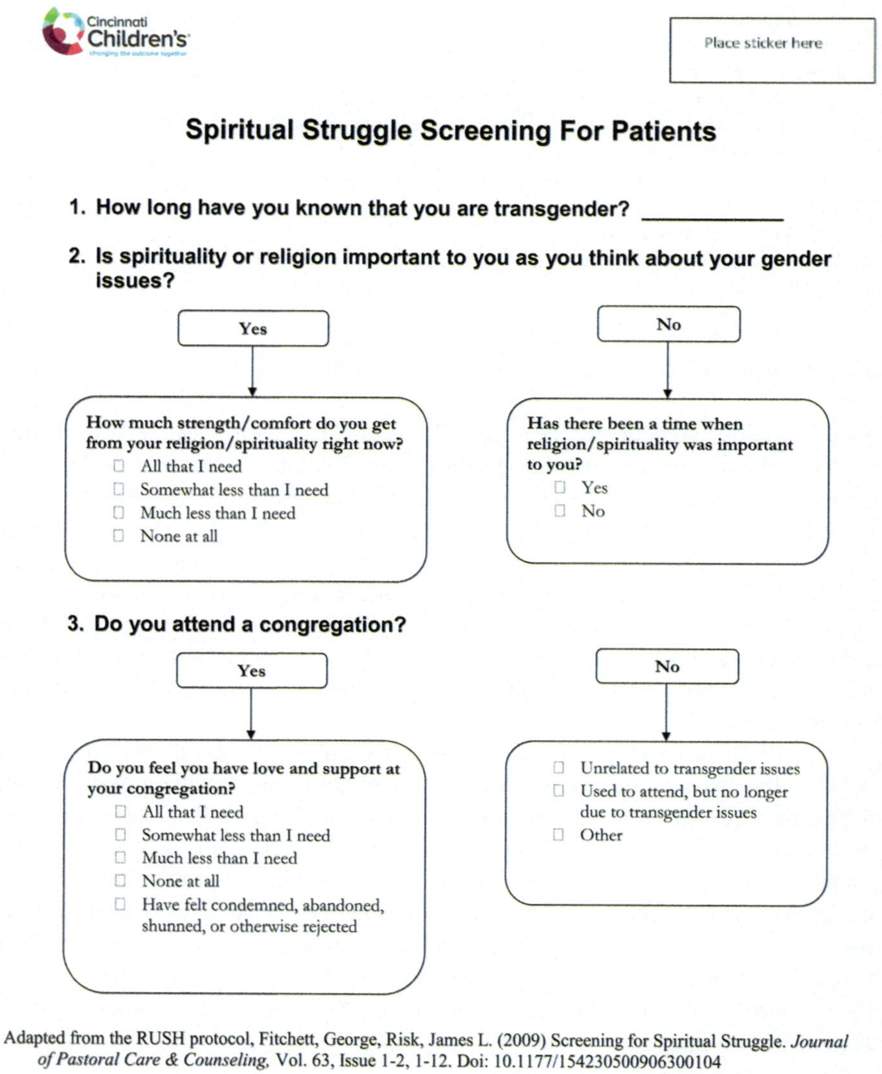
Cincinnati Children's
changing the outcome together

Place sticker here

Spiritual Struggle Screening For Patients

1. **How long have you known that you are transgender?** ____________

2. **Is spirituality or religion important to you as you think about your gender issues?**

Yes

How much strength/comfort do you get from your religion/spirituality right now?

- ☐ All that I need
- ☐ Somewhat less than I need
- ☐ Much less than I need
- ☐ None at all

No

Has there been a time when religion/spirituality was important to you?

- ☐ Yes
- ☐ No

3. **Do you attend a congregation?**

Yes

Do you feel you have love and support at your congregation?

- ☐ All that I need
- ☐ Somewhat less than I need
- ☐ Much less than I need
- ☐ None at all
- ☐ Have felt condemned, abandoned, shunned, or otherwise rejected

No

- ☐ Unrelated to transgender issues
- ☐ Used to attend, but no longer due to transgender issues
- ☐ Other

Adapted from the RUSH protocol, Fitchett, George, Risk, James L. (2009) Screening for Spiritual Struggle. *Journal of Pastoral Care & Counseling*, Vol. 63, Issue 1-2, 1-12. Doi: 10.1177/154230500906300104

Fig. 18.1 Spiritual struggle screening for patients. Adapted from the RUSH protocol [32]

delineates these six forms of R/S struggle and provides examples of what might constitute each one. This scale has the potential to be used as an assessment tool by chaplains, who are trained to recognize signs of each of these forms of struggle.

Before returning to these tools with cases that illustrate their practical application in clinical settings, we will summarize key themes in the small body of research that looks at the R/S lives of transgender people.

Table 18.2 Summary of Exline et al.'s categories of R/S struggle

Type of struggle	Examples
Divine struggle	Feeling let down by God, angry with God, abandoned by God
Demonic struggle	Feeling tormented by the devil/evil spirits or that these forces are trying to turn one away from what is good
Interpersonal struggle	Feeling hurt, mistreated, misunderstood, rejected, or offended by religious/spiritual people
Intrapersonal struggle: moral	Feeling guilty, feeling torn between what one wants and what one knows is morally right
Intrapersonal struggle: doubt-related	Struggling to figure out what one really believes, feeling confused about one's beliefs
Intrapersonal struggle: struggle around ultimate meaning	Questioning whether one's life has meaning in the world, having concerns about whether there is ultimate purpose to life or existence

Transgender People's R/S Lives: An Overview of the Literature

As already described, religiosity can function in people's lives in both positive and negative ways, a theme that recurs throughout the small literature about transgender people's religious and spiritual (R/S) lives. This section summarizes the findings of literature that focuses on the R/S lives of *transgender adults* (including overarching themes applicable to all age groups and also including some content about young adults); *transgender children, adolescents, and young adults*; and *older transgender people*.

Adults

The United States Transgender Survey reveals a cycle of belonging to, leaving, and finding religious communities. The survey, which collected responses from more than 27,000 transgender people, found that two-thirds of respondents had belonged to a faith community at some time in their lives and almost a third had belonged to one in the past year. Of these, almost two-thirds were members of communities in which they reported that leaders/members thought or knew the respondent was transgender. However, more than a third (39%) of respondents had left a faith community because of the fear of rejection and 19% reported that they had been rejected. While some faith communities are welcoming—or at least tolerant—of transgender people, others are unsupportive and even hostile. This dual reality might be reflected in respondents' reports about finding new faith communities. Of those who were rejected by a faith community, 42% subsequently found a new community that welcomed them as a transgender person [36].

Reinforcing the notion that religion can be both a positive and negative force in transgender people's lives, a study of 92 young transgender women found that "God Consciousness," a subscale of the Religious Background and Behaviors (RBB) questionnaire, can protect against HIV risk. However, the same relationship was not found to exist between HIV risk and "Formal Religious Practices," [37]. Similarly, a study of 75 transgender women asked participants about several forms of stress-related growth and found that religious beliefs and behaviors were not supportive forces in respondents' lives. Instead, they were predictors of unprotected anal sex, especially for respondents who also reported low levels of social support. But in contrast to religious beliefs and behaviors, religious stress-related growth, defined as perceptions of positive personal or life changes associated with stressful events, was a negative predictor of unprotected anal sex. The authors offer the following interpretation of these findings: "[I]t appears that translating the stresses associated with being a transgender woman into a stronger religious identity allows these individuals to avoid sexual risk-taking as a negative coping strategy." [38].

The work of Dowshen et al. and Golub et al. might fall into the category of studies that Stanton and colleagues describe as focusing on negative outcomes and risk reduction [39]. A relatively smaller number of studies focus on resilience, strengths, and identity development and allow us to hear transgender people describing their R/S lives in their own words. A phenomenological study that involved semi-structured interviews with six MTFs and five FTMs drew out six key elements of resilience in response to traumatic life events, including "cultivating spirituality and hope for the future." In this study, a 26-year-old Latina MTF described God as a source of self-assurance. She reported, "I loved God—knew he didn't make me transgender for no reason at all—this was my journey in life." Referring to a time in her life when her mother perceived her as a gay man, a 27-year-old multiracial MTF described how religion was initially a negative and later a positive force in her life. She said, "A punishment from my mom was being forced to read passages condemning homosexuals to hell … I am a very spiritual person though. Eventually, I established my own relationship with my creator that I don't have to justify to anyone who I am." [40].

In another study, case vignettes taken from one author's therapy practice illustrate how "spiritual discernment or awakening" can help "integrate body and spirit" during the process of coming out as transgender [41]. In a summary of studies about the R/S lives of LGBT people, Dahl and Galliher identify four avenues by which sexual-minority adults resolve religious conflicts: identifying as spiritual rather than religious, modifying religious beliefs, abandoning religious contexts, and joining "gay-friendly" religious communities [42].

Fostering practices and beliefs outside traditional religious frameworks appears to be a strategy employed by at least some transgender people. A 2008 study of 33 FTMs intended to look at how spirituality and religiosity might mitigate the effects of violence and abuse during the life course. However, the authors unintentionally found that existing psychometric instruments that draw on Christian, Jewish, or Islamic monotheistic concepts did not seem to resonate for at least some of their respondents [43]. Similarly, the U.S. Transgender Survey shows disproportionately high percentages of people seeking spiritual connections outside the three major monotheistic religions. In this study, 13% of respondents identified as Pagan or Wiccan and 6% as Buddhist, which is much greater than the representation in the general population, polling at .3 and .7%, respectively [44]. This theme is reinforced by Witten and Eyler, who report that in one study "over half of respondents had moved from one of the more traditional Western religions to a more personalized spiritual perspective, often considered a fusion of the best principles of the faiths in which the individual believes" [45].

At the time of writing, there is no published research about the provision of spiritual care to transgender adults. However, an unpublished small case series that documents a chaplain's visits to six inpatients following gender affirmation surgeries found that the patients tended to identify as "spiritual but not religious," did not outwardly exhibit negative transference towards the chaplain conducting the visits, and welcomed the chaplain as someone who witnessed their gratitude and, if appropriate, honored their ambivalence [46].

Children/Adolescents/Young Adults

There is very little published research about any aspect of TGNB children's development. However, a qualitative study of 110 transgender adults asked them to reflect on their experiences as gender-variant children and on interventions that may have been helpful for them and their parents. Participants identified their parents' rigid religious beliefs as a barrier to acceptance [47]. Echoing this, a qualitative study of 19 LGBT adolescents and young adults, three of whom identified as transgender and all of whom had been raised in Christian contexts, identified "religious-related guilt" as a risk factor for negative outcomes [48]. Similarly, a series of focus groups among transgender youth ages 15–21 found that some respondents believe themselves to be at "high risk of self-harm because of their religious backgrounds and the pressures their families and communities put on them to conform to traditional gender behaviors" [49].

However, the lead author of this focus group study led another study eight years later that found lower rates of suicidal ideation among respondents with more frequent religious service attendance. This qualitative study involved 129 transgender youth ages 15–21 and showed relatively low levels of religious involvement, with 68% reporting they did not have a religion and had never attended services. Of those who were religiously involved, only 11% attended services weekly or more frequently [50].

Grossoehme and colleagues conducted a QI project in an outpatient adolescent transgender clinic in Cincinnati to determine whether the Rush screening protocol is an effective means of screening for spiritual distress among adolescent patients and their caregivers. The authors developed this project after noticing patients and their parents describe what they interpreted as spiritual or religious struggles connected to coming out as a transgender person or to being the parent of a transgender child.

The project demonstrated that using the Rush protocol in this setting was acceptable to adolescents, their caregivers, and clinic staff nurses who administered the screening. Used in tandem with another set of screening questions, the protocol revealed a high level of spiritual struggle among this patient population [33].

Older Transgender People

Witten and Eyler write that it's common for transgender people to find community and support outside traditional religious structures. They also report findings of gerontological research that show "a strong correlation between faith, spirituality or religiosity and reduced morbidity and enhanced sense of wellbeing" [45]. However, when Porter and colleagues conducted an exploratory study of the religious affiliations of 289 transgender people over the age of 51, the data did not support the expectation that religious affiliation would predict successful aging [51]. The respondents in this study, who were predominantly white, highly educated, and high income, were more likely to affiliate with an LGBT-affirming religion than was the general population. However, echoing a theme reiterated throughout this literature review, the largest affiliation category was "nonspecific spirituality." Of those who did affiliate with a formal religion, only 23% were out as transgender within their religious community, compared to 94% who were out in most other parts of their lives. The authors note that this may echo Witten and Eyler's finding that transgender older adults are fearful about how they will be treated by faith-based agencies.

Summary

Overall, limited studies of R/S in transgender populations show that transgender people have complex R/S lives and that further research is needed. The following four case studies illustrate how transgender people's beliefs, behaviors, and senses of belonging might present in clinical settings.

Case Studies

By presenting four cases drawn from adult, geriatric, and pediatric patients, this section brings together themes from earlier sections of the chapter and utilizes some of the screening/assessment tools presented above. We offer approaches to the cases that could be utilized by a spiritual care specialist (i.e., a chaplain) or by a spiritual care generalist (i.e., clinicians from any other discipline).

Case 1: Adult Medicine

"Dinah" is a 32-year-old white Jewish woman who began transgender medical treatment 7 years ago and has been taking hormone therapy since that time. She hopes to undergo vaginoplasty surgery at an academic medical center that has a strong commitment to transgender healthcare. As part of the process of preparing for surgery, she meets with one of the nurse practitioners at the clinic. The NP has received some basic training on spirituality and religion and listens for these themes, among many others, as he takes Dinah's history.

As Dinah gives a brief account of her life, she reports she is Jewish and grew up attending a Conservative synagogue. She had a bar mitzvah ceremony at age 13 but knew at the time that she was transgender. She struggled with the idea that her bar mitzvah ostensibly marked her coming of age as a Jewish man and stopped attending synagogue at that time. However, she finds comfort in practicing some Jewish rituals at home.

In the first version of this case, there are no chaplains available to serve patients at this clinic. In this situation, the NP or any other spiritual care generalist could:

- Identify Dinah's Jewish upbringing as *both* a possible source of R/S struggle *and* a potentially supportive resource.
- Invite Dinah to talk at greater length about how her connection to Judaism may be helpful to her as she prepares for and recovers from surgery. As described above, a majority of patients welcome the opportunity to discuss their spiritual needs with their physicians and other caregivers. In addition, there may be a chaplain available at the hospital where Dinah will have surgery and the NP could make a referral to facilitate this.
- Maintain a list of local and national houses of worship and religious networks/ organizations that are LGBT-welcoming. (A list of online resources is included at the end of this chapter.) This list can assist spiritual care generalists in referring patients to resources outside the clinic or hospital.

In the second version of this case, the NP makes a referral to a chaplain to conduct a more thorough spiritual assessment. When the chaplain meets with Dinah, he draws on Exline et al.'s model of spiritual struggle and makes the following assessments (Table 18.3).

The chaplain meets with Dinah twice and, with the chaplain's guidance, Dinah uses these sessions to grieve the losses and give voice to the pain associated with the feeling that she doesn't "belong" in a synagogue. At the same time, Dinah describes and articulates a relationship with God that is rooted in love, acceptance, and welcome. Dinah's conversations with the chaplain strengthen her overall feelings of emotional and spiritual wellbeing as she prepares for surgery. Having established this relationship with Dinah prior to her surgery, the chaplain makes a follow-up postsurgical visit, which deepens Dinah's sense that she is well supported by an interdisciplinary team. Additionally, the chaplain consults with some

Table 18.3 Application of Exline et al.'s categories to "Dinah's" case

Type of struggle	Examples	Chaplain's assessment of Dinah
Divine struggle	Feeling let down by God, angry with God, abandoned by God	**No.** Has consistently experienced God as a loving presence over the course of her life
Interpersonal struggle	Feeling hurt, mistreated, misunderstood, rejected, or offended by religious/spiritual people	**Yes.** Feels hurt and rejected by the rigid gender binary of the Judaism with which she grew up
Intrapersonal struggle	Struggling to figure out what one really believes, feeling confused about one's beliefs	**Yes.** Struggling to reconcile her personal experiences of a loving God with the painful experiences of her bar mitzvah

colleagues and refers Dinah to some written and online resources developed by LGBT Jews. These resources expand Dinah's understanding of how others have integrated the transgender and Jewish parts of themselves.

Case 2: Geriatric Medicine

"James" is a 71-year-old African American transgender man who used street hormones intermittently, beginning at age 40. Two years ago, he began receiving hormone therapy from a provider at a transgender health clinic. James has not undergone any transgender-specific surgeries. For the past two years, James has been experiencing increasing pain and immobility in his right hip. His primary care provider, whom he sees at the transgender health clinic, referred him to an orthopedist, who recommended hip replacement surgery. James grew up Baptist and now attends a Presbyterian church, where he and his partner, Kiara, an African American cisgender woman who identifies as a lesbian, have a strong community of support.

James does not want to have hip replacement surgery because he is fearful about a postsurgical stay in a skilled nursing facility. He has heard upsetting stories about older transgender people "de-transitioning" in LTC facilities. However, his concerns about pain and immobility are also mounting. He and Kiara make an appointment with James's PCP at the transgender health clinic to discuss their options.

James' PCP recently read about the FICA model and has begun employing it when taking patients' histories. By using the FICA tool with James and Kiara, James' PCP learns the following:

- F—Faith and Belief
- "Do you consider yourself spiritual or religious? Is spirituality something important to you? Do you have spiritual beliefs that help you cope with stress/ difficult times? What gives your life meaning?"
  - *James and Kiara use the terms "religious" and "spiritual" to describe themselves. They report that they use prayer to cope with stress. They pray to God on their own behalf and they add their names to their church's communal prayer list during times of sickness. They regularly attend worship services and report that liturgy and the cycle of religious holidays provide them with "meaning," "community," and "structure." They are grateful to belong to a religious community that includes a number of LGBT members and they report that they are "out" to their pastor.*
- I—Importance
- "What importance does your spirituality have in your life? Has your spirituality influenced how you take care of yourself, your health? Does your spirituality influence you in your healthcare decision-making? (e.g., advance directives, treatment, etc.)"
  - *The PCP learns that James's identity as a transgender man is affecting his decision-making process with regard to this surgery. As James and Kiara talk about their fears of long-term care facilities, they report that it would be meaningful to receive a visit from their pastor in the event that James goes to a SNF for rehab. James and Kiara's R/S beliefs and practices are very important to them and help them cope during stressful times. While their religious beliefs aren't influencing their decision-making, the possibility that they could receive support from their pastor in a rehab setting may contribute to them leaning towards choosing the surgery.*
- C—Community
- "Are you part of a spiritual community? Is this of support to you and how? Is there a group of people you really love or who are important to you?"
  - *The PCP has already gathered answers to these questions.*
- A—Address/Action in Care
- "How would you like me, your healthcare provider, to address these issues in your healthcare?"
  - *The PCP lets James and Kiara know that his clinic has a relationship with a SNF that has invested in educating its staff on how to provide culturally-effective care to LGBT patients. James and Kiara say they would like to look at the SNF's webpage in order to learn more about it. They also report that they are comforted by the prospect of requesting a visit from their pastor. While James still hasn't made a final decision, he feels more hopeful that he could receive good and affirming care in a rehab setting.*

Case 3: Pediatric Medicine

"Sarah" is an 18-year-old Latina transgender woman. She began appearing as female while in high school and has been taking hormone therapy for about 18 months. She is attending college and doing well. She receives her healthcare at an adolescent transgender clinic. At one of her clinic visits, she agrees to take the spiritual distress screening that was adapted from the Rush protocol. Sarah scored positive for being at risk for spiritual struggle. The chaplain made an initial follow-up contact per the protocol and then met with Sarah a second time. She answered the prompts on the screening protocol as follows:

- How long have you known that you are transgender? *At least 12 years, although I didn't learn the word "transgender" until I was about ten.*
- Is spirituality or religion important to you as you think about your gender issues? *No.*
  - Has there been a time when religion/spirituality was important to you? *Yes.*
- Do you attend a congregation? *No.*
  - *Used to attend, but no longer attends for reasons described in more detail below.*

In their first visit, the chaplain learned that Sarah's spiritual history includes being raised in a Roman Catholic family and serving as an altar boy when in grade school. She attended religious services regularly with her mom and siblings and found comfort and support from her beliefs while in grade school and junior high. As Sarah continued to mature and began identifying herself as transgender, she began to have more struggles with the teachings of the church. She struggled to reconcile these beliefs with her lived experience of being transgender. When Sarah came to the realization that she was transgender, she initially used her faith as a way to avoid the topic. She prayed for God to "heal" her from being transgender, used the sacrament of confession to be forgiven and cleansed, and at one point considered talking to her priest about an exorcism. As time went on, however, she realized she could no longer use her faith as a way to avoid being transgender and that the faith she held at that time was not helpful to her in planning the next steps. She found the teachings of the church to be incompatible with her experience of being transgender.

During their second visit, the chaplain explored where Sarah currently was spiritually and religiously. Since leaving the church, she's become increasingly agnostic. While she initially missed the sense of community that her church provided, she has also found that she doesn't need her Catholic faith to help her cope with being transgender. The chaplain and Sarah explore what does help her cope and uncover themes that echo those in Hirschmann et al.'s unpublished small case series, cited above.

- Sarah is beginning to describe herself as "*spiritual but not religious*." She finds support in talking with some family members and several close friends, and she finds meaning in making music.
- Sarah expresses gratitude for the medical team that cares for her and also for simple things she enjoys doing with friends, such as being in nature. She also expresses gratitude that her life has gotten better over time. It is meaningful to Sarah to share these vignettes with the chaplain and to have her *gratitude witnessed by the chaplain*.
- Sarah describes how her medical team at the clinic, as well as the clinic's chaplain, have *honored her ambivalence* as she has wrestled with her beliefs about God and the teachings of the Catholic church. She appreciates being listened to without being judged and being asked helpful clarifying questions, even when she doesn't have an answer. Sarah also reports that it has been helpful for the medical team to check in about spiritual struggle during her clinic appointments, even if she doesn't want to talk about it at that time.

Case 4: Pediatric Medicine

"Miriam" is a 20-year-old Muslim transgender woman of Pakistani descent. Her parents emigrated from Pakistan before Miriam and her sisters were born; Miriam was born in the United States. She began appearing in more gender-neutral clothing about a year ago and is not on hormone therapy. She is attending college and lives with her family. She and her family practice Islam and attend a local mosque regularly.

Miriam comes to a new patient visit in an adolescent transgender clinic and brings her parents with her. During the intake interview, Miriam tells the APN that her parents will accompany her to appointments because this is customary for young unmarried adults, according to her family's culture. She also reports she has been hesitant to dress in a more feminine way around her parents because, in her words, to do so would be "disrespectful." When the APN asks what this has been like for Miriam, she becomes tearful and says she feels torn between wanting to respect her parents and inviting them to accept her as a woman. She reports feeling stuck and unsure of the "right" thing to do. The APN identifies Miriam's sadness and moral confusion as forms of distress that indicate she may benefit from seeing a chaplain.

The APN then meets with Miriam and her parents together. During this time, Miriam's parents say that they do not understand the changes they perceive in "Hassan" (Miriam's birth name). During the clinic's standard screen for spiritual distress, Miriam's father reports he is worried about Miriam's soul because she will have no place to pray when they go to the mosque. Miriam won't be able to pray with the men downstairs if she doesn't present as male and nor will she be "welcome" upstairs with the women. From Miriam's father's perspective, this leaves

Table 18.4 Application of Exline et al.'s categories to "Miriam's" case

Type of struggle	Examples	Miriam	Miriam's parents
Divine struggle	Feeling let down by God, angry with God, abandoned by God	**Yes.** She is unsure how to maintain her relationship to God without a communal place to pray	**Somewhat.** They aren't experiencing struggle in their own relationship with God but are saddened as they watch Miriam's struggle
Interpersonal struggle	Feeling hurt, mistreated, misunderstood, rejected, or offended by religious/spiritual people	**Yes.** With her parents and, to some extent, with her imam	**Yes.** With Miriam because her gender identity and presentation are at odds with their religious values
Intrapersonal struggle	Struggling to figure out what one really believes, feeling confused about one's beliefs	**Yes.** Struggling to reconcile values learned at home and in her mosque with her current gender identity	**Yes.** Struggling to reconcile their values with their love for their child

Miriam praying in isolation without community or support. Miriam is similarly unsure how to maintain her relationship with God without a communal place to pray.

The APN asks if Miriam has spoken with her imam; Miriam reports she has but this hasn't been helpful to her. While Miriam isn't comfortable speaking with the chaplain, particularly because no Muslim chaplain is available, she begins using the APN as a resource person. She asks the APN if the chaplain has any resources about transgender identity and experience from an Islamic perspective and the chaplain supplies a list of trans-affirming websites and contacts. Miriam isn't able to find a way in which she can pray at her family's mosque but, with the help of these resources, she begins to form friendships with young Muslims who share her values.

In the meantime, the APN consults with the chaplain and, together, they use Exline's model to identify the following sources of R/S distress (Table 18.4).

This framework provides the APN with useful context as she continues to provide medical care to Miriam.

Conclusion

We began this chapter with the recommendation that all those who work with transgender people in healthcare settings integrate an assessment of their patients' R/S needs and resources into their overall work flow. As the research literature shows, transgender people's R/S lives are complex, with religion and spirituality functioning in both harmful and supportive ways. As the four cases illustrate, thoughtful engagement by a spiritual care generalist or specialist can help transgender people access supportive religious resources and, with the help of a chaplain, transgender people may be able to work through some of the grief and pain associated with religious rejection.

Resource List

The following is a list of Internet-based resources that address the R/S lives and needs of LGBT people.

- Catholic
  - DignityUSA—www.dignityusa.org
- Christian
  - Believe Out Loud—www.believeoutloud.com
- Jewish
  - Keshet—www.keshetonline.org
  - Eshel—www.eshelonline.org
- Muslim
  - Muslim Alliance for Gender and Sexual Diversity—www.muslimalliance.org
- Multifaith
  - TransFaith—www.transfaithonline.org/

References

1. Steinhauser KE, Fitchett G, Handzo GF, Johnson KS, Koenig HG, Pargament KI, Puchalski CM, Sinclair S, Taylor EJ, Balboni TA. State of the science of spirituality and palliative care research part I: definitions, measurement, and outcomes. J Pain Symptom Manage. 2017;54(3):428–40.
2. Ammerman NT. Spiritual but not religious? Beyond binary choices in the study of religion. J Sci Study Relig. 2013;52(2):258–78.
3. Puchalski C, Ferrell B, Virani R, Otis-Green S, Baird P, Bull J, Chochinov H, Handzo G, Nelson-Becker H, Prince-Paul M, Pugliese K. Improving the quality of spiritual care as a dimension of palliative care: the report of the Consensus Conference. J Palliat Med. 2012;12(10):885–904.

4. Fitchett G, Murphy PE, Stein K, Portier K, Crammer C, Peterman AH. Racial/ethnic differences in spiritual well-being among cancer survivors. J Behav Med. 2013;36(5):441–53.
5. Tuck I, McCain NL, Elswick RK Jr. Spirituality and psychosocial factors in persons living with HIV. J Adv Nurs. 2001;33(6):776–83.
6. Vallurupalli MM, Lauderdale MK, Balboni MJ, Phelps AC, Block SD, Ng AK, Kachnic LA, VanderWeele TJ, Balboni TA. The role of spirituality and religious coping in the quality of life of patients with advanced cancer receiving palliative radiation therapy. J Support Oncol. 2012;10(2):81–7.
7. Wang CW, Chan CLW, Ng SM, Ho AHY. The impact of spirituality on health-related quality of life among Chinese older adults with vision impairment. Aging Ment Health. 2008;12 (2):267–75.
8. Pargament KI, Murray-Swank NA, Magyar GM, Ano GG. Spiritual struggle: a phenomenon of interest to psychology and religion. In: Miller WR, Delaney HD, editors. Judeo-Christian perspectives on psychology: human nature, motivation, and change, 1st ed. Washington, DC: American Psychological Association; 2005. p. 245–68.
9. Johnson M, Bulechek GM, Dochterman JM, Maas M, Moorhead S, editors. Nursing diagnoses, outcomes, and interventions: NANDA, NOC, and NIC linkages. St. Louis: Mosby; 2001.
10. Pargament K, Feuille M, Burdzy D. The brief RCOPE: current psychometric status of a short measure of religious coping. Religions. 2011;2(1):51–76.
11. Fitchett G, Murphy PE, Kim J, Gibbons JL, Cameron JR, Davis JA. Religious struggle: prevalence, correlates and mental health risks in diabetic, congestive heart failure, and oncology patients. Int J Psychiatry Med. 2004;34(2):179–96.
12. King SD, Fitchett G, Murphy PE, Pargament KI, Harrison DA, Loggers ET. Determining best methods to screen for religious/spiritual distress. Support Care Cancer. 2017;25(2):471–9.
13. McCord G, Gilchrist VJ, Grossman SD, King BD, McCormick KF, Oprandi AM, Schrop SL, Selius BA, Smucker WD, Weldy DL, Amorn M. Discussing spirituality with patients: a rational and ethical approach. Ann Fam Med. 2004;2(4):356–61.
14. Best M, Butow P, Olver I. Do patients want doctors to talk about spirituality? A systematic literature review. Patient Educ Couns. 2015;98(11):1320–8.
15. Astrow AB, Wexler A, Texeira K, He MK, Sulmasy DP. Is failure to meet spiritual needs associated with cancer patients' perceptions of quality of care and their satisfaction with care? J Clin Oncol. 2007;25(36):5753–7.
16. Balboni TA, Vanderwerker LC, Block SD, Paulk ME, Lathan CS, Peteet JR, Prigerson HG. Religiousness and spiritual support among advanced cancer patients and associations with end-of-life treatment preferences and quality of life. J Clin Oncol. 2007;25(5):555–60.
17. Balboni MJ, Sullivan A, Amobi A, Phelps AC, Gorman DP, Zollfrank A, Peteet JR, Prigerson HG, VanderWeele TJ, Balboni TA. Why is spiritual care infrequent at the end of life? Spiritual care perceptions among patients, nurses, and physicians and the role of training. J Clin Oncol. 2012;31(4):461–7.
18. Phelps AC, Lauderdale KE, Alcorn S, Dillinger J, Balboni MT, Van Wert M, VanderWeele TJ, Balboni TA. Addressing spirituality within the care of patients at the end of life: perspectives of patients with advanced cancer, oncologists, and oncology nurses. J Clin Oncol. 2012;30(20):2538–44.
19. Robinson MR, Thiel MM, Shirkey K, Zurakowski D, Meyer EC. Efficacy of training interprofessional spiritual care generalists. J Palliat Med. 2016;19(8):814–21.
20. Zollfrank AA, Trevino KM, Cadge W, Balboni MJ, Thiel MM, Fitchett G, Gallivan K, VanderWeele T, Balboni TA. Teaching health care providers to provide spiritual care: a pilot study. J Palliat Med. 2015;18(5):408–14.
21. Handzo G, Koenig HG. Spiritual care: whose job is it anyway? South Med J. 2004;97 (12):1242–4.
22. Handzo GF, Flannelly KJ, Murphy KM, Bauman JP, Oettinger M, Goodell E, Hasan YH, Barrie DP, Jacobs MR. What do chaplains really do? I. Visitation in the New York chaplaincy study. J Healthc Chaplain. 2008;14(1):20–38.

23. Handzo GF, Flannelly KJ, Kudler T, Fogg SL, Harding SR, Hasan YH, Ross AM, Taylor BE. What do chaplains really do? II. Interventions in the New York chaplaincy study. J Healthc Chaplain. 2008;14(1):39–56.
24. Idler EL, Grant GH, Quest T, Binney Z, Perkins MM. Practical matters and ultimate concerns, "doing", and "being": a diary study of the chaplain's role in the care of the seriously ill in an urban acute care hospital. J Sci Study Relig. 2015;54(4):722–38.
25. Massey K, Barnes MJ, Villines D, Goldstein JD, Pierson ALH, Scherer C, Vander Laan B, Summerfelt WT. What do I do? Developing a taxonomy of chaplaincy activities and interventions for spiritual care in intensive care unit palliative care. BMC Palliat Care. 2015;14(1):10.
26. Piderman KM, Marek DV, Jenkins SM, Johnson ME, Buryska JF, Shanafelt TD, O'Bryan FG, Hansen PD, Howick PH, Durland HL, Lackore KA. Predicting patients' expectations of hospital chaplains: a multisite survey. Mayo Clin Proc. 2010;85(11):1002–10.
27. Bay PS, Beckman D, Trippi J, Gunderman R, Terry C. The effect of pastoral care services on anxiety, depression, hope, religious coping, and religious problem solving styles: a randomized controlled study. J Relig Health. 2008;47(1):57–69.
28. Kestenbaum A, Shields M, James J, Hocker W, Morgan S, Karve S, Rabow MW, Dunn LB. What impact do chaplains have? A pilot study of spiritual AIM for advanced cancer patients in outpatient palliative care. J Pain Symptom Manage. 2017;54(5):707–14.
29. Williams JA, Meltzer D, Arora V, Chung G, Curlin FA. Attention to inpatients' religious and spiritual concerns: predictors and association with patient satisfaction. J Gen Intern Med. 2011;26(11):1265–71.
30. Marin DB, Sharma V, Sosunov E, Egorova N, Goldstein R, Hando GF. Relationship between chaplain visits and patient satisfaction. J Healthc Chaplain. 2015;21(1):14–24.
31. Sharma V, Marin DB, Sosunov E, Ozbay F, Goldstein R, Handzo GF. The differential effects of chaplain interventions on patient satisfaction. J Healthc Chaplain. 2016;22(3):85–101.
32. Fitchett G, Risk JL. Screening for spiritual struggle. J Pastoral Care Counsel. 2009;63(1–2): 1–12.
33. Grossoehme DH, Teeters A, Jelinek A, Dimitriou SM, Conard LA. Screening for spiritual distress in an adolescent transgender clinic: feasibility and acceptability. J Healthc Chaplain. 2016;22(2):54–66.
34. Fitchett G, Murphy P, King SDW. Examining the validity of the Rush Protocol to screen for religious/spiritual struggle. J Healthc Chaplain. 2017;23(3):98–112.
35. Exline JJ, Pargament KI, Grubbs JB, Yali A. The religious and spiritual struggles scale: development and initial validation. Psychol Relig Spiritual. 2014;6(3):208–22.
36. National Center for Transgender Equality. The report of the 2015 U. S. transgender survey. Washington, DC: 2016.
37. Dowshen ND, Forke CM, Johnson AK, Kuhns LM, Rubin D, Garofalo R. Religiosity as a protective factor against HIV risk among young transgender women. J Adolesc Health. 2011;48(4):410–4.
38. Golub SA, Walker JJ, Longmire-Avital B, Bimbi DS, Parsons JT. The role of religiosity, social support, and stress-related growth in protecting against HIV risk among transgender women. J Health Psychol. 2010;15(8):1135–44.
39. Stanton MC, Ali S, Chaudhuri S. Individual, social and community-level predictors of wellbeing in a US sample of transgender and gender non-conforming individuals. Cult Health Sex. 2017;19(1):32–49.
40. Singh AA, McKleroy VS. "Just getting out of bed is a revolutionary act": the resilience of transgender people of color who have survived traumatic life events. Traumatology. 2011;17 (2):34–44.
41. Bockting WO, Cesaretti C. Spirituality, transgender identity, and coming out. J Sex Educ Ther. 2001;26(4):291–300.
42. Dahl A, Galliher RV. The interplay of sexual and religious identity development in LGBTQ adolescents and young adults: a qualitative inquiry. Identity. 2012;12(3):217–46.

43. Kidd JD, Witten TM. Understanding spirituality and religiosity in the transgender community: implications for aging. J Relig Spiritual Aging. 2008;20(1–2):29–62.
44. Pew Research Center. America's changing religious landscape. 2015 May 12.
45. Witten TM, Eyler AE. Transgender and aging: beings and becomings. In: Gay, lesbian, bisexual and transgender aging: challenges in research, practice and policy. Baltimore: Johns Hopkins University Press; 2012.
46. Hirschmann J, Rapport Y, Sharma V, Reich D, Freeman R, Goldstein Z, Warren B, Marin D. Spiritual care for gender affirmation patients: themes and issues in a small case series. 2017 World Professional Association for Transgender Health meeting, oral presentation 0852-000086.
47. Rile EA, Clemson L, Sitharthan G, Diamond M. Surviving a gender-variant childhood: the views of transgender adults on the needs of gender-variant children and their parents. J Sex Marital Ther. 2013;39(3):241–63.
48. Dahl AL, Galliher RV. LGBTQ adolescents and young adults raised within a Christian religious context: positive and negative outcomes. J Adolesc. 2012;35(6):1611–8.
49. Grossman A, D'augelli AR. Transgender youth. J Homosexual. 2008:51(1):111–28.
50. Grossman A, Park JY, Russell ST. Transgender youth and suicidal behaviors: applying the interpersonal psychological theory of suicide. J Gay Lesbian Ment Health. 2016;20(4): 329–49.
51. Porter KE, Ronneberg CR, Witten TM. Religious affiliation and successful aging among transgender older adults: findings from the Trans MetLife Survey. J Relig Spiritual Aging. 2013;25(2):112–38.

Chapter 19
Resources for Transgender Individuals: Transgender Organizations and Services

Deeangelys Colón, Samantha Goldstein and Leonid Poretsky

Introduction

Individuals who identify as transgender are often faced with social, economic, medical, and political barriers that require guidance from knowledgeable organizations. Such organizations have experience in providing medical care, counseling, support groups, legal assistance, and social services. We have therefore compiled a list of some of the notable national and international resources for transgender individuals. Here we describe some of these in more detail.

In the ***United States***, the National Center for Equality (NCTE) was founded in 2003 by transgender activists who recognized the urgent need for policy change to advance transgender equality. They set out to accomplish what no one had yet done: provide a powerful transgender advocacy presence in Washington, D.C. The organization works in many areas, including public advocacy, media activism, discrimination in employment, access to public accommodations, fair housing, identity documents, hate crimes and violence, criminal justice reform, federal surveys and census, and healthcare access. Today, NCTE is a team of hardworking staff members supported by a nationwide community of transgender people, allies, and advocates with an extensive record of winning lifesaving changes for transgender people.

D. Colón (✉)
Department of Endocrinology, Lenox Hill Hospital, Northwell Health, New York, NY, USA
e-mail: dcolon32@northwell.edu

S. Goldstein
Department of Internal Medicine, Lenox Hill Hospital, Northwell Health, New York, NY, USA

L. Poretsky
Friedman Transgender Health and Wellness Program, Division of Endocrinology, Lenox Hill Hospital, Donald and Barbara Zucker School of Medicine at Hofstra/Northwell, New York, NY, USA

L. Poretsky and W. C. Hembree (eds.), *Transgender Medicine*, Contemporary Endocrinology, https://doi.org/10.1007/978-3-030-05683-4_19

The Human Rights Campaign (HRC) has a division that works to educate the public on transgender issues and to advocate for full inclusion and equality. Through the use of surveys, research, and reporting, the HRC enlightens the public on gender identity and the various forms of gender expression. HRC provides a range of resources on such issues like workplace discrimination, securing identity documents, finding culturally competent health care, family and parenting issues, and combating violence. HRC advocates on behalf of transgender and gender nonconforming community for equal rights.

The mission of the Transgender Law Center (TLC) is to change law, policy, and attitudes so that all people can live safely, authentically, and free from discrimination regardless of their gender identity or expression. TLC is the largest national trans-led organization advocating self-determination for all people. Grounded in legal expertise and committed to racial justice, TLC employs a variety of community-driven strategies to keep transgender and gender nonconforming people alive, thriving, and fighting for liberation.

The Trevor Project was established with the goal of providing crisis intervention and suicide prevention services to LGBTQ young people whose ages vary from 13 to 24. Some of the services, including Trevor Lifeline, TrevorChat, and TrevorText, are available only in the United States. The project operates the toll-free Trevor Lifeline, a confidential service with trained counselors. They provide crisis intervention, guidance, and resources for parents and educators to foster safe, accepting, and inclusive environment for all youth at home, school, and society at large. Nationwide, they offer an around-the-clock crisis and suicide prevention helpline for LGBTQ youth in the United States. In order to provide support for the international transgender population, a website was created, TrevorSpace.org, which promotes safe and secure social networking. This website can be accessed from anywhere; however, users are warned that visiting the website may leave a record on the individual's computer.

The Trans Youth Equality Foundation (TYEF) is a national nonprofit foundation that advocates for transgender, gender nonconforming, and intersex youth whose ages vary from 2 to 18. The organization was founded by the mother of a transgender person. Along with support from friends, transgender individuals, and youth healthcare providers, she began to build programs. Because of her own struggle to find resources for her child between 2002 and 2007, she realized the great need for high-quality resources and support services for youth and their families. TYEF seeks to address this need through yearly youth retreats, including a popular summer and fall camp; TransWaves, an educational podcast program; trainings for educational and medical professionals; youth workshops; and social media presence. TYEF was founded upon the principle that no family and no child have to be alone on their transition journey. TYEF provides education, advocacy, and support for transgender children, youth, and their families. Its mission is to share information about the unique needs of the transgender community, and to partner with families, educators, and service providers in order to help foster a healthy, caring, and safe environment for all transgender children.

Parents, Families and Friends of Lesbian and Gays Inc., PFLAG, is a national organization with over 400 chapters nationwide. Uniting people who are lesbian, gay, bisexual, transgender, and queer (LGBTQ) with families, friends, and allies, PFLAG is committed to advancing equality through support, education, and advocacy. PFLAG has 200,000 members crossing multiple generations of American families in major urban centers, small cities, and rural areas in all 50 states, the District of Columbia and Puerto Rico. This vast grassroots network is cultivated, resourced, and serviced by PFLAG National, located in Washington, D.C., the National Board of Directors and 13 volunteer Regional Directors.

The Transgender Veterans Association (TAVA) works to collaborate proactively with other concerned gay, lesbian, bisexual, and transgender (GLBT) organizations to ensure that transgender veterans receive appropriate care for their medical conditions in accordance with the Veterans Health Administration's Customer Service Standards' promise to "treat you with courtesy and dignity as the first class citizen that you are." Further, TAVA helps education efforts of the Department of Veterans Affairs (DVA) and the Department of Defense (DoD) on issues regarding fair and equal treatment of transgender and transsexual individuals. In addition, TAVA also provides help to the general transgender community on a variety of issues.

The United States-based Suicide.org is a nonprofit organization which has a comprehensive list of suicide hotlines nationally and for 61 countries. Befrienders Worldwide, a suicide prevention website, offers support services by gay, lesbian, bisexual, and transgendered people and can offer guidance through personal experience.

Many ***international*** organizations exist to promote gender equality.

The International Lesbian, Gay, Bisexual, Trans and Intersex Association (ILGA) is an organization dedicated to achieving equal rights for LGBTI people across the globe. It is the voice of the LGBTI community in the United Nations and is funded by governments, private foundations, and private donors. ILGA speaks and lobbies on behalf of more than 1200 member organizations from 132 countries with the goal to raise awareness of the transgender community through advocacy, research, and education.

Another organization, the International Lesbian, Gay, Bisexual, Transgender, Queer and Intersex (LGBTQI) Youth & Student Organization (IGLYO), supports young people who identify as LGBTQI. It is the largest LGBTQI youth and student network in the world, with over 95 chapters in more than 40 countries. The objective of this organization is to encourage international cooperation and partnership.

Global Action for Trans Equality (GATE) is a group that supports the global initiative for gender equality. Some of its recent work includes promoting awareness about gender identity and gender expression for the international human rights campaign as well as advocating for transgender and intersex access to funding. GATE is also hoping to contribute to the new ICD-11 classification system. Current categories exclude transgender people from the right to identity and self-determination, and ICD diagnoses are required to grant access to legal gender recognition and to transition-related health care.

Seventy-eight nations criminalize same-sex relations and seven use the death penalty for consensual same-sex conduct. As a result, many LGBT individuals are forced to flee their countries. Organization for Refuge, Asylum and Migration (ORAM) works to protect these vulnerable refugees via advocacy and education. This effort has resulted in faster consideration of LGBTIs applying for refugee status and publication of a training guide for adjudicators to help assess the credibility and eligibility of LGBTI refugee claims.

Health care for the transgender population requires a multidisciplinary team of well-educated professionals to develop best practices for this underserved group. Transgender patients have unique healthcare needs, such as hormonal therapy and gender reassignment surgeries. The World Professional Association for Transgender Health (WPATH) aims to advance clinical and academic research to develop evidence-based medicine for high-quality care. The WPATH website offers a search engine to find qualified medical professionals all around the world that specialize in transgender-specific health care.

The transgender community has made immense progress in the last decade. Through hotline services, advocacy groups, and trained medical specialists, the United States offers a variety of services for the transgender and gender nonconforming population. On an international front, many countries also offer some means of support. However, there are still countries that continue to criminalize gender dysphoria, thereby forcing residents of those countries to hide their gender identity or flee the country for their safety. Hopefully, with the continued progress of the gender equality movement, more countries will provide protection for transgender people and develop the support networks they so desperately need.

ASSOCIATIONS—UNITED STATES OUTREACH PROGRAMS AND RESOURCES

Alabama

Central Alabama Pride, Inc.
205 32nd Street S
Birmingham, AL 35233
Phone: (256) 813-4227
Internet: https://www.centralalabamapride.org

ALGBTICAL-
Association for Lesbian, Gay, Bisexual and Transgender Issues in Counseling of Alabama—Alabama Counseling Association
217 Darryl Street
Livingston, AL 35470
Phone: (205) 625-1712
Internet: http://www.algbtical.org

Free2be
8210 Stephanie Drive, Suite A
Huntsville, AL 35902
Phone: (256) 886-1150
Internet: https://www.free2be.org

Parents & Friends of Lesbians and Gays—PFLAG Birmingham
Unitarian Universalist Church
4300 Hampton Heights Drive
Birmingham, AL 35209
Phone: (205) 915-0629
Internet: http://www.pflagbham.org

Alaska

Identity Alaska
336 East 5th Avenue
Anchorage, AK 99501
Phone: (907) 929-4528
Fax: (907) 334-1992
Internet: http://www.identityalaska.org

Alaskan T People
c/o Bobbie Wendy Tucey
P.O. Box 670349
Chugiak, AK 99567
Internet: http://alaskan-transcendentalist.blogspot.com

Arizona

LGNTO Resource Center University of Arizona
Program Director for LGBTIQ Affairs
Student Union, Room 404
PO BOX 210017
Tucson, AZ 85721
Phone: (520) 626-1996
Internet: http://lgbtq.arizona.edu/transgender-resources

Arizona Trans Youth & Parent Organization
Email: contact@aztypo.org
Internet: http://www.aztypo.org/contact

Southern Arizona Gender Alliance—SAGA
PO Box 41863
Tucson, AZ 85717
Phone: (520) 477-7096
Internet: http://www.sagatucson.org

Trans Spectrum of Arizona
First Church
1407 North 2nd Street
Phoenix, AZ 85004
Phone: (480) 382-3757
Internet: https://www.transspectrum.org

Arkansas

River Valley Equality Center
215 North 6th Street
Fort Smith, AK 72901
Phone: (479) 274-0825
Internet: http://www.rvecark.org/support

Diverse Youth for Social Change
First Presbyterian Church
800 Scott Street
Little Rock, AR 72201
Phone: (501) 244-9690
Internet: https://www.car4ar.org

Lucie's Place
300 South Spring Street, Suite 715
Little Rock, AR 72201
Phone: (501) 508-5005
Internet: http://www.luciesplace.org

California

Bakersfield Transgender Services and Support
Email: bakotsslg@gmail.com
Internet: http://www.bakotranssupport.weebly.com

Los Angeles LGBT Center
McDonald/Wright Building
1625 North Schrader Blvd.
Lost Angeles, CA 90028
Phone: (323) 993-7400
Fax: (323)-993-7699
Internet: https://www.lalgbtcenter.org/social-service-and-housing/transgender

Los Angeles LGBT Center-We Ho
8745 Santa Monica Blvd, 2nd Floor
West Hollywood, CA 90069
Phone: (323) 993-7440
Internet: https://www.lalgbtcenter.org/about-the-cente

The Village at Ed Gould Plaza
1125 North McCadden Place
Los Angeles, CA 90038
Phone: (323) 993-7400
Internet: https://www.lalgbtcenter.org/about-the-center

The LGBT Center Long Beach
2017 East 4th Street
Long Beach, CA 90814 Phone: (562) 434-4455
Fax: (562) 433-6428
Internet: https://www.centerlb.org/transservices

Parents & Friends of Lesbians and Gays—PFLAG Los Angeles
PO Box 24565
Los Angeles, CA 90024
Phone: (888) 735-2488
Internet: http://www.pflaglosangeles.org/transgender.html

Stonewall Alliance Center
358 East 6th Street
Chico, CA 95928
Phone: (580) 893-3336
Internet: http://www.stonewallchico.org

Transgender San Francisco
3543 18th Street #30 San Francisco, CA 94110
Phone: (415) 839-9448
Internet: http://www.tgsf.org

San Diego LGBT Community Center
3909 Centre Street San Diego, CA 92103
Phone: (619) 692-2077 Fax: (619) 260-3092
Internet: http://www.thecentersd.org

The Source LGBT Bakersfield—Transgender Program
Montgomery Square
208 West Main Street, Suite B
Visalia, CA 93279
Phone: (559) 429-4277
Internet: http://www.thesourcelgbt.org/transgender

TRANZ Central Coast
1060 Palm Street San Luis Obispo, CA 93401
Phone: (805) 242-3821
Internet: http://www.tranzcentralcoast.org

TRANS THRIVE—Asian & Pacific Islander Wellness Center (API)
730 Polk Street
San Francisco, CA 94109
Phone: (415) 292-3400 Fax: (415) 292-3404
Internet: http://apiwellness.org/transthrive

Trans-E-Motion
P.O. BOX 16272 Fresno, CA 93755-6272
Phone: 559 464-5806
Internet: https://www.transemotion.com

Intersex Society of North America 979 Golf Course
Drive #282 Rohnert Park CA 94928
Fax: (801) 348-5350
Internet: http://www.isna.org/about/contact

Colorado

The Gender Identity Center of Colorado
120 Bryant Street
Denver, CO 80219
Phone: (303) 202-6466
Internet: https://www.giccolorado.org

The GLBT Community Center
1301 East Colfax Avenue
Denver, CO 80218
Phone: (303) 733-7743
Fax: (303)-282-9399
Internet: http://www.glbtcolorado.org/transgender

PAGE—Peak Area Gender Expressions
Pikes Peak Metropolitan Community Church
1102 South 21st Street, Colorado Springs, CO 80904
Website: http://www.ppmcc.org

Trans-Youth Education & Support of Colorado (TYES)
Phone: (720)443-7708
http://www.tyes-colorado.org/contact

It Takes A Village—TransAction
1477 Lima Street
Aurora, CO 80010
Phone: (720) 262-6313
Internet: http://www.ittakesavillagecolorado.org/programs/transaction.htm

Out Boulder County—Transgender Programs
2132 14th Street
Boulder, CO 80302
Phone: (303) 499-5777
Internet: http://www.outboulder.org/trans

Connecticut

Connecticut Outreach Society
P.O. Box 163 Farmington, CT 06034
Phone: (860) 294-4392
Internet: http://www.ctoutreach.org

New Haven Pride Center
84 Orange Street
New Haven, CT 06510
Phone: (203) 387-2252
Fax: (203) 387-2252
Internet: http://www.newhavenpridecenter.org

Triangle Community Center
618 West Avenue, Suite 205
Norwalk, CT 06850
Phone: (203)853-0600
Internet: http://www.ctpridecenter.org

Delaware

Delaware Pride
PO Box 9834
Newark, DE 19714
Internet: http://www.delawarepride.org

Camp Rehoboth
37 Baltimore Avenue Rehoboth Beach, DE, 19971
Phone: (302) 227-5620
Fax: (302) 227-5604
Internet: http://www.camprehoboth.com

Delaware Renaissance
First Unitarian Church 730 Halstead Road Wilmington, DE 19803
Internet: http://www.delren.org

Florida

Metro Health, Wellness & Community Center
3251 3rd Ave. North, Ste. 125 St. Petersburg, FL 33713
Phone: (727) 321-3854 Fax: (727) 327-7670
http://www.metrotampabay.org

Metro Health, Wellness & Community Center
1315 East 7th Avenue, Ste. 201 Tampa, FL 33605
Phone: (813) 232-3808 Fax: (813) 234-3075
http://www.metrotampabay.org

Metro Health, Wellness & Community Center
4747 US Hwy. 19 New Port Richey, FL 34652
Phone: (727) 494-7625 Fax: (727) 494-7629
http://www.metrotampabay.org

Metro Health, Wellness & Community Center
2349 Sunset Point Rd #405 Clearwater, FL 33765
Phone: (727) 321-3854 Fax: (727) 327-7670
http://www.metrotampabay.org

Gulf Coast Transgender Alliance Phone: (850) 332-8416
Internet: https://www.gulfcoasttransgenderalliance.com

SunServe
2312 Wilton Drive Wilton Manors, FL, 33305
Phone: (954) 764-5150
Fax: (954) 764-5143
Internet: https://www.sunserve.org/programs/transgender-services

Trans Miami
777 Brickell Avenue, Suite 500
Miami, FL 33131
Phone: (305) 423-9326
Internet: https://www.facebook.com/pg/TransMiamiCtr
http://unitycoalition.org/TransNews.html

Transgender Tallahassee-The Family Tree Community Center
PO Box 38477
Tallahassee, FL 32315
Phone: (850) 222-8555
Internet: http://transgender.familytreecenter.org

Georgia

PFLAG Atlanta 2480 Briarcliff Road North East, Suite 6-252 Atlanta, GA 30329
Phone: (678) 561 7354
Internet: http://www.pflagatl.org

The Phillip Rush Center—Atlanta 1530 Dekalb Avenue, Suite A Atlanta, Georgia, 30307 Phone: (678) 362-4084 Internet: http://www.rushcenteratl.org

Savannah LGBT Community Center/FCN
1515 Bull Street Savannah, Georgia, 31401
Phone: (912) 547-4543
Internet: https://www.savannahlgbtcenter.org

Hawaii

The LGBT Center-Waikiki
310 Paoakalani Avenue, Suite 206E
Honolulu, HI 96815
Phone: (808) 369-2000
Internet: http://hawaiilgbtlegacyfoundation.com/lgbt-center-in-waikiki

The Lavender Clinic
1345 South Beretania Street, Suite 101
Honolulu, HI 96814
Phone: (808) 445-539
Fax: (866) 793-8372
Internet: http://www.lavenderclinichawaii.com

Parents & Friends of Lesbians and Gays—PFLAG Kauai
Phone: (808) 634-0127
Email: pflagkauai@gmail.com
Parents & Friends of Lesbians and Gays—PFALG Kona/Big Island
Internet; https://www.pflag.org/chapter/pflag-konabig-island

Idaho

All Under One Roof LGBT Advocates
234 N Main Street
Pocatello, ID 83204
Phone: (208) 251-1661
Internet: http://www.allunderoneroof.org

The Community Center Inc.
1088 North Orchard Street
Boise, ID 83706
Phone: (208)-336-3870
Internet: http://tccidaho.org/trans

IFPLAG—Eastern Idaho Chapter
P.O. Box 52242
Idaho Falls, ID 83405
Phone: (208)538-9217/(208) 522-1057
Internet: http://www.ifpflag.com

Illinois

The Phoenix Center
109 East Lawrence Ave Springfield, IL, 62704
Phone: (217) 528-5253 Fax: (217) 528-5260
Internet: http://www.phoenixcenterspringfield.org/resources

The Center on Halsted 3656 North Haltsted Street Chicago, IL 60613
Phone: (773) 472-6469 Fax: (773) 472-6643
Internet: http://www.centeronhalsted.org

Chicago Gender Society PO Box 66595 Chicago, IL 60666
Email: chigendersoc@aol.com Internet: http://chicagogender.com

Ann & Robert H. Lurie—Gender & Sex Development Program Children's Hospital of Chicago 225 E. Chicago Avenue Chicago, IL 60611 Phone: (773) 303-6056 Internet: https://www.luriechildrens.org/en-us/care-services/specialties-ser-vices/gender-program

Howard Brown Health 4025 North Sheridan Road Chicago, IL 60613
Phone: (773)-388-1600 Fax: (773) 388-1602 Internet: https://howardbrown.org/programs-services/transgender-health/support

Parents & Friends of Lesbians and Gays—PFLAG of Northern Illinois P.O. Box 734 Elmhurst, IL 60126 Phone (630) 415-0622 Internet: http://www.pflagillinois.org

Pinwheels Arlington Heights—Parents & Youth Support Groups Reconciling Ministries Network 123 West Madison Street, Suite 2150 Chicago, Il 60602
Phone: (773) 736-5526 Internet: http://www.pinwheels.us

Indiana

Trans Indy
Life Journey Church 2950 E 55th Place Indianapolis, IN 46220
Internet: http://www.transindy.org
Riley Gender Health Program
705 Riley Hospital Dr. Indianapolis, IN 46202
Phone: (317) 274-8812
Internet: https://www.rileychildrens.org/departments/gender-health-program

Transcend Support Group
Kane Loveridge Wellness Group
3900 South Memorial Drive
New Castle, IN 47362
Phone (765) 388-2671
Internet: https://www.klwellness.com/group-therapy

Gender Nexus
1100 West 42nd Street, Suite 315
Indianapolis, IN 46208
Phone: (317) 650-5988
Internet: http://gendernexus.org

inTRANSit Support Group
Rainbow Serenity, Ltd c/o InTRANSit P.O. Box 9221 Highland, IN 46322
Phone: (219) 595-2321
Fax: (219) 513-3280
Internet: http://rainbowserenity.org/programs/intransit

Trans Lafayette
Pride Lafayette
640 Main Street Lafayette, IN 47901 Phone: (765) 423-7579
Internet:http://indianatransgendernetwork.com/resources/support/support-groups/trans-lafayette

Iowa

Transcend North Iowa
1948 Gil Avenue,
Charles City, IA 50616
Phone: (319) 359-7774
Internet: http://transcendnorthiowa.com

OneIowa
950 Office Park Road, Suite 240
West Des Moines, IA 50265
Phone: (516) 288-4019
Internet: https://oneiowa.org/work/transgender-iowans

Kansas

The Center of Wichita Inc.
800 N Market Wichita, KS, 67214 Phone: (316) 285-0007 Fax: (316) 243-5358
Internet: http://www.thecenterofwichita.org

Wichita Transgender & Community Network
200 North Broadway, Suite 220
Wichita, KS 67202
Internet: https://www.facebook.com/witconwichita

Kansas State Transgender Education Project—KSTEP
P.O. Box 13
Topeka, KS 66601
Phone: (785) 215-7436
Internet: http://kstep.org

Kentucky

TransKentucky
Internet: http://www.transkentucky.co/
Phone: (859) 448-5428

Pride Community Services Organization
389 Waller Ave #100
Lexington, KY 40504
Phone: (859) 253-3233
Internet: https://pcsoky.org

Lexington Fairness, Inc. PO Box 417
Lexington KY 40588
Phone: (859) 951-8565
Internet: http://lexingtonfairness.org

Parents, Families & Friends of Lesbians and Gays—PFLAG Louisville
First Lutheran Church
417 East Broadway
Louisville, KY 40202
Phone: (502) 233-1323
Internet: http://www.pflaglouisville.org

Louisiana

Louisiana Trans Advocates—Support Groups
Administrative Office
650 North 6th Street
Baton Rouge, LA 70802
Internet: http://www.latransadvocates.org/support-groups
Baton Rouge Last Saturday of the month from 2:00 PM to 4:00 PM.

Metropolitan Community Church 7747 Tom Drive Baton Rouge, LA 70806 Lafayette Second Saturday of the month from 2:00 PM to 4:00 PM.

Acadiana Center for the Arts 101 W. Vermillion Street Lafayette, LA 70501 Metairie Third Sunday of the month from 2:00 PM to 4:00 PM. 4721 Loveland Street Metairie, LA 70006

Shreveport First Sunday of the month from 1:30 PM to 3:00 PM. Contact: shreveport@latransadvocates.org

All Souls Unitarian Universalist Church 9449 Ellerbe Road Shreveport, LA 71106

LGBT Center of New Orleans 2727 S. Broad Street, Suite 102 New Orleans, LA 70125 Phone: (504) 407-5428
Internet: https://www.lgbtccneworleans.org

BreakOUT
1001 South Broad Street, Suite 217
New Orleans, LA 70125
Phone: (504):522-5435
Internet: http://www.youthbreakout.org

Louisiana Trans Advocates—Providers List
Administrative Office
650 North 6th Street
Baton Rouge, LA 70802
Internet: http://www.latransadvocates.org/support-groups

Parents, Family & Friends of Lesbians and Gays—PFLAG Louisiana
Congregation Gates of Prayer
4000 West Esplanade
Metairie, LA 70002
Phone: (504) 862-5912
Internet: http://pflagno.org

Maine

Maine Trans Net
511 Congress Street
Portland, ME 04101
Phone: (207) 370-0359
Internet: http://www.mainetransnet.org

Maine Family Planning—Open Door Transgender Health Care
P.O. Box 587
Augusta, ME 04332
Phone: (207) 622-7524
Internet: http://www.mainefamilyplanning.org

Mabel Wadsworth Center
700 Mount Hope Avenue, Suite 420
Bangor, Maine, 04401
Phone: (207) 947-5337
Fax: (207) 947-9163
Internet: https://www.mabelwadsworth.org

SAGE Maine
P.O. Box 10844
Portland, ME 04104
Phone: (207) 809-7015
Internet: http://www.sagemaine.org

Trans Youth Equality Foundation
P.O. Box 7441
Portland, ME 04112
Phone: (207) 478-4087
Internet: http://www.transyouthequality.org

Maryland

The Gay, Lesbian, Bisexual and Transgender Community Center of Baltimore and Central Maryland
The Baltimore Transgender Alliance
2530 North Charles Street 3rd Floor—Room 1 Baltimore, MD 21218
Phone: (410) 777-8145
Internet: http://www.glccb.org

FreeStateJustice—Legal Services
2526 St. Paul Street Baltimore, MD 21218
Phone: (410) 625-5428
Internet: https://freestate-justice.org

Rainbow Youth Alliance
Unitarian Universalist Congregation of Rockville 100 Welsh Park Drive Rockville, MD 20850
Phone: (240) 324-7823
Internet: http://www.rainbowyouthalliancemd.org

Parents, Families & Friends of Lesbians and Gays—PFLAG
Adult Transgender Group
Owen Brown Interfaith Center
7246 Cradlerock Way
Columbia, MD 21045
Phone: (443) 718-0474
Internet: https://www.pflaghoco.org

Massachusetts

Fenway Health—The Fenway Institute
Ansin Building
1340 Boylston Street
Boston, MA 02215
Phone: (617) 927-6400
Internet: http://fenwayhealth.org/the-fenway-institute

Tiffany Club of New England
30 Guinan Street
Waltham, MA 02451
Phone: (781) 891-9325
Internet: http://tcne.org

Trans4mations—Youth 85 Green Street
Worcester, MA 01604
An educational drop-in group for transgender, gender variant, and questioning individuals. This group is limited to individual's age range: 18–35.
Phone: (508) 755-3773 Internet: http://aidsprojectworcester.org

New Horizons 85 Green Street
Worcester, MA 01604 An educational drop-in group for transgender, gender variant, and questioning individuals age range: 35+
Phone: (508) 755-3773
Internet: http://aidsprojectworcester.org

Parents, Family & Friends of Lesbians and Gays—PFLAG of Greater Worcester
4 Mann Street
Worcester, MA 01602
Phone: (508) 631-2699
Internet: https://www.worcesterpflag.org

Michigan

Transgender Michigan
23211 Woodward Avenue #309
Ferndale, MI 48200
Phone: (800) 842-2854
Fax: (800) 842-2954
Internet: https://transgendermichigan.org

Affirmations
Transgender Support
290 West Nine Mile Road
Ferndale, MI 48220
Phone: (248) 398-7105
Fax: (248) 541-1943
Internet: http://www.goaffirmations.org

Michigan Medicine—University of Michigan
Transgender Support Groups
2025 Traverwood Dr. Suite A1 Ann Arbor, MI 48105
Phone: 734-998-2150
Internet: http://www.uofmhealth.org

Jim Toy Community Center
FTM A2-YPSI Trans Men Group
319 Braun Court
Ann Arbor, MI 48104
Phone: (734) 995-9867
Internet: https://www.jimtoycenter.org

Stand With Trans—Youth Programs
Phone: 248-579-8996
Internet: http://standwithtrans.org

Trans Sistas of Color Project
19641 West 7 Mile Road
Detroit, MI 48219
Phone: (313) 537-7000 Ext.107
Internet: https://www.facebook.com/TSCOPD

Minnesota

University of Minnesota—Program in Human Sexuality
Transgender Health Services
Center for Sexual Health 1300 South 2nd Street, Suite 180
Minneapolis, MN 55454
Phone (612) 625-1500 Fax: (612) 626-8311
Internet: https://www.sexualhealth.umn.edu

Minnesota Transgender Health Coalition
3405 Chicago Avenue S, Suite 103
Minneapolis, MN 55407
Phone: (612) 823-1152
Internet: http://www.mntranshealth.org

Parents, Family & Friends of Lesbians and Gays—PFLAG Twin Cities
Box 1920
Minneapolis, MN 55419
Phone: (612) 825-1660
Internet: http://www.pflagtc.com

Reclaim Youth Services
771 Raymond Avenue
St. Paul, MN 55114
Phone: (612)235-6743
Fax: (612) 524-5527
Internet: https://reclaim.care/contact

Mississippi

Mississippi Rainbow Center
P.O. Box 66
Biloxi, MS 39533
Phone: (601) 336-0162
Internet: https://www.msrainbowcenter.org

The Spectrum Center
210 South 25th Avenue
Hattiesburg, MS 30401
Phone: (601) 310-6185
Internet: https://hattiesburgpride.com

Southern Miss PRISM LGBTQ
118 College Drive
Hattiesburg, MS 39406
Phone: (601) 266-5716
Internet: https://www.facebook.com/RainbowCenterJxn

Parents, Families & Friends of Lesbians and Gays—PFLAG Jackson, MS
P.O. Box 13092
Jackson, MS 39236
Phone: (601) 842-2274
Internet: https://pflagjacksonms.wordpress.com/lgbt-youth-resources

Missouri

The Transgender Institute
8080 Ward Parkway, Suite 400
Kansas City MO 64111
Phone: (816) 305-0843
Internet: http://transinstitute.org/contact

Metro Trans Umbrella Group
438 N Skinker Blvd St. Louis, MO 63130
Internet: https://www.stlmetrotrans.com

The Center Project
P.O. Box 521
Columbia, MO 65205
Phone: (573) 449-1189
Internet: http://www.thecenterproject.org

The GLO Center—Gay & Lesbian Community Center of the Ozarks
P.O. Box 225
Springfield, MO 65801
Phone: (417) 869-3978
Fax: (417) 831-6063
Internet: http://www.glocenter.org

LGBTO Resource Center—University of Missouri
TRANS at MIZZOU
G225 MU Student Center Columbia, MO 65211 Phone: (573) 884-7750
Internet: https://lgbtq.missouri.edu/trans

The Transgender Institute
8080 Ward Parkway, Suite 400 Kansas City, MO 64114
Phone: (816) 305-0943
Internet: http://transinstitute.org/contact

Parents, Family & Friends of Lesbians and Gays—Kansas City PFLAG
PO Box 414101 Kansas City, MO 64141 Phone: (816) 765-9818
Internet: http://pflagkc.org

Children's Mercy—Kansas City
Gender Pathway Services
2401 Gillham Road Kansas City, MO 64108
Phone: (816) 960-413
Internet: https://www.childrensmercy.org/gender-pathway-services/

Gender Inc.
520 West 103 Street, Suite 252
Kansas City, MO 64114
Phone: (800) 513-1715
Internet: http://genderinc.com

The Transgender Institute
8080 Ward Parkway, Suite 400 Kansas City, MO 64114
Phone: (816) 305-0943
Internet: http://transinstitute.org/contact

Montana

Western Montana Gay & Lesbian Community Center
Gender Expansion Project
127 North Higgins Avenue, Suite 202
Missoula, MT 59801
Phone: (406) 848-1220
Internet: http://genderexpansionproject.org

Blue Mountain Clinic Family Practice—Transgender Health Care
610 N. California Street Missoula, MT 59802
Phone: (406) 721-1646
Internet: http://www.bluemountainclinic.org

Montana Two Spirit Society
P.O. Box 7514
Missoula, MT 59807
Phone: (406) 829-8075
Internet: https://www.mttwospirit.org

Parents, Family & Friends of Lesbians and Gays—PFLAG Hamilton-Bitterroot
456 Whisperidge Drive
Corvallis, MT 59828
Phone: (406) 360-6796
Internet: http://pflaghamiltonbitterroot.org

Nebraska

The Nebraska Medicine Transgender Clinic
Nebraska Medicine—Specialty Care Clinic
Attn: Dr. Jean Amoura
804 South 52nd Street
Omaha, NE 68106
Phone: (402) 559-2666
Fax: (402) 553-5963
Internet: https://www.nebraskamed.com/transgender-care

River City Gender Alliance
P.O. Box 284
Boys Town, NE 68010
Phone: (402) 476-8091
Internet: http://rcga.co

Common Root Mutual Aid Center
Trans + Support Group
3140 O Street, Suite 202
Lincoln, NE 68510
Email: contaact@commonroot.net
Internet: https://www.commonroot.net

Imperial Court of Nebraska
P.O. Box 3772
Omaha, NE 68103

Parents, Family & Friends of Lesbians and Gays—PFLAG Omaha
P.O. Box 390064
Omaha, NE 68139
Phone: (402) 291-6781
Internet: http://pflag-omaha.org

Open Arms Trans Social Group
Second Unitarian Church
3012 South 119th Street
Omaha, NE 68144
Phone: (402) 334-0537
http://www.openarmsomaha.com

Proud Horizons Youth Group
Heartland Pride
Attn: Proud Horizons
P.O. Box 8273
Omaha, NE 68108
Internet: https://proudhorizons.wordpress.com

Inclusive Life Center
4501 South 96ht Street
Omaha, NE 68127
Phone: (402) 575-7006
Internet: https://inclusivelife.org

Youth Emergency Services—YES
2679 Farnam Street, Suite 205
Omaha, NE 68131
Phone: (402) 345-5187
Fax: (402) 345-6704
Internet: http://www.yesomaha.org

Nevada

Transgender Allies Group—Resources
1745 South Wells Avenue
Reno, NV 89502
Internet: http://www.transgenderalliesgroup.org

The Center—LGBTQ Community of Nevada
Identi-T*
401 South Maryland Parkway
Las Vegas, NV 8901
Phone: (702) 733-9800
Internet: http://thecenterlv.org/programs/tran s

OUR Center
1745 South Wells Avenue
Reno, NV 89502
Phone: (775) 624-3720
Internet: http://www.ourcenterreno.org/gender

New Hampshire

Transgender New Hampshire—TG-NH
Resources & Community Organizing
Internet: http://www.tg-nh.org
A Peaceful Balance—Transgender Support Groups
154 Broad Street, Suite 1511
Nashua, NH 03063
Phone: (603) 577-5551
Fax: (603) 577-5576
Internet: http://www.apeacefulbalance.com

Seacoast Outright—Youth
206 Court Street
Portsmouth, NH 03801
Phone: (603) 552-5824

Internet: http://www.seacoastoutright.org

Equality Health Center
38 South Main Street
Concord, NH 03301
Phone: (603) 225-2739
Internet: http://equalityhc.org

Parents, Family & Friends of Lesbians and Gays—PFLAG New Hampshire
PO Box 957
Concord, NH 03302
Phone: 211 (A clearinghouse run by United Way)
Internet: http://www.pflagnh.org

New Jersey

The Pride Center of New Jersey
Transgender Support
85 Rariton Avenue, Suite 100
Highland Park, NJ 08904
Phone: (732) 846-2232
Internet: http://www.pridecenter.org

Hudson Pride Center
Trans View Support Group
CarePoint Health, Christ Church
176 Palisade Avenue, 3 East
Jersey City, NJ 07306
Phone: (201) 963-4779
Fax: (201 963-7983
Internet: https://www.hudsonpride.org

True Colors Center for Creative Therapy
Transgender Support Groups
93 Main Street
Newtown, NJ 07860
Phone: (973) 222-3750
Internet: http://jenwhitlock.com

Newark LGBT Center
11 Halsey Street Newark, NJ, 07102 Phone: (973) 424-9555 Fax: (973) 424-0037
Internet: http://newarklgbtqcenter.org

Parents, Family & Friends of Lesbians and Gays—PFLAG Jersey City St. Paul's Evangelical Church 440-480 Hoboken Avenue Jersey City, NJ 07306
Phone: (571) 969-3015 Internet: https://www.pflag.org

HiTOPS
Adolescent Health & Well Being
Transgender Youth Groups
21 Wiggins Street
Princeton, NJ 08540
Phone: (609)683-5155 x219
Internet: https://www.hitops.org

QSpot—LGBT Community Center
Jersey Shore Transgender—JSTSURF Group
66 Main Street
Ocean Grove, NJ 07756
Phone: (732) 455-3373
Fax: (732) 556-6332
Internet: http://qspot.org

New Mexico

Transgender Resource Center of New Mexico
149 Jackson Street North East
Albuquerque, NM 87108
Phone: (505) 200-9086
Internet: http://www.tgrcnm.org

Alianza of New Mexico—Health Care
1615 N Solano Drive
Las Cruces, NM 88001
Phone: (575) 915-1770
Internet: http://www.alianzanm.org

Allianza of New Mexico—Health Care
311 West 2nd Street
Roswell, NM 88203
Phone: (575) 623-1995
Internet: http://www.alianzanm.org

Engender, Inc.
Counseling services
2632 Pennsylvania Street North East
Suite E
Albuquerque, NM 87110
Phone: (505) 242-4400
Fax: (505) 242-4595
Internet: http://www.engenderwellness.com

Rainbow Village-LGBTQ Grant County
211B North Texas Street
Silver City NM 88061
Phone: (575) 519-5562
Internet: http://gaysilver.org

New York

The Anti-Violence Project (AVP)
116 Nassau Street, 3rd Floor
New York, NY 10038
Phone: (212) 714-1184
Internet: https://www.avp.org

Audra Lorde Project
147 West 24th Street, 3rd Floor
New York, NY 10011
Phone: (212) 463-0342
Fax: (212) 463-0344
Internet: https://www.alp.org

Audra Lorde Project
85 South Oxford Street
Brooklyn, NY 11217
Phone: (718) 596-0342
Fax: (718) 596-1328
Internet: https//www.alp.org

American Indian Community House
39 Eldridge Street, 4th Floor
New York, NY 10002
Phone: (212) 966-4227
Fax: (212) 966-4963
Internet: http://www.aich.org

Brooklyn Community Pride Center
1360 Fulton Street, Ground Floor
Brooklyn, NY 11216
Phone: (347) 889-7719
Internet: http://www.lgbtbrooklyn.org

Center Lane—Ages 13–21
34 South Broadway, 6th Floor Room 7
Yonkers, NY 10701
Phone: (914) 4223-0610
Internet: http://www.wjcs.com/center-lane-locations

Center Lane-The Loft
252 Bryant Avenue
White Plains, NY 10605
Phone: (914) 423-0610
Internet: http://www.wjcs.com/center-lane-locations

Cometfire—Jewish Community Center—Youth Services ages 11–14
334 Amsterdam Avenue
New York, NY 10023
Phone: (646) 505-4444
Internet: http://www.pflagnyc.org/support/cometfire

Community Kinship Life (CK Life)
1276 Fulton Avenue, 3rd Floor
Bronx, NY 10456
Phone: (347) 881-0075
Internet: http://www.cklife.org

The Door—Youth Services ages 12–21
555 Broome Street
New York, NY 10013
Phone: (212) 941-9090
Internet: http://www.door.org

FIERCE NYC—Youth Services ages 13–24
2427 Morris Avenue
Bronx, NY 10468
Phone: (929) 246-5237
Internet: http://www.fiercenyc.org

GRIOT Circle
25 Flatbush Avenue, 5th Floor
Brooklyn, NY 11217
Phone: (718) 246-2775
https://www.griotcircle.org

Hetrick Martin Institute—Youth Services ages 13–24
2 Astor Place, 3rd Floor
New York, NY 10003
Phone: (212) 674-2400
Internet: http://www.him.org

Identity House
208 West 13th Street
New York, NY 10011
Phone: (212) 243-8181
Internet: http://www.identityhouse.org

Lesbian, Gay, Bisexual & Transgender Community Center
Center Wellness-Gender Identity Project
208 West 13th Street
New York, NY 10011
Phone: (212) 620-7310
Internet: http://www.gaycenter.org

Lesbian, Gay, Bisexual & Transgender Community Center
Youth Enrichment Services (YES)—ages 13–21
208 West 13th Street
New York, NY 10011
Phone: (212) 620-7310
Internet: http://www.gaycenter.org

Long Island Gay & Lesbian Youth (LEGALY)—ages 13–21
34 Park Avenue
Bay Shore, NY 11706
Phone: (631) 665-2300
Fax: (631) 665-7874
Internet: http://www.lgbtnetwork.org

Make the Road New York
Internet: http://www.maketheroadny.org
Borough sites:
Bushwick: 301 Grove Street Brooklyn, New York 11237 Phone: (718) 418-7690 Fax: (718) 418-9635
Queens: 92-10 Roosevelt Avenue Jackson Heights, New York 11372 Phone: (718) 565-8500 Fax (718) 565-0646
Staten Island: 161 Port Richmond Avenue SI, New York 10302 Phone: (718) 727-1222 Fax: (718) 981-8077
Long Island: 1090 Suffolk Avenue Brentwood, NY 11717 Phone: (631) 231-2220 Fax: (631) 231-2229

New Alternatives for LGBTQ + Homeless Youth—ages 16–24
410 West 40th Street
New York, NY 10018
Phone: (718) 300-0133
Fax: (888) 568-3033
https://www.newalternativesnyc.org

Parents, Families & Friends of Lesbians and Gays—PFLAG NYC
TransFamilies Project
334 Amsterdam Avenue
New York, NY 10023
Phone: (646) 505-4444
Email: transgender@pflagnyc.org
Internet: http://www.pflagnyc.org/support/transfamiliesproject

Positive Health Project
301 West 37th Street 2nd Floor
New York, NY 10018
Phone: (212) 465-8304 Ext.4822
Fax: (212) 465-8306
Internet: https://www.housingworks.org

PRIDE CENTER OF Staten Island
25 Victory Blvd., 3rd Floor
Staten Island, NY 10301
Phone: (718) 808-1360
Fax: (718) 808-1397
Internet: https://www.pridecenterssi.org

Queens Pride House
76-11 37th Avenue, Suite 206
Jackson Heights, NY 11372
Phone: (718) 429-5309
Fax: (718) 429-5013
Internet: https://www.queenspridehouse.org

Queens LGBT Community Center (Q Center)
37-18 Northern Blvd. Suite 107
Long Island City, NY 11101
Phone: (718) 514-2155
Fax: (718) 750-4715
Internet: https://lgbtnetwork.org

Edie Windsor SAGE Center (Services and Advocacy for LGBT Elders)
305 7th Avenue, 15th Floor
New York, NY 10001
Phone: (212) 576-8669
Internet: https://www.sageusa.org

Sylvia Rivera Law Project
147 West 24th Street, 5th Floor
New York, NY 10011
Phone: (212) 337-8558
Fax: (212) 337-1972
Internet: http://www.srlp.org

Pride Center of the Capital Region
Transgender Support Groups
332 Hudson Avenue
Albany, NY 12210
Phone: (518) 462-6138
Fax: (518) 462-2101
Internet: http://www.capitalpridecenter.org

In Our Own Voices, Inc.
245 Lark Street
Albany, NY 12210
Phone: (518) 432-4288
Fax: (518) 432-4123
Internet: http://inourownvoices.org

Pride Center of Western New York
Transgeneration
200 South Elmwood Avenue
Buffalo, NY 14201
Phone: (716) 852-7743
Fax: (716) 541-0673
Internet: http://www.pridecenterwny.org

Hudson Valley LGBTQ Community Center
Transgender Support Groups
300 Wall Street
Kingston, NY 12401
Phone: (845) 331-5300
Internet: http://www.lgbtqcenter.org

Rockland County Pride Center
Transgender Support Groups
P.O. Box 505
Nyack, NY 10960
Phone: (845) 353-6300
Internet: http://rocklandpridecenter.org

Out Alliance of the Genesee Valley
100 College Avenue # 100
Rochester, NY 14607
Phone: (585) 244-8640
Fax: (585) 244-8246
Internet: http://www.gayalliance.org

North Carolina

LGBT Center of Raleigh—Transgender Initiative
324 South Harrington Street
Raleigh, NC 27603
Phone: (919) 832-4484
Internet: https://www.lgbtcenterofraleigh.com

Planned Parenthood Raleigh Health Center
100 South Boylan Avenue
Raleigh, NC 27603
Phone: (919) 833-7526

Fax: (919) 832-9061
Internet: https://www.plannedparenthood.org/planned-parenthood-south-atlan-tic/for-patients

Western NC Community Health Services
257 Biltmore Avenue
Asheville, NC 28801
Phone: (828) 285-0622
Internet: http://www.wncchs.org

Blue Ridge Pride
417 Biltmore Avenue
Asheville, NC 28801
Phone: (917) 822-9085
Internet: https://www.blueridgeprice.org

Time Out Youth
3800 Monroe Road
Charlotte, NC 28206
Phone: (704) 344-8335
Fax: (704) 344-8166
Internet: https://www.timeoutyouth.org

LGBTQ Center of Durham
114 Hunt Street
Durham, NC 27701
Phone: (919) 827-1436
Internet: https://www.lightcenterofdurham.org

North Star LGBTQ Community Center
930 Burke Street
Winston-Salem, NC 27101
Phone: (336) 893-9353
Internet: http://www.northstarlgbtcc.com

North Dakota

DOR Dakota OutRight
P.O. Box 3064
Bismarck, ND 59502
Internet: http://dakotaoutright.org

Pride Collective and Community Center
1105 1st Avenue
South Fargo, ND 58103
Phone: (218) 287-8034
Internet: http://pridecollective.com

Tri State Transgender
Phone: (701) 404-9955
Internet: http://tristatetransgender.weebly.com/

Ohio

TransAlive Akron Support Group
2095 West Market Street
Akron, OH 44133
Phone: (330) 240-1600
Internet: https://sites.google.com/a/transfamily.org

Kaleidoscope Youth Center
P.O. Box 8104
Columbus, OH 43201
Phone: (614) 294-5437
Internet: http://www.kycohio.org

Toledo Area Transgender Support (TATS) Group
2413 Collingwood Blvd 419 Pride Center
Toledo OH 43620
Phone: (419) 619-6810
Internet: http://www.equalitytoledo.org/transgender-resources

TransFamily—LGBT Center of Cleveland
6600 Detroit Avenue
Cleveland, OH 44102 Phone: (216) 691-4357
Internet: https://www.transfamily.org

Gatlyn Dame Group Inc.
The Greater Dayton LGBT Center
24 North Jefferson Street, Suite 200
Dayton, OH 45402
Phone: (513) 571-1874
Internet: http://gatlyndamegroup.com

Parents, Families & Friends of Lesbians and Gays—PFLAG Dayton
P.O. Box 3721
Dayton, OH 45401
Phone: (937) 640-333
Internet: http://pflagdayton.org

Oklahoma

Trans Peer Support Group
4001 North Classen Blvd. Suite 116
Oklahoma City, OK 73118
Phone: (405) 802-8229
Internet: http://www.okeq.org/transgender-support

Trust Women—South Wind Women's Center
1240 South West 44th Street
Oklahoma City, OK 73109
Phone: (405) 429-7940
Internet: http://www.southwindwomenscenter.org

Dennis R. Neill Equality Center—Transgender Support Groups
621 East 4th Street
Tulsa, OK 74119
Phone: (918) 743-4297
Fax: (918) 295-6885
Internet: https://www.okeq.org

Parents, Family & Friends of Lesbians and Gays—PFLAG Oklahoma City
4001 North Classen Blvd
Oklahoma City, OK 73118
Phone: (405) 593-8868
Internet: https://www.pflagoklahomacity.org

Expressions Community Center-ECC
Transgender Support Group
2245 North West 39th Street
Oklahoma, OK 73112
Phone: (405) 528-2210
Internet: http://eccokc.org

Oregon
Q Center—Transgender Programs
4115 North Mississippi Avenue
Portland, OR 97217
Phone: (503) 234-7837
Internet: http://www.pdxqcenter.org

North West Gender Alliance—NWGA
P.O. Box 4928
Portland, OR 97208
Phone: (503) 533-8787
Internet: http://www.nwgenderalliance.org

TransActive Gender Center
1631 North East Broadway Street 355-T
Portland, OR 97232
Phone: (503) 252-3000
Internet: http://www.transactiveonline.org

Sexual & Gender Minority Youth Resource Center—SMYRC
1220 South West Columbia Street
Portland OR 97201

Phone: (503) 872-9664
Internet: http://www.smyrc.org

The Lower Columbia Q Center—Gender Alliance
1636 Exchange Street
Astoria, OR 92103
Internet: https://www.lcqcastoria.org

Intersex Initiative
P.O. Box 40570
Portland, OR 97240
Internet: http://www.ipdx.org/contact.html

Pennsylvania

Mazzoni Center—Trans Care
1349 Bainbridge Street
Philadelphia, PA 19147
Phone: (215) 563-0652
Internet: https://www.mazzonicenter.org

Trans Central PA
c/o MCC of the Spirit
2973 Jefferson Street
Harrisburg, PA 17110
Phone: (717) 831-8142
Internet: http://transcentralpa.org

Central PA LGBT Center—Transgender Support Group
Alder Health Services
1891 Santa Barbara Drive, Suite 104
Lancaster, PA 17601
Phone: (717) 509-6349
Internet: http://www.centralpalgbtcenter.org

Renaissance of the Leigh High Valley—Transgender Support Group
Metropolitan Community Church of Leigh High Valley
1401 Greenview Drive
Bethlehem, PA 18018
Internet: https://www.renaissancelv.org

Youth Trans and Unified at the Attic Youth Center
255 South 16th Street
Philadelphia, PA 19102
Phone: (215) 545-4331
Internet: https://www.atticyouthcenter.org

Bradbury-Sullivan LGBT Community Center
522 West Maple Street
Allentown, PA 18101
Phone: (610) 347-9988
Internet: http://www.bradburysullivancenter.org

TriVersity-Center for Gender & Sexual Diversity
Upper Delaware GLBT Center Inc.
201 West Harford Street
P.O. Box 1295
Milford, PA 18337
Phone: (570) 832-4955
Internet: http://www.udglbt.org

Puerto Rico

Igual Que Tu—Centro Comuntario LGBBTT DE PR
Transgender Support Group
Urb. Perez Morris Calle Mayaguez #37
San Juan, PR 00917
Phone: (787) 294-9850
Internet: http://www.centrolgbttpr.org

Rhode Island

TGI Network of Rhode Island
PO Box 40365
Providence, RI 02940
Phone: (401) 441-5058
Internet: http://www.tginetwork.org

Thundermist Health Center
Trans Health Access Team
450 Clinton Street
Woonsocket, RI 02895
Phone: (401) 767-4100 ext. 4303
Internet: http://www.thundermisthealth.org

Youth Pride Inc.
743 Westminster Street
Providence, RI 02903
Phone: (401) 421-5626
Fax: (401) 274-1990
Internet: http://youthprideri.org

Parents, Family & Friends of Lesbians and Gays-PFLAG Greater Providence
P. O. Box 41344 Providence, RI 02940 Phone: 401-307-1802
Internet: http://www.pflagprovidence.org

South Carolina

Midlands Area Transgender Support
Harriet Hancock LGBT Center
1108 Woodrow Street
Columbia, SC 29201
Phone: (803) 771-7713
Internet: http://harriethancockcenter.org

We Are Family—Trans Love Fund
P.O. Box 21806
Charleston, SC 29413
Internet: http://wearefamilycharleston.org/tlf

Parents, Family & Friends of Lesbians and Gays-PFLAG Spartanburg
Spartanburg Community College Downtown Campus
220 East Kennedy Street
Spartanburg, SC 29302
Phone: (864) 381-8187
Internet: http://pflagupstatesc.org

Upstate Pride South Carolina
P.O. Box 9128
Greenville, SC 29604
Phone: (864) 735-0023
Internet: http://www.upstatepridesc.org

South Dakota

Black Hills Center for Equality—True Colors Support Group
P.O. Box 1558 Rapid City, SD 57709
Phone: (605) 348-3244
Internet: https://www.bhcfe.org

Sioux Falls Pride
Transgender Resources
P.O. Box 2403
Sioux Falls, SD 57101
Phone: (605) 610-9206
Internet: http://www.siouxfallspride.org

Queer Gender South Dakota
1430 Haines Avenue, Suite 108277
Rapid City, SD 57701
Phone: (605) 519-8097
Internet: https://www.queersd.org

TransAction South Dakota
PO Box 91614 Sioux Falls SD 57106 Phone: (605) 681-6506
Internet: https://www.transactionsd.org

Tennessee

The Tennessee Vals
P.O. Box 331006
Nashville, TN 37203
Phone: (615) 664-6883
Internet: http://www.tvals.org

Pride Community Center of the Tri-Cities
P.O. Box 5277
Johnson City, TN 37602
Internet: http://pridetricities.com

Chattanooga Pride
Trans Support
1100 Market Street Chattanooga, TN 37402
Internet: http://www.tennesseevalleypride.com

Tennessee Valley Transgender Support Group
2002 Oak Street
Chattanooga, TN 37404
Phone: (423) 591-5147
Internet: www.facebook.com/TennValleyTGsupportgrp

Transgender, Gender Variant & Crossdressing Group
Axiom Associates 108 W Summit Hill Drive Knoxville, TN 37902 Phone: (865) 245-4713
Internet: https://www.groupaxiom.com/ShanaVHamiltonLockwoodPhD

CHOICES Memphis Center for Reproductive Health & Transgender Services
1726 Poplar Avenue Memphis, TN 38104 Phone: (901) 274-3550
Internet: https://www.memphischoices.org

Vanderbilt Health Medical Center
1211 Medical Center Drive Nashville, TN 37232 Phone: (615) 322-5000
Internet: https://www.vanderbilthealth.com/lgbtihealthprogram

Texas

Transgender Education Network of Texas
Operations Office 102 Wonder World Dr. #304-174
San Marcos TX 78666
Internet: http://www.transtexas.org/

Trans Pride Initiative
614 West Davis Street, Suite 208
Dallas, TX 75208 Phone: (214) 449-1439
Internet: http://tpride.org

Trans-Cendence International
P.O. Box 13476
Arlington, TX 76094
Phone: (682) 305-7686
Internet: https://www.transcendint.org

OutYouth
909 East 49th ½ Street
Austin, TX 78751
Phone: (512) 419-1233
Internet: https://www.outyouth.org

Montrose Center
401 Branard Street
Houston, TX 77006
Phone: (713) 529-0037
Fax: (713) 526-4367
Internet: http://www.montrosecenter.org/hub

Transgender Foundation of Houston
604 Pacific Street
Houston, TX 77006
Internet: http://www.tfahouston.com/

Kind Clinic—Gender Affirming Care
1101 West 40th Street #102
Austin, TX 78756
Phone: (512) 853-9547
Internet: https://kindclinic.org

Resource Center—GenderBrave
5750 Cedar Springs Road Dallas, Texas 75235
Phone: 214) 540-4415
Internet: https://www.genderbrave.org

Parents, Families & Friends of Lesbians and Gays—PFLAG Dallas Northaven United Methodist Church Room 250 11211 Preston Rd Dallas, TX 75230 Phone: (972) 849-0383
Internet: https://www.pflag.org/chapter/pflag-dalla s

Parents, Families & Friends of Lesbians and Gays PFLAG Austin
P.O. Box 49417
Austin, TX 78765
Phone: (512) 302-3524
Internet: https://pflagaustin.org

Pride Center San Antonio—Transgender Support Groups
3010 N. St. Mary's Street San Antonio, TX 78212
Phone: (210) 370-7743
Internet: http://pridecentersa.org

Utah

Equality Utah—Transgender Resources
175 West 200 South, Suite 1004
Salt Lake City, UT 8401
Phone: (801) 355-3479
Internet: https://www.equalityutah.org/issues/transgender

Authentic Awareness
597 West 800 North
Orem, UT 84057
Phone: (208) 357-9268
Internet: https://www.psychologytoday.com/us/groups/authentic-awareness

UTAH Pride Center—Transgender Support Groups
P.O. Box 1078
Salt Lake City, UT 84110
Phone: (801) 539-8800
Internet: https://www.utahpridecenter.org

University of Utah Health—Transgender Health Program
50 North Medical Drive
Salt Lake City, UT 84132
Phone: (801) 581-2121
Internet: https://healthcare.utah.edu/transgender-health

Parents, Families & Friends of Lesbians and Gays—PFLAG Salt Lake City
Utah Pride Center
255 East 400 South
Salt Lake City, 84111
Phone: (801) 688-2281
Internet: http://pflag-saltlakecity.org

Encircle LGBTQ Family & Youth Resource Centers
91 West 200 South
Provo, UT 94601

331 South 600 E
Salt Lake City, UT 84102
Internet: https://encircletogether.org

Vermont

Pride Center of Vermont
Transgender Programs
255 Champlain Street, Suite 12
Burlington, VT 05401
Phone: (802) 860-7812
Internet: https://www.pridecentervt.org

Outright Vermont
Transgender Groups
241 North Winooski Avenue
Burlington, VT 05401
Phone: (802) 865-9677
Internet: http://www.outrightvt.org

Green Mountain Crossroads
P.O. Box 1685
Brattleboro, VT 05302
Internet: http://www.greenmountaincrossroads.org

The University of Vermont Medical Center
Transgender Youth Program
111 Colchester Avenue
Main Campus
Burlington, VT 05401
Phone: (802) 847-3811
Internet: https://www.uvmhealth.org

Virginia

Health Brigade—Transgender Health Services
1010 North Thompson Street
Richmond, VA 23220
Phone: (804) 358-6343 ext. 143
Fax: (804) 521-0809
Internet: http://www.healthbrigade.org

Richmond Transformers Transmasculine Spectrum
1010 North Thompson Street
Richmond, VA 23220
Phone: (804) 358-6343
Internet: https://groups.yahoo.com/neo/groups/RichmondTransformers/info

He, She, Ze, and We
2111 Westwood Avenue
Richmond, VA 23230
Phone: (804) 644-4800
Email: heshezeandwe@gmail.com

Side by Side—Trans Youth Group
P.O. Box 5542
Richmond, VA 23230
Phone: (888)644-4390
Internet: http://www.sidebysideva.org

James River Transgender Society
Diversity Richmond
1407 Sherwood Avenue
Richmond, VA 21220
Phone: (804) 404-2425
Internet: http://jrts.org

Serenity, Inc. –Transgender Support
114 North Union Street
Petersburg, VA 23803
Phone: (804) 861-9977
Internet: http://www.serenity-crater.org

Gender Expression Movement—Support Services
LGBT Center of Hampton Roads
247 W. 25th Street
Norfolk, VA 23517
Phone: (757) 200-9198
Website: http://www.accessaids.org

Transgender Assistance Program of Virginia (TAP)
5906 Beachwalk Drive
Virginia Beach, VA 23464
Phone: 757-933-1504
Email: transactivista@gmail.com
Website: https://www.tapvirginia.org

Metro Area Gender Identity Connection (MAGIC)
Meets at Falls Church Presbyterian Church
225 Broad Street
Falls Church, VA 22041
Website: www.magicdc.org

PFLAG T* Families Support Group/TransFormation Ministry
Meets at Metropolitan Community Church NOVA
10383 Democracy Lane

Fairfax, VA 22030
Phone: (202) 460-6002
Email: transfamiliesva@gmail.com
Internet: http://www.mccnova.com

Transgender Education Association (TGEA)
Metropolitan Community Church of Northern Virginia
10383 Democracy Lane
Fairfax, VA 22030
Mailing Address: 5765F Burke Centre Parkway, Suite 167
Burke, Virginia 22015
Internet: http://www.tgea.org

PFLAG Blue Ridge: Charlottesville Transgender Support Groups
The Women's Initiative; Facilitators: Jane Cornelius, Circe Strauss
1101 East High Street
Charlottesville, Virginia 22902
Internet: www.pflagblueridge.org/charlottesville.html

Teen and Young Adult Health Center—UVA Transgender Health Services
University of Virginia
1204 W. Main Street
Charlottesville, VA 22903
Phone: (434) 982-0090
Fax: (434) 924-9983
Internet: https://childrens.uvahealth.com/services/teen-health

Ladies and Gents of the Blue Ridge—Transgender Alliance, LLC (LGBR-TA)
Meets at Roanoke Diversity Center
806 Jamison Avenue SE
Roanoke, Virginia 24013
Internet: https://www.facebook.com/groups/LBRTA

Lynchburg Diversity Center
901 Jefferson Street, Suite 201
Lynchburg VA 24504
Phone: (434) 515-1143
Internet: https://www.lynchburgdiversity.org

Washington

Gay City-LGBT Center
Transgender Parents of Washington—TPOW
517 East Pike Street
Seattle, WA 98122
Phone: (206) 860-6969
Fax: (206) 860-0196
Internet: https://www.gaycity.org

Ingersoll Gender Center
1425 Broadway # 509
Seattle, WA 98122
Phone: (206) 849-7859
Internet: http://ingersollgendercenter.org

Gender Diversity Education & Support Services
6523 California Avenue South West # 360
Seattle, WA 98136
Phone: (855) 443-6337
Internet: http://www.genderdiversity.org/contact

Gender Alliance of the South Sound
The Oasis Rainbow Center—Transgender Support Groups 2215 Pacific Ave. Tacoma, WA 98402 Phone: (253)-383-2318
Internet: http://www.southsoundgender.com

The Emerald City Trans Social Group
P.O. Box 59893
Renton, WA 98058
Phone: (425) 827-9494
Internet: http://www.theemeraldcity.org

Washington Gender Alliance Support Group at Walla Walla
Glover Alston Center 26 Boyer Avenue
Walla Walla, WA 99362
Phone: (509) 522-4410
Internet: http://www.washingtongenderalliance.com/index.html?content=walla-walla

Parents, Family & Friends of Lesbians and Gays-PFLAG Olympia
First United Methodist Church
1224 Legion Way South East
Olympia, WA 98501
Phone: (360) 207-1608
Internet: http://pflag-olympia.org

Lambert House
Transgender Support Group
1818 15th Avenue Seattle, WA 98122
Phone: (206) 322-2515
Internet: http://www.lamberthouse.org/contact

Metro Area Gender Identity Connection—MAGIC of Washington DC
Falls Church, Presbyterian Church
225 East Broad Street

Falls Church VA 22046
Phone: (703) 606-4936
Internet: http://www.magicdc.org

Washington D.C.

D.C Area Trans Masculine Society (DCATS)
Meets at Whitman Walker Health
1701 14th Street NW
Washington, D.C. 20009
Phone: (571) 293-2287
Website: http://www.dcatsinfo.org

TransLAW
Meets at Whitman Walker Health
1701 14th Street, NW
Washington DC 20009
Phone: 202.939.7627
Internet: https://www.translawdc.org

Casa Ruby
2822 Georgia Avenue North West
Washington, DC 20001
Phone: (202) 355-5155
Internet: http://www.casaruby.org

Supporting & Mentoring Youth Advocates and Leaders—SMYYAL
Trans & Non-Binary Group
410 7th Street South East
Washington, DC 20003
Phone: (202) 546-5940
Internet: https://www.smyal.org

The DC Center for the LGBT Community
2000 14th Street NW # 105
Washington, DC 20009
Phone: (202) 682-2245
Internet: http://thedccenter.org

Whitman-Walker Health—Transgender Health Care
1525 14th Street, N.W.
Washington, D.C. 20005
Phone: 202-745-7000
Fax: 202-332-1049
Website: http://www.whitman-walker.org

West Virginia

Eastern Panhandle LGBTQ Alliance
P.O. Box 1431
Charles Town, WV 25414
Phone: (304) 728-0247
Internet: http://panhandlealliance.wixsite.com/panhandle-alliance

West Virginia University
SPECTRUM—LGBTQ Support
c/o Student Organization Services
P.O. Box 6444
Morgantown, WV 26506
Phone: (304) 293-8200
Internet: https://spectrum.orgs.wvu.edu

Fairness West Virginia—Advocacy
405 Capitol Street, Suite 405
Charleston, WV 25301
Phone: (681) 265-9062
Internet: http://fairnesswv.org/

Wisconsin

FORGE
P.O. Box 1272
Milwaukee, WI 53201
Phone: (414) 559-2123
Internet: http://forge-forward.org

Madison Area Transgender Association Support Group
2701 International Lane, Suite 101
Madison, WI 53704
Phone: (608) 255-8582
Internet: http://isthmus.com/events/madison-area-transgender-social-support-group-Outreach/

OutReach
South Central Wisconsin LGBT Community Center
2701 International Lane
Madison, WI 53704
Phone: (608) 255-8582
Internet: https://www.outreachmadisonlgbt.org

Transgender Transformations c/o Positive Voice, Inc. PO Box 1381 Green Bay, WI 54305 Email: tg@pvinc.org

Transgender Youth Resource Network of Wisconsin
Pediatric & Adolescent Transgender Health Clinic
1675 Highland Avenue
Madison, WI 53792
Phone: (608) 890-5437
Internet: http://www.uwhealthkids.org/pediatric-diabetes/transgender-youth-resource-networkh

GSAFE—Gay Straight Alliance for Safe Schools
122 East Olin Avenue, Suite 290
Madison, WI 53713
Phone: (608) 661-4141
Fax: (608) 661-1360
Internet: https://www.gsafewi.org/links/

Wyoming

Wyoming GSA Network
Trans Support Group
1603 Capitol Avenue, Suite 405
Cheyenne, WY 82001
Phone: (307) 778-7645 Ext. 2
Internet: http://www.wygsanetwork.org/event/trans-support-group

University of Wyoming
Rainbow Resource Center
1000 East University Avenue
Laramie, WY 82071
Phone: (807) 766-1121
Internet: http://www.uwyo.edu/rrc/resources/

Wyoming Equality
P. O. Box 2531
Cheyenne, WY 82003
Phone: (866) 881-2742
Internet: http://wyomingequality.org/

Sheridan Support LGBTQ
Phone: (866) 881-2742 Ext. 705
Internet: http://www.lgbtqsheridanwy.net/contact

Parents, Family & Friends of Lesbians and Gays-PFLAG Jackson Wyoming
PO Box 2683
Jackson, WY 83001
Phone: (307) 733-8349
Internet: http://www.jacksonpflag.com

Parents, Family & Friends of Lesbians and Gays—PFLAG Casper Wyoming 1511 S Melrose Street Casper, WY 82609 Phone: (307) 265-5449 Internet: http://www.casperpflag.com

Health Reach
2030 Blue Grass Circle
Cheyenne, WY 82009
Phone: (307) 635-3500
Internet: http://healthreachwyo.com

Transgender/Gender Non-Conforming Community Resource Guides

Alabama

Transvivor
http://transvivor.com/alabama-transgender-doctors.html

Alaska
http://alaskan-transcendentalist.blogspot.com/2014/09/resource-list-for-trans-people-in-alaska.html

Arizona
Resources for Transgender Community Phoenix Arizona
https://tsaz.org/wp-content/uploads/2016/06/Trans-Resource-Guide-6-13-16-edited.pdf

Arkansas
http://www.luciesplace.org

California
http://www.acphd.org/media/269820/transgender_resource_guide.pdf

Colorado
https://giccolorado.org/the-gic/resources-2/transgender-in-colorado/

Connecticut
https://www.gay-therapy-ct.com/HealthCareCT.html

Delaware
https://www.static1.ssquarespace.com

Florida
http://www.eqfl.org/sites/default/files/.images/TransGuide_071517.pdf

Georgia
http://georgiaequality.org/wp-content/uploads/2015/08/GA-Trans-Resource-Guide-DIGITAL-1.pdf

Hawaii
http://hawaiilgbtlegacyfoundation.com/resources
https://lgbtresourceshawaii.com/hawaii-resource-contacts

Idaho
http://tccidaho.org/trans/
https://genderequity.boisestate.edu/lgbtqia/lgbtqia-resources

Illinois
https://www.luriechildrens.org/en-us/care-services/conditions-treatments/gender-development/resources/Documents/gender-resource-list1.pdf

Indiana
http://indianatransgendernetwork.com/category/resources/

Iowa
http://www.thiowa.org/resources.html

Kansas
http://kstep.org/resources/rxc.html

Kentucky
http://www.transkentucky.com/other-resources/

Louisiana
http://www.latransadvocates.org/providerlist/
http://www.latransadvocates.org/support-groups

Maine
https://umaine.edu/lgbtq/resources-and-services/lgbt-resources-in-maine/

Maryland
https://www.hagerstownhopesmd.org/lgbtq-resource-list
https://studentaffairs.jhu.edu/lgbtq/trans-resources

Massachusetts
COMPASS
F-M resources in Massachusetts-New England
http://www.compassftm.org/mission.html

Michigan
http://www.transgendermichigan.org/Index.html
http://standwithtrans.org/248-579-8996

Minnesota
https://www.outfront.org/resources

Missouri
https://www.transgenderhealthnetwork.org/trans-friendly-health-provider-list.html

Montana
http://www.genderexpansionproject.org/resources&publica-tions/GEP%20Trans%20Resource%20Booklet%20-%20Montana.pdf

Nebraska
Professional Transgender Resource Network—PTRN
Internet: http://www.ptrnnebraska.com/

Nevada
https://issuu.com/nnhopes/docs/northern_nevada_transgender_resourc

New Hampshire
http://www.tg-nh.org/resources.html

New Jersey
http://njgsaforum.com/resources
http://pflagjerseyshore.org/resources/lgbt-related-services-organizations

New Mexico
https://cyfd.org/docs/I_Am_Me_Resource_Guide.pdf

New York
http://nytransguide.wikidot.com/
https://www1.nyc.gov/site/doh/health/health-topics/transgender-support.page

North Carolina
http://faithaction.org/wp-content/uploads/2015/05/LGBTQ-Resource-Guide-Jan-2015.pdf

North Dakota
https://djcorganization.wordpress.com/transgender/resources/state/nd
http://dakotaoutright.org/resources

Ohio
http://www.transohio.org/?page_id=268
https://stonewallcolumbus.org/trans-resource-directory
http://transwellness.org/resources/health-resources/local-doctors-and-healthcare-professionals/ohio/

Oklahoma
http://www.okeq.org/transgender-support.html

Oregon
https://oregontranshealth.com/2016/04/22/ohp-providers/

Pennsylvania
Resource: https://translawhelp.org/states/pennsylvaniaLegalservicesthroughoutUS

Rhode Island
http://www.tginetwork.org

South Carolina
http://wearefamilycharleston.org/tlf/south-carolina-resources
https://www.ghs.org/diversity/lgbt/medicalresource

South Dakota
https://tgguide.com/transgender-resources/support-groups/us-states-o-s/south-dakota/

Tennessee
https://www.vanderbilt.edu/lgbtqi/resources/nashville-resources

Texas
http://renee-baker.com/transgender-counseling-dallas/transgender-hormone-therapy/
https://www.texastransgenderhealth.org/for-patients/
http://centexmcc.com/transgender-resources/

Utah
https://www.equalityutah.org/resources/transgender-resource-guide
https://tgguide.com/transgender-resources/support-groups/us-states-t-w/utah

Vermont
https://www.pridecentervt.org/resources/trans-resources

Virginia
http://www.vdh.virginia.gov/content/uploads/sites/10/2016/12/TransRRList.pdf
https://www.equalityvirginia.org/resources/transgenderresources/

Washington
Resource Washington Gender Alliance-State
Phone: (360) 445-2411
Internet: http://washingtongenderalliance.com/

West Virginia
Resources—WV Transgender Resources'
https://www.wvtransresources.org/contact.html

Wisconsin
https://witranshealth.org/

Wyoming
http://wyomingequality.org/resources/wyoming/

Mid-Western States
http://transwellness.org/resources/support-and-community-resources/midwest-state-links/

Southern States
http://www.southernequality.org/wp-content/uploads/2016/09/Transinthe-South_September2016.pdf

Medical Care/Behavioral Health Services

Alabama

Magic City Wellness Center
2500 4th Avenue South
Birmingham, AL 35233
Phone: (205) 877-8677
Internet: http://www.magiccitywellnesscenter.org

UAB LGBT Mental Health & Wellness Center
Sparks Building, 9th Floor 1720 7th Avenue South
Birmingham, AL 35233
Phone (205) 934-7008
Internet: https://www.uab.edu/medicine/psychiatry/patient-care/lgbtq-mental-health-wellness

Alaska

Avante Medical Center
915 West Northern Lights Blvd
Anchorage, AK 99503
Phone: (907) 770-6700
Internet: https://www.avantemedicalcenter.com/

Avante Medical Center
Providence Health Park
3851 Piper Street, Suite U-464
Anchorage, AK 99504
Phone: (907) 212-3631
Internet: https://alaska.providence.org/

White Raven Center—TGNC Counseling
511 Jordt Circle
Anchorage, AK 99504
Phone: (907) 333-4478
Internet: https://www.whiteravencenter.org

Arizona

Spectrum Medical Group, P.C.
52 East Monterey Way
Phoenix, AZ 85012
Phone: (602) 631-604-9500
Fax: (602) 631-9303
Internet: http://www.spectrummedgroup.com

Phoenix Children's Hospital Gender Management Service
1919 E. Thomas Road
Phoenix, AZ 85016
Phone: (602) 933-0659
http://www.phoenixchildrens.org

Arkansas

Freeway Medical Center
Dr. Janet Cathey
5800 West 10th Street, Suite 510
Little Rock, AK 72204
Phone: (501) 526-4740
Internet: http://transcaresite.org/?p=1773

California

Los Angeles LGBT Center—Transgender Health Program
McDonald/Wright Building
1625 North Schrader Blvd.
Lost Angeles, CA 90028
Phone: (323) 993-7500
Fax: (323)-993-7699
Internet: https://lalgbtcenter.org/health-services/medical-services/transgender-health-program

AEGIS TREATMENT CENTERS, LLC-Substance Abuse Program
1018 21st St.
Bakersfield, CA 93301
Phone: (661) 861-9967
http://aegistreatmentcenters.com

Clinica Sierra Vista
34th Street Community Health Center 2000 Physicians Plaza Bakersfield, CA 93301
Phone: (661) 324-1455
Internet: https://www.clinicasierravista.org/location/locationDetail/34th-street-community-health-center

CENTENNIAL MEDICAL GROUP
1801 16th Street, Suite A
Bakersfield, CA 93301
Phone: (661) 326-8989
Fax: (661) 326-8991
Internet: http://www.cmg.md/

Lyon Martin Transgender Health Services
1735 Mission Street
San Francisco, CA 94103

Phone: (415) 565-7667
Fax: (415) 252-7512
Internet: http://lyon-martin.org

Gender Health Center
2020 29th Street, Suite 201
Sacramento, CA 95817
Phone: (916) 455-2391
Fax: (916) 455-2393
Internet: http://www.thegenderhealthcenter.org/

Colorado

Denver Health
Transgender Health Services
777 Bannock Street
Denver, CO 80204
Phone: (303) 436-4949
Internet:http://www.denverhealth.org/for-patients-and-visitors/amenities-and-experience/lgbt-health-services/transgender-health-services

Boulder Endocrinology
Dr. Lindsey Rentschler
892 West South Boulder Road
Louisville, CO 80027
Phone: (303) 586-5200
Internet: https://www.boulderendo.com/

Rocky Mountain Hospital for Children
Pediatric Endocrine Associates
Dr. Sunil Nayak
Greenwood Village
8200 East Bellevue Avenue, Suite 510 E
Greenwood Village, CO 80111
Phone: (303) 783-3883
Internet: https://rockymountainhospitalforchildren.com

Connecticut

Circle Care Center
618 West Avenue
Norwalk, CT 06850
Phone: (203) 852-9525
Internet: http://circlecarecenter.org/services/transgender-care

Stamford Health Medical Group—Endocrinology
Dr. Melissa Goldstein
292 Longridge Road, Suite 206
Stamford, CT 06902

Phone: (203) 276-7212
Fax: (203) 276-4975
Internet: https://www.stamfordhealthmedicalgroup.org

Anchor Health Initiative
Dr. Adrian Demidont
54 Meadow Street, 1st Floor
New Haven, CT 06519
Phone: (203) 903-8303
Fax: (203) 599-3927
Internet: http://www.anchorhealthinitiative.org/

Delaware
Christiana Care Health System
P.O. Box 1668
Wilmington, DE 19899
Phone: (302) 733-1227
Internet: https://christianacare.org/services/lgbtqhealth

Florida
University of Miami—LGBTQ Center for Wellness, Gender & Sexual Health
West Building, 1321 NW 14th Street
Miami, FL 33136
Phone: (305) 689-3100
Internet: https://surgery.med.miami.edu/plastic-and-reconstructive/gender-affirmation

University of Miami—Miller School of Medicine
Gender Affirmation Surgeries
Clinical Research Building
1120 NW 14th Street, 4th Floor
Miami, FL 33136
Phone: (305) 243-6713
Fax: (305) 243-4535
Internet: http://med.miami.edu/

Georgia

Intown Primary Care—Transgender Health
2215 Cheshire Bridge Road NE
Atlanta,, GA 30324
Phone: (404) 541-0944
Internet: http://intownprimarycare.com/contact

Feminist Women's Health Center—Trans Health Initiative
1924 Cliff Valley Way

Atlanta, GA 30329
Phone: (404) 728-7900
Internet: http://www.feministcenter.org/en/health-wellness-services/trans-health-initiative

Equality Clinic of Augusta Inc.
987 Sebastian Way
Augusta, GA 30901
Phone: (762) 218-2226
Internet: https://www.equalityclinicaugusta.com

Hawaii

Hawk Health Clinic
1345 South Beretania Street, Suite 101
Honolulu, HI 96814
Phone: (808) 744-2543
Fax: (866) 451-4608
Internet: http://www.hawkhealthclinic.com

Idaho

Davis Family Medicine
222 North 2nd Street, Suite 204
Boise, ID 83702
Phone: (208) 429-9100
Fax: (208) 429-9118
Internet: http://davisfamilymedicine.net/lgbtq.aspx

Illinois

Howard Brown Health 4025 North Sheridan Road Chicago, IL 60613 Phone: (773)-388-1600 Fax: (773) 388-1602 Internet: https://howardbrown.org/programs-services/transgender-health/sup-port-groups/

Chicago Women's Health Center—Trans Health Services
1025 West Sunnyside Avenue
Chicago, IL, 60640
Phone: (773) 935-6125
Internet: http://www.chicagowomenshealthcenter.org/services/tgap-trans-greater-access-project

Indiana

Eskenazi Health
720 Eskennazi Avenue
Indianapolis, IN 46202
Phone: (317) 880-60442
Internet: http://www.eskenazihealth.edu/health-services/transgender-care

Riley Gender Health Program
705 Riley Hospital Drive
Indianapolis, IN 46202
Phone: (317) 274-8812
Internet: https://www.rileychildrens.org/departments/gender-health-program

MOSAIC Health & Healing Arts
330 Lakeview Drive
Goshen, Indiana 46528
Phone: (574) .537-2680
Fax: (574) .533-0218
Internet: http://mosaichha.org

Iowa

The University of Iowa LGBTQ Clinic
Iowa River Landing, 105 East 9th Street
Coralville, IA 52241
Phone: (319) 467-2000
Fax: (319) 456-2512
Internet: http://www.uilgbtqclinic.com

United Community Services—UCS Healthcare
LGBT Medical Services 4908 Franklin Avenue Des Moines, IA 50310 Phone: (515) 280-3860
Internet: https://www.ucsonline.org/who-we-are/locations/des-moines

Kansas

The University of Kansa Physicians
2000 Olathe Blvd
Kansa City, KS 66160
Phone: (913) 588-2229
Internet: http://www.kansashealthsystem.com/WomensHealth

South Wind Women's Center
5108 East Kellogg Drive
Wichita, KS 67218
Phone: (316) 260-6934
Internet: http://www.southwindwomenscenter.org/patient-care-services/lgbtqia-services

Family Health Care-Transgender Health Services
300-340 Southwest Blvd
Kansas City, KS 66103
Phone: (913) 722-3100
Fax: (913) 722-2542
Internet: http://www.swbfhc.org

Kentucky

University of Kentucky—UK Health Care
Transform Health Clinic
1000 South Limestone
University of Kentucky
Lexington, KY 40536
Phone: (859) 323-2778
Internet: https://ukhealthcare.uky.edu/services/transform-health

University of Louisville-LGBT Care
Internal Medicine
401 East Chestnut Street, Suite 370
Louisville, KY 40202
Phone: (502) 588-4500
Internet: http://www.uoflphysicians.com/lgbtq-care?

Louisiana

Louisiana Trans Advocates—Providers List
Administrative Office
650 North 6th Street
Baton Rouge, LA 70802
Internet: http://www.latransadvocates.org/support-groups

Maine

Maine Family Planning—Open Door Transgender Health Care
P.O. Box 587
Augusta, ME 04332
Phone: (207) 622-7524
Internet: http://www.mainefamilyplanning.org

Maine Medical Partners—The Gender Clinic
887 Congress Street, Suite 100
Portland, ME 04102
Phone: (207) 662-5522
Fax: (207) 662-5526
Internet:https://mainehealth.org/maine-medical-partners/practices/pediatric-specialty-care/endocrinology-diabetes/the-gender-clinic

Open Door Transgender Program
179 Lisbon Street
Lewiston, ME 04240
Phone: (207) 795-4007
Internet: www.mainefamilyplanning.org/page/958-881/transgender-health-care

Maryland

Chase Brexton Health Care
1111 North Charles Street
Baltimore, MD 21201
Phone: (410) 837-2050
Internet: https://www.chasebrexton.org/about-us/locations/mt-vernon

Your Trans Care at Star Track Adolescent Health
120 Penn Street,
Baltimore, MD 21230
Phone: (410) 706-4789
Internet: http://www.startrackhealth.org

University of Maryland Medical Center
Midtown Campus
827 Linden Avenue
Baltimore, MD 21201
Phone: (443) 682-6800
Internet: https://www.umm.edu/programs/childrens/services/adolescent-and-young-adult/transgender-family-health-services

The Center for Transgender Health
Johns Hopkins Medicine
1800 Orleans Street
Baltimore, MD 211287
Phone: (844) 546-5645
Internet: https://www.hopkinsmedicine.org/center_transgender_health

Massachusetts

Fenway Health –The Fenway Institute
Ansin Building
1340 Boylston Street
Boston, MA 02215
Phone: (617)-927-6400
Internet: http://fenwayhealth.org/the-fenway-institute

Boston Medical Center
Center for Transgender Medicine & Surgery
One Boston Medical Center Place
Boston, MA 02118
Phone: (617) 638-1833
Internet: https://www.bmc.org/center-transgender-medicine-and-surgery

Baystate Health—Transgender Services
South Hadley Adult Medicine

470 Granby Road
South Hadley, MA 01075
Phone: 413-533-3926
Internet: https://www.baystatehealth.org/services/transgender-services

Michigan

Michigan Medicine—University of Michigan
The Comprehensive Gender Services Program
2025 Traverwood Drive, Suite A1
Ann Arbor, MI 48105
Phone: 734-998-2150
Internet: http://www.uofmhealth.org

C.S. Mott Children's Hospital
Gender Management Program (GeM)
1540 East Hospital Drive
Ann Arbor, MI 48109
Phone: (734) 764-5175
Internet: http://www.mottchildren.org/conditions-treatments/gender-manage-ment

Henry Ford Medical Center—New Center One
Transgender Health Program
3031 West Grand Blvd.
Detroit, MI 48202
Phone: (313) 916-9517
Internet: https://www.henryford.com/services/transgender-health

Minnesota
University of Minnesota—Program in Human Sexuality
Transgender Health Services
Center for Sexual Health
1300 South 2nd Street, Suite 180
Minneapolis, MN 55454
Phone: (612) 625-1500
Fax: (612) 626-8311
Internet: https://www.sexualhealth.umn.edu

Minnesota Transgender Health Coalition
3405 Chicago Ave S, Suite 103
Minneapolis, MN 55407
Phone: (612) 823-1152
Internet: http://www.mntranshealth.org

Park Nicollet Health Partners
2001 Blaisdell Avenue S.
Minneapolis, MN 55404
Phone: (962) 993-8052

Internet: http://www.parknicollet.com/Medical-Services/Gender-Transgender-Services

Family Tree—Trans Health Services
1619 Dayton Avenue #205
St. Paul, MN 55104
Phone: (651) 645-0478
Fax: (651) 624-2523
Internet: https://www.familytreeclinic.org/contact

Mississippi

The Open Arms Healthcare Center
Transgender Health
805 East River Place
Jackson, MS 39202
Phone: (601) 500-7660
Fax: (601) 957-3625
Internet: http://oahcc.org

Missouri

The Transgender Institute
8080 Ward Parkway, Suite 400
Kansas City, MO 64114
Phone: (816) 305-0943
http://transinstitute.org/contact

KC Care Clinic—Transgender Clinic
3515 Broadway
Kansas City, MO 64111
Phone: (816) 753-5144
Internet: http://www.kccareclinic.org/news/kc-care-clinic-transgender-clinic

Missouri State Health Provider List
Internet: https://www.transgenderhealthnetwork.org/trans-friendly-health-provider-list.html

Montana

Blue Mountain Clinic Family Practice—Transgender Health Care
610 N. California Street
Missoula, Montana 59802
Phone: (406) 721-1646
Internet: http://www.bluemountainclinic.org

Nebraska

The Nebraska Medicine Transgender Clinic
Nebraska Medicine—Specialty Care Clinic
Attn: Dr. Jean Amoura
804 South 52nd Street
Omaha, NE 68106
Phone: (402) 559-2666
Fax: (402) 553-5963
Internet: https://www.nebraskamed.com/transgender-care

Heartland Trans Wellness Group
Leslie A. Epstein, MA, LMHP, CPc
11942 Elm Street, Suite 109
Omaha, NE 68144
Phone: (402) 547-0533
Internet: http://transwellness.org/resources/health-resources/local-doctors-and-healthcare-professionals/nebraska

Nevada

Northern Nevada HOPES 580 West 5th Street Reno, NV 89503 Phone: (775) 786-4673
Internet: https://www.nnhopes.org
Huntridge Family Clinic
1830 East Sahara Avenue, Suite 201
Las Vegas, NV 89104
Phone: (702) 979-1111
Internet: https://huntridgefamilyclinic.org/contact

New Hampshire

Equality Health Center
38 South Main Street
Concord, NH 03301
Phone: (603) 225-2739
Internet: http://equalityhc.org

Dartmouth Hitchcock Medical Center
1 Medical Center Drive
Lebanon, NH 03756
Phone: (603) 650-8630
Internet: http://www.dartmouth-hitchcock.org

University of New Hampshire
Health & Wellness—Transgender Care
4 Pettee Brook Lane

Durham, NH 03824
Phone: (603) 862-9355
Fax: (603) 862-4259
Internet: https://www.unh.edu/health/services/transgender-health

New Jersey

Robert Wood Johnson University Hospital Somerset (RWJUH PROUD Family Health Center)
110 Rehill Avenue
Somerville, NJ 08876
Phone: (855) 776-8334
Internet: https://www.rwjbh.org/rwj-university-hospital-new-brunswick

Healthy Transitions
50 Church Street, Suite L3
Montclair, NJ 07042
Phone: (718) 894-0301
Internet: http://healthytransitionsllc.org/montclair-nj

New Mexico

Alianza of New Mexico—Health Care
1615 A.N. Solano
Las Cruces, NM 88001
Phone: (575) 915-1770
Internet: http://www.alianzanm.org

Allianza of New Mexico—Health Care
311 West 2nd Street
Roswell, NM 88201
Phone: (575) 623-1995
Internet: http://www.alianzanm.org

New York

APICHA Community Health Center
400 Broadway
New York, NY 10011
Phone: (212) 334-6029
Fax: (212) 334-7957
Internet: http://www.apicha.org

Ackerman Institute for the Family—Counseling Services
936 Broadway
New York, NY 10010
Phone: (212) 879-4900
Fax: (212) 744-0006
Internet: http://www.ackerman.org

Callen-Lorde Community Health Center
256 West 18th Street
New York, NY 10011
Phone: (212) 271-7200
Fax: (212) 271-7225
Internet: http://www.callenlorde.org

CK Life—Community Kinship—Trans Clinic
1276 Fulton Avenue
Bronx, NY 10456
Phone: (347) 886-9002
Internet: http://cklife.org

Community Health Network—CHN
975 Westchester Avenue
Bronx, NY 10459
(718) 320-4466
90-04 161st Street
Jamaica, NY 11432
(718) 523-2123
Internet: http://www.chnnyc.org

Gerald J. Friedman Transgender Program for Health & Wellness
Northwell Health Physicians Partners
110 East 59th Street, Suite 8B
New York, NY 10022
Phone: (212) 434-3556
Fax: (212) 434-4974
Internet: http://www.northwell-edu/gerald-j-friedman-transgender-health-wellness-program
Internet: https://www.friedmantransgenderprogram.org

Center for Transgender Care
Northwell Health
865 Northern Blvd. Suite 101
Great Neck, NY 11021
Phone: (516) 622-5195
Internet: https://www.northwell.edu/find-care/services-we-offer/lgbt/clinical-services

Institute for Contemporary Psychotherapy (PCGS)
Psychotherapy Center for Gender & Sexuality
1841 Broadway, 4th Floor
New York, NY 10023
Phone: (212) 333-3444
Fax: (212) 333-5444
Internet: http://www.icpnyc.org/pcgs

Mount Sinai Center for Transgender Medicine & Surgery
Institute for Advanced Medicine
275 Seventh Avenue
New York, NY 10011
Phone: (212) 604-1730
Internet: http://www.mountsinai.org

Washington Heights Corner
566 West 181st Street, 2nd Floor
New York, NY 10033
Phone: (212) 923-7600
Fax: (888) 977-1617
Internet: http://www.cornerproject.org

North Carolina

Western NC Community Health Services
257 Biltmore Avenue
Asheville, NC 28801
Phone: (828) 285-0622 ext. 2144
Internet: http://www.wncchs.org

Duke Health
Child & Adolescent Gender Care
2301 Erwin Road
Durham, NC 27710
Phone: (919) 684-8361
Internet: https://www.dukehealth.org/locations/duke-child-and-adolescent-gender-care

Planned Parenthood—Charlotte Health Center
4822 Albermarle Road #103
Charlotte, NC 28205
Phone: (704) 556-7581
Internet: https://www.plannedparenthood.org

Charlotte Transgender Health Group
Internet: http://cthcg.org

North Dakota

Mid Dakota Clinic-Center for Women
Dr. Janice Bury/Dr. Thomas Hutchens
1000 East Rosser Avenue
Bismarck, ND 58501
Phone: (701) 530-6000
Internet: https://www.middakotaclinic.com

Sanford Diabetes Center
Dr. David Newman/Dr. Luis Casas
2400 32nd Avenue S
Fargo, ND 58103
Phone: (701) 234-7980
Fax: (701) 234-3838
Internet: http://www.sanfordhealth.org

Altru Family Medicine Residency
Dr. William Zaks
725 Hamline Street
Grand Forks, ND 58203
Phone: (701) 780-6800
Fax: (701) 780-6817
Internet: https://www.altru.org

Ohio

Pride Clinic –Thomas McCafferty Health Center
4242 Lorain Avenue
Cleveland, OH 44113
Phone: (216) 957-4905
Internet: https://www.metrohealth.org/pride-clinic

Equitas Health
King-Lincoln Medical Center
750 E. Long Street, Suite 3000
Columbus OH 43203
Phone: (614) 340-6700
Fax: (614) 340-6787
Internet: http://equitashealth.com/locations-and-staff/

Short North Medical Center
1033 N. High Street
Columbus OH 43201
Phone: (614) 340-6777
Fax: (614) 572-0859
Internet: http://equitashealth.com/locations-and-staff

Dayton Medical Center
1222 S. Patterson Blvd., Suite 230
Dayton OH 45402
Phone: (937) 853-3650
Fax: (937) 853-4367
Internet: http://equitashealth.com/locations/dayton-medical-center

Oklahoma

South Wind Women's Center
1240 South West 44th Street
Oklahoma City, OK 73109
Phone: (405) 429-7940
Internet: http://www.southwindwomenscenter.org/patient-care-services/lgbtqia-services

Planned Parenthood of the Heartland
Midtown Health Center
1007 South Peoria Avenue
Tulsa, OK 74120
Phone: (855)-841-7526
Fax: (918) 587-0589
Internet: www.plannedparenthood.org/planned-parenthood-heartland

Oklahoma City VA Health Care System
Transitions Support
921 North East 13th Street
Oklahoma City, OK 73104
Phone: (405) 456-5183
Internet: https://www.oklahoma.va.gov/services/LGBTQ_Services.asp

Oregon

Oregon Health & Science University—OHSU—Transgender Health Program
Dillehunt Hall, Room 1007
3181 S.W. Sam Jackson Park Rd.
Portland, Oregon 97239
Phone: (503) 494-7970
Internet: http://www.ohsu.edu/xd/health/services/transgender-health

Kaiser Permanente—Gender Pathways
Interstate Medical Office East
3550 North Interstate Avenue
Portland, OR 97227
Phone: (503) 249-6748
Internet: https://multco.us/benefits/kaiser-gender-affirming-services

Oregon Trans Health
https://oregontranshealth.com/2016/04/22/ohp-providers

Pennsylvania

Mazzoni Center—Trans Care
1349 Bainbridge Street
Philadelphia, PA 19147
Phone: (215) 563-0652
Internet: https://www.mazzonicenter.org

Allenton Women's Center
31 South Commerce Way, Suite 100
Bethlehem, PA 18017
Phone: (877) 342-5292
Internet: https://allentownwomenscenter.com

Puerto Rico

Centro Ararat—Translucent Project
HUB Clinic
1507 Calle Prof. Augusto Rodriguez
Condominio Asia, Suite 600
San Juan, PR 00909
Phone: (787)-497-0800
Internet: http://centroararat.org/

Rhode Island

Thundermist Health Center—Trans Health Access
450 Clinton Street
Woonsocket, RI 02895
Phone: (401) 767-4100 Ext 4303
Internet: http://www.thundermisthealth.org/Services/TransHealthAccess

Lifespan Physician Group, Adolescent Health Care Center.
Dr. Michelle Forcier
245 Chapman Street, Suite 100
Providence, RI 02905.
Phone: (401)-444-5980
Fax: (401)-444-3873
Internet: https://www.lifespan.org

South Carolina

Planned Parenthood—Charleston Health Center
1312 Ashely River Road
Charleston, SC 29407
Phone: (843) 937-6497
Internet: https://www.plannedparenthood.org

Springwood Lake Family Medicine
Dr. Kimberly Williams
1721 Horseshoe Drive, Columbia, SC 29223
Phone: (803) 788-7884
Internet: http://harriethancockcenter.org/trans-support-resource-guide

Grace Medical Group Llc.
Michelle Rojas, MD
1333 Taylor Street, Suite 3B,
Columbia, SC 29201
Phone: (803) 933 0288
3025 Farrow Road
Columbia, SC 29203
Phone: (803) 933-0288
Internet: http://harriethancockcenter.org/medical-resourcesservices

South Dakota

Regional Health Medical Clinic
Dr. Sonalika G Khachikian, MD
640 Flormann Street
Rapid City, SD 57701
Phone: (605) 755-3300
Fax: 605 755-3123
Internet: https://www.regionalhealth.com/location/regional-health-medical-clinic-flormann-street

Sanford Health Fertility and Reproductive Medicine
Dr. Keith Hansen
1500 W 22nd Street, Suite 102
Sioux Falls, SD 57105
Phone: (605) 328-8800
Fax: (605) 328-8801
Internet: http://www.sanfordhealth.org/locations/sanford-health-fertility-and-reproductive-medicine

Bach Counseling
Mahala Bach
2218 Jackson Blvd Suite 13, Rapid City, SD 57702
Phone: (605) 431-4106
Internet: https://www.bachcounseling.com

Tennessee

Vanderbilt Health Medical Center
1211 Medical Center Drive Nashville, TN 37232 Phone: (615) 322-5000
Internet: https://www.vanderbilthealth.com/lgbtihealthprogram

Connectus Health
601 Benton Avenue
Nashville, TN 37204
Phone: (615) 292-9770
Internet: https://www.connectus.org/transgender-health/

CHOICES Memphis Center for Reproductive Health & Transgender Services
1726 Poplar Avenue
Memphis, TN 38104
Phone: (901) 274-3550
Internet: https://www.memphischoices.org

Texas

Resource Center Transgender Health Clinic at Nelson Tebedo Clinic
4012 Cedar Spring 4483
Dallas. TX 75219
Phone: (214) 540-4446
Fax: (214) 528-3436
Internet: https://www.rcdallas.org/what-we-do/health/transgender-health

Resource Center Community Center—Transgender Counseling Services
5750 Cedar Springs Rd.
Dallas TX 75235
Phone: 214-393-3680
Internet: https://www.rcdallas.org

Kind Clinic—Gender Affirming Care
1101 West 40th Street #102
Austin, TX 78756
Phone: (512) 853-9547
Internet: https://kindclinic.org

Legacy Community Health
Montrose Clinic
1415 California Street
Houston, TX 77006
Phone: (713) 665-8800
Fax: (713) 559-3268
Internet: https://www.legacycommunityhealth.org/region/montrose

Branard Clinic
401 Branard Street, Level 3
Houston, TX 77006
Phone: (713) 366-7444
Fax: (713) 559-3260
Internet: https://www.legacycommunityhealth.org/region/montrose/

Utah

University of Utah Health—Transgender Health Program
50 North Medical Drive

Salt Lake City, UT 84132
Phone: (801) 581-2121
Internet: https://healthcare.utah.edu/transgender-health

Rebirth OB/GYN Clinic + Gender Center
2180 East 4500 South
Holladay, UT 84117
Phone: (801) 272-3909
Internet: http://www.rebirthobgyn.com/transgender-health/gender-center/

Vermont

Pride Center of Vermont
Transgender Programs
255 Champlain Street, Suite 12
Burlington, VT 05401
Phone: (802) 860-7812
Internet: https://www.pridecentervt.org

The University of Vermont Medical Center
Transgender Youth Program
111 Colchester Avenue
Main Campus
Burlington, VT 05401
Phone: (802) 847-3811
Internet: https://www.uvmhealth.org

Brattleboro Retreat—Mental Health
Central Intake and Ambulatory Services
Anna Marsh Lane
P.O. Box 803
Brattleboro, VT 05302
Phone: 1-800-258-3700
Admission Fax: 802-258-3791
Internet: https://www.brattlebororetreat.org

Community Health Centers of Burlington
Dr. Rachel Inker
Pearl Street Youth Health Center
179 Pearl Street
Burlington, Vermont, 05401
Phone: (802-864-6309
Internet: https://www.chcb.org/locations-providers/pearl-street-youth-health-cen-ter

Riverside Health Center
617 Riverside Avenue
Burlington, Vermont, 05401

Phone: (802-864-6309
Internet: https://www.chcb.org/locations-providers/riverside-health-center

Virginia

Health Brigade—Transgender Health Services
1010 North Thompson Street
Richmond, VA 23220
Phone: (804) 358-6343 Ext. 143
Fax: (804) 521-0809
Internet: http://www.healthbrigade.org

Teen and Young Adult Health Center—UVA Transgender Health Services
University of Virginia
1204 W. Main Street
Charlottesville, VA 22903
Phone: (434) 982-0090
Fax: (434) 924-9983
Internet: https://childrens.uvahealth.com/services/teen-health

The Transgender Health Alliance of Central Virginia
P.O. Box 5057
Charlottesville, VA 22905
Internet: http://www.thacva.org

Washington

Virginia Mason Hospital & Seattle Medical Center
1100 Ninth Avenue
Seattle, WA 98101
Phone: (206) 223-6600
Internet: https://www.virginiamason.org/Seattle

The PolyClinic Downtown Seattle
509 Olive Way, Suites 200 & 900
Seattle, WA 98101
Phone: (206) 329-1760
Internet: https://polyclinic.com/locations/downtown

Queen Anne Medical Associates PLLC
200 West Mercer #104
Seattle, WA 98119
Phone: (206) 281-7163
Fax: (206) 281-5088
Internet: http://queenannemedicalassociates.com/transgender-care

Washington DC-National

GLMA: Health Professionals Advancing LGBT Equality
1100 H Street, NW Suite 540 Washington, DC 20005 Phone: (202) 600-8037

Internet: http://www.glma.org

Ace Lipson, MD
Transgender Health Care
1120 19th Street, NW, Suite 200
Washington, D.C. 20036
Phone: (202) 296-3443
Fax: (202) 296-8760
Hours of Operation: Monday–Friday 8:00 AM–5:00 PM
Internet: http://www.dracelipson.com

Mark Sklar, MD
3 Washington Circle, NW, Suite 303
Washington, D.C. 20037
Phone: 202-887-4769
Fax: 202-223-2552
Internet: http://www.sklarendocrinology.com

Whitman-Walker Health
1525 14th Street, NW
Washington, DC 20005
Phone: (202) 745-7000
Internet: https://www.whitman-walker.org/service/medical/transgender-care

West Virginia

Persad Transgender Resources-LGBTQ Center
P.O. Box 6201
Morgantown, WV 26506
Phone: (304) 293-0111
Internet: https://www.wvu.edu

Wisconsin

Froedtert & Medical College of Wisconsin\
Transgender Services
9200 West Wisconsin Avenue
Milwaukee, WI 53226
Phone: (414) 805-3666
Internet: https://www.froedtert.com/endocrinology/transgender-hormonal-therapy

Pathways Counseling Center
13105 West Bluemound Road, #100
Brookfield, WI 53005
Phone: (262) 640-9790
Fax: (262) 641-9791
Internet: https://www.pathwayscounseling.com

University of Wisconsin—Gender Services
University Hospital
600 Highland Avenue
Madison, WI 53792
Phone: (608) 263-7502
Internet: https://www.uwhealth.org/gender-transgender-services/gender-services

Transformations
2349 Deming Way
Middleton, WI 53562
Phone: (608) 836-9990
Internet: https://www.uwhealth.org/gender-transgender-services

Wyoming

Health Reach
2030 Blue Grass Circle
Cheyenne, WY 82009
Phone: (307) 635-3500
Internet: http://healthreachwyo.com

Gender Affirming Surgeons

Gary Alter, MD
461 Park Avenue South, 7th Floor
New York, NY 10016
Phone: (310) 2775-5566
Fax: (310) 271-0521
Consultations available in NY. Surgery performed in LA only.
Internet: https://www.altermd.com/contact-us/

Rachel Bluebond-Langner MD
NYU Langone Medical Center
305 East 33rd Street
New York, NY 10016
Phone: (212) 263-3030
Internet:http://nyulangone.org/doctors/1902867393/rachel-bluebond-langner#credentials

Marci Bowers, MD
San Mateo Surgery Center
345 Lorton Avenue, Suite 101
Burlingame, CA 94010
Phone: (650) 570-2270
Fax: (650) 570-2283
Internet: https://marcibowers.com/

Jordan Deschamps –Braly MD, FACS
Deschamps-Braly Clinic of Plastic & Craniofacial Surgery
Facial Feminization/Masculinization Surgery
450 Sutter Street, Suite 1520
San Francisco, CA 94108
Phone: (415) 624-3922
Internet: https://deschamps-braly.com

Beth Drzewiecki MD
Montefiore Medical Center
1280 Waters Place
Bronx, NY 10461
Phone: (718) 920-7479
Internet: http://www.montefiore.org/lgbtqcare

Curtis N. Crane, MD
Thomas Satterwhite, MD
Brownstein & Crane Surgical Services
575 Sir Francis Drake Blvd., Suite 1
Greenbrae, CA 94904
Phone: (415) 625-3230
Fax: (415) 461-3233
Internet: http://brownsteincrane.com/

Charles Garromone, DO, FACOS
The Garramone Center—FTM Top Surgery
4725 Volunteer Road, Suite 202
Davie, FL 33330
Phone: (954) 752-7842
Fax: (954) 473-2454
Internet: http://drgarramone.com/

Alexis Hazen, MD
NYU Langone Medical Center
305 East 33rd Street
New York, NY 10016
Phone: (646) 501-4480263-3030
Internet: https://nyulangone.org/doctors/1003820366/alexes-hazen

Sherman Leis, MD
19 Montgomery Avenue
Bala Cynwyd, PA 19004
Phone: (610) 667-1888
Internet: http://www.thetransgendercenter.com/

Christine McGinn, MD
The Papillon Center
18 Village Row, Suite 43

New Hope, PA 18938
Phone: (215) 693-1199
Internet: http://drchristinemcginn.com/

Daniel Medalie, MD
Cleveland Plastic Surgery
25700 Science Park Drive
Landmark Centre, Suite 190
Beachwood, OH 44122
Phone: (216) 393-9924
Fax: (216) 3893-9925
Internet: http://www.clevelandplasticsurgery.com

Toby R. Meltzer, MD, PC
Plastic and Reconstructive Surgery
7025 North Scottsdale Road, Suite 302
Scottsdale, AZ 85253
Phone: (480) 657-7006
Fax: (480) 657-7020
Internet: http://www.tmeltzer.com

Kathy L. Rumer, MD
Rumer Cosmetic Surgery
105 Ardmore Ave
Ardmore, PA 19003
Phone: (855) 782-5665
Fax: (484) 413-1700
Internet: http://www.rumercosmetics.com/

Jeffrey Spiegel, MD FACS
The Spiegel Center—Advanced Facial Aesthetics
335 Boylston Street
Newton, MA 02459
Phone: (617) 566-3223
Fax: (617) 566-3220
Internet: http://www.drspiegel.com/

Jess Ting, MD
Zoe Rodriguez, MD
Aaron Grotas, MD
The Mount Sinai Center for Transgender Medicine and Surgery
275 7th Avenue
New York, NY 10011
Phone: (212) 604-1730
Internet: http://www.mountsinai.org/locations/center-transgender-medicine-surgery/team

Luis M. Capitan, MD, PHD, OMFS
Daniel Simon, DMD, MA Oral Surgery
FACIALTEAM –Facial Feminization Surgery
HC Marbella International Hospital
Ventura del Mar 11
29660 Nueva Andalucía, Marbella (Malaga)—Spain
Phone: 00 34952 898 842
Internet: https://facialteam.eu

Pierre Brassard, MD, FRCSC
Maud Belanger, MD, FRCSC
Eric Bensimon, MD, FRCSC
GRS Montreal
995 De Salaberry
Montreal, (Quebec), Canada
H3L 1L2
Phone: (514) 288-2097
Fax: (514) 288-3547
Internet: https://www.grsmontreal.com/

Rados Djinovic, MD
Sava Perovic Foundation Surgery
Tirsova, 10, Belgrade, Serbia
Phone: (216) 220-4220
Internet: https://www.savaperovic.com/rados-djinovic.htm

Miroslave L. Djordjevic, MD, PhD
Belgrade Center for Genital Reconstructive Surgery
Belgrade, Serbia
Internet: http://www.genitalsurgerybelgrade.com/

Stan Monstrey, MD
University Hospital 2K12 IC
Department of Plastic Surgery
De Pintelaan, 185
B 9000 Ghent, Belgium
Phone: +32 (0) 9 332 32 78
Fax: +32 (0) 9 332 38 99
Internet: http://www.plastischechirurgiegent.be/en/how-to-contact-us/contact-details/index.html

Preecha Tiewtranon, MD
PAI Preecha Aesthetic Institute
898/1 Sukumvit Soi (Thon Lor)

Wattana, Bangkok, 10110 Thailand
Phone: (662) 715-0111
Fax: (602) 715-0113
Internet: http://pai.co.th

Suporn Watanyusakul MD
The Suporn Clinic
938 Sukumvit Road
Bangplasoi, Muang District
Chonburi, 20000 Thailand
Phone; +66 38273360
Fax: +66 38273370
Internet: http://www.supornclinic.com

Intersex Resources

Intersex Initiative
P.O. Box 40570
Portland, OR 97240
Internet: http://www.ipdx.org/contact.html

Intersex Society of North America 979 Golf Course Drive #282 Rohnert Park CA 94928
Fax: (801) 348-5350
Internet: http://www.isna.org/about/contact

Hotline Resources

Trans Lifeline (877) 565-8860
2443 Fillmore Street # 380-9468
San Francisco, CA 94115
Internet: http://www.translifeline.org

Trans Lifeline is dedicated to the wellbeing of transgender people. The hotline is staffed by transgender people for transgender people.

The Trevor Project
(866) 488-7386
PO Box 69232
West Hollywood, CA 90069
Internet: https://www.thetrevorproject.org

The National Suicide Prevention Lifeline
(800) 273-8255
Internet: https://suicidepreventionlifeline.org

Internet Support Services

Transsexual & Transgender Road Map
http://www.tsroadmap.com/index.html

Susan's Place Transgender Resources
https://www.susans.org/

Trans Pulse Transgender Resources
http://www.lauras-playground.com/

Lynn Conway Transgender Resources
http://www.ai.eecs.umich.edu/people/conway/conway.html

Transgender Universe
https://www.themaven.net/transgenderuniverse

National/Government Agencies

Transgender Law Center
PO Box 70976
Oakland, CA 94612
Phone: (510) 587-9696
Fax: (510) 587.9699
Internet: https://transgenderlawcenter.org

Transgender Legal Defense Fund
20 West 20th Street, Suite 705
New York, NY 10011
Phone: (646-862-9396
Fax: (646) 930-5654
Internet: http://www.transgenderlegal.org

Trans Women of Color Collective
Phone: (202) 643-7631
Internet: http://www.twocc.u
Trans Latin@ Coalition
3055 Wilshire Blvd. Suite 350
Los Angeles, CA 90010
Internet: https://www.translatinacoalition.org

TransYouth Family Allies
P.O. Box 1471
Holland, MI 49422
Phone: (888) 462-8932
Internet: http://www.imatyfa.org

Transgender American Veteran's Association
P.O. Box 4513
Akron, OH 44310

Phone: (516) 838-2911
Internet: http://transveteran.org/contact-us-page/

Parents Friends of Lesbians and Gays Inc.—PFLAG National Office
1828 1 Street, NW Suite 660
Washington, DC 20036
Phone: (202) 467-8180
Fax: (202) 467-8194
Internet: https://www.pflag.org

Gender Spectrum
National Child and Youth Advocacy
Phone: (510) 788-2
Internet: https://www.genderspectrum.org

FORGE
P.O. Box 1272
Milwaukee, WI 53201
Phone: (414) 559-2123
Internet: http://forge-forward.org

Human Rights Campaign
1640 Rhode Island Avenue, N.W.
Washington, DC 20036
Phone: (202) 628-4160
Fax: (202) 347-5323
Internet: http://www.hrc.org/hrc-story

National Center for Transgender Equality
1133 19th St NW Suite 302 Washington D.C. 20036
Phone: (202) 642-4542
Internet: https://transequality.org

National LGBT Health Education Center—Transgender Health
The Fenway Institute
Anain Building, 8th Floor
1340 Boylston Street
Boston, MA 02215
Phone: (617) 927-6354
Internet: http://www.lgbthealtheducation.org/publication/transgender-sod/

World Professional Association for Transgender Health—WPATH
2575 Northwest Parkway
Elgin, IL 60124
Internet: https://www.wpath.org/

International Transgender Resources

AFRICA

Botswana

Rainbow Identity Association Address: Gaborone Botswana Website: http://rainbowidentitybotswana.blogspot.com

Nigeria

Trans and Intersex People for Human Rights in Nigeria Address: Nigeria—Federal Capital Territory—Abuja
South Africa Social, Health and Empowerment Feminist Collective of Transgender Women of Africa (S.H.E.) Website: http://transfeminists.org/

South Africa

Gender DynamiX Email: info@genderdynamix.org.za Address: Unit 21, Collingwood Building, 10 Anson Street, Observatory, Cape Town Telephone: +27 (0)21 447 4797 Website: www.genderdynamix.org.za

ASIA

China

Transgender Resource Center
Email: info@tgr.org.hk Address: Shop 7, G/F, Hip Fai Building, 9 Station Lane, Hung Hom, Hong Kong
Telephone: +852-8230-0838
Website: http://transchina.org.cn

India

Sahodari Foundation
Email: reachsahodari@gmail.com, aurokalki@gmail.com
Address: Tamilnadu, India
Telephone: 91 + 7639741916

Japan

Stonewall Japan
Website: http://stonewalljapan.org

Kyrgyzstan

Labrys
Email: kyrgyzlabrys@gmail.com
Address: p/o box 1969, Glavpochtamt 720000, Bishkek, Kyrgyz Republic
Telephone: +996 (312) 902 963
Website: http://www.labrys.kg/

Mongolia

The LGBT Centre
Email: info@lgbtcentre.mn Address: 4th floor, 10/5, Undur Gegeen Zanabazar street, Ulaanbaatar (6,315.62 mi) Ulaanbaatar, Mongolia Telephone: +976 7740 0323 Website: www.lgbtcentre.mn
Pacific Islands National Queer Asian Pacific Islander Alliance (NQAPIA) Email: info@nqapia.org Address: NQAPIA PO Box 1277 Old Chelsea Station New York, NY 10113 Telephone: 917-439-3158 Website: http://www.nqapia.org/wpp/

Pakistan

Wajood
Telephone: +92 333 5180668
Philippines
Society of Transsexual Women of the Philippines (STRAP)
Email: strapmanila@gmail.com

Thailand

Asia Pacific Transgender Network
Email: hello@weareaptn.org
Address: 3/29, 3rd fl (W District), Soi Sukhumvit 71 Phra Khanong Nuea, Wat-thana, Bangkok 10110
Telephone: +66 2 108 8855
Thai Transgender Alliance
Email: thaitga@gmail.com

OCEANIA

Australia

New South Wales

The Gender Centre
Email: reception@gendercentre.org.au
Address: 41-43 Parramatta Road, Annandale NSW 2038
Telephone: (02) 9519 7599
Website: https://gendercentre.org.au

Northern Territory

Northside Health
Email: admin@northsidehealthnt.com.au
Address: The Clock Tower—4/1 Caryota Court, Coconut Grove
Telephone: 7999 7448
Website: http://www.northsidehealthnt.com.au/

Queensland

Australian Transgender Support Association of Queensland
Email: atsaq.inc@gmail.com
Address: PO Box 212 New Farm QLD 4005 Australia
Telephone: 07 3843 5024
Website: http://www.atsaq.com/

South Australia

Chameleons
Telephone: (08) 8293 3700
Address: P.O. Box 2603 Kent Town S.A. 5071

Tasmania

Working it Out
Address: 278 Argyle St North Hobart, Tasmania 7002 03 6231 1200 Telephone: (03) 6231 1200
Website: https://www.beingproud.org.au

Victoria

Transgender Victoria Address: 100 Drummond St, Carlton, 3053 Telephone: +61 3 9020 4642
Website: https://www.transgendervictoria.com

Western Australia

Living Proud
Email: admin@livingproud.org.au
Address: Living Proud City West Lotteries House 2 Delhi Street West Perth WA 6005
Telephone: (08) 9486 9855/1800 184 527
Website: http://www.livingproud.org.au/

New Zealand

Agender NZ
Email: admin@agender.org.nz
Telephone: 027 280-6466

CENTRAL/SOUTH AMERICA

Brazil
Rede Trans Brasil
Telephone: sayonara@redetransbrasil.org
Website: www.redetransbrasil.org

Grupo Gay da Bahia
Email: ggb@ggb.org.br
Address: Rua Frei Vicente, 24—Pelourinho—Caixa Postal 2552
Telephone: (71) 3322-2552-71 9989 4748
Website: www.ggb.org.br

Chile

Organizando Trans Diversidades Address: Dominica 14, Recoleta, Providencia, Region Metropolitana, Chile Website: http://otdchile.org/

Colombia

Santamaría Fundación
Email: equipofucsia@sfcolombia.org
Address: Carrera 35 No. 19–32 Barrio Cristóbal Colón Cali (Valle del Cauca)—Colombia
Telephone: 057-2-325 31 67
Website: http://www.sfcolombia.org/

Costa Rica

Mulabia
Email: natasha@mulabi.org
Address: Guancaste, Costa Rica
Website: http://www.mulabi.org/

Dominican Republic

Trans Siempre Amigas
Email: transsadominicana@gmail.com
Address: C/Josefa Brea #94, Mejoramiento Social Santo Domingo, D.N.
Telephone: 809-686-1949
Website: http://transsadominicana1.blogspot.com/

Honduras

Cattrachas
Address: Tegucigalpa, Honduras
Website: http://www.cattrachas.org/quienes-somos.php

Mexico

Centro de Apoyo a las Identidades Trans A.C.
Website: http://centroapoyoidentidadestrans.blogspot.mx

Peru

Instituto Runa
Email: runa@runa.org.pe
Address: Eugenio de la Torre N° 191 1er. Piso, San Miguel, Lima 32, Perú

St Lucia

United and Strong Email: unitedandstrongslu@yahoo.com
Address: Massade, Gros Islet P O Box 772, Castries Saint Lucia Telephone: 1(758) 450 0976 Website: https://unitedandstrongstlucia.wordpress.com

EUROPE

Austria

TransX
Email: transx@transgender.at
Address: 1060 Wien, Linke Wienzeile 102
Telephone: 0680/24 14 748
Website: www.transx.at

Belgium

Genres Pluriels
Email: contact@genrespluriels.be
Address: Pluriels genres—rue marché au Charbon, 42-1000 Brussels
Telephone: +32 (0) 487 63 23 43
Website: http://www.genrespluriels.be/?lang=en

Croatia

Trans Aid
Email: info@transaid.hr
Address: Zagreb, Croatia Telephone: +385 (1) 5514 207
Website: http://www.transaid.hr/english/

Germany

TransInterQueer Email: triq@transinterqueer.org Address: Hermannstr. 51 12049 Berlin Telephone: (030) 62 90 13 55
Website: www.transinterqueer.org

Ireland

Clonmel Transgender Adult Support Group
Email: Gerard@clonmelcrc.i.e.
Address: Clonmel Community Resource Centre
Telephone: (052) 612 9143
The last Thursday of every month from 7 to 9 pm

Dublin Trans Peer Support Group
Email: tpsgdublin@gmail.com
Address: Outhouse, 105 Capel Street, Dublin 1
Telephone: (01) 873 4932
Website: www.facebook.com/Transpeersupportdublin Every first and third Wednesday of the month, 7:30 pm–9:30 pm

IndividualiTy (run by BeLonG To Youth Services)
Email: info@belongto.org
Address: Ombudsman for Children's Office, 52 Strand Street Great, North City, Dublin
Telephone: (01) 6706223
Every second Wednesday, 5:30 pm–7:30 pm
LGBT Helpline
Telephone: 1890 929 539
Website: www.lgbt.ie

Poland

Trans-Fuzja Foundation Email: kontakt@transfuzja.org
Address: Warsaw, Poland
Website: http://transfuzja.org/

Serbia

Gayten-LGBT
Website: www.transserbia.org

Slovenia

Trans Akcija
Email: transakcijaslo@gmail.com
Address: Ljubljana, Slovenia
Website: http://transakcija.si/index.php/english/

Spain

Barnacclinic + Grup Hospital Clinic
Gender Identity Clinic
Calle Villaroel, 170
08036 Barcelona
Tel: 93 227 93 91
Fax: 93 227 93 55
Website: https://www.barnaclinic.com/en/specialties/44/gender-identity-clinic

United Kingdom

All About Trans
Email: info@onroadmedia.org.uk
Address: Development House 56-64 Leonard Street London EC2A 4LT UK
Telephone: 020 7065 0790
Website: http://www.allabouttrans.org.uk/

Press For Change
Email: office@pfc.org.uk
Address: BM Network London WC1 N 3XX UK
Website: http://www.pfc.org.uk/

The Gender Identity Research and Education Society (GIRES)
Email: info@gires.org.uk
Address: Melverley The Warren Ashtead Surrey KT21 2SP UK
Telephone: 01372 801554
Website: http://www.gires.org.uk/

The Gender Trust
Email: info@gendertrust.org.uk
Address: 76 The Ridgeway, Astwood Bank, Worcestershire B96 6LX UK
Telephone: 01527 894 838
Website: http://www.gendertrust.org.uk/

Transgender Law & Policy Institute
Bradley Chapman 86 Friar Street CLEETON ST MARY DY14 7RZ United Kingdom info@transgenderlaw.org
Trans Media Watch
Email: transmediawatch@googlemail.com
Address: BM TMW London WC1 N 3XX UK
Website: http://www.transmediawatch.org/

MIDDLE EAST

Turkey

Istanbul LGBTI Solidarity Association
Email: istanbulgbtt@gmail.com Address: Şehit Muhtar Mah. Atıf Yılmaz Cad. Öğüt Sk. 18/4 Telephone: (212) 252 10 88
Website: http://www.istanbullgbti.org/

Pembe Hayat
Email: bilgi@pembehayat.org
Telephone: 0312 433 85 17
Website: www.pembehayat.org
Red Umbrella (Kırmızı Şemsiye)
Email: kirmizisemsiye@kirmizisemsiye.org Telephone: +90 312 419 29 91

NORTH AMERICA

Canada

CAMH Gender Identity Clinic
Telephone: 416-535-8501, press 2
Address: 100 Stokes Street, 3rd floor, Toronto, ON
Positive Space Network
Email: psncoordinator@rockonline.ca

Address: 504 Iroquois Shore Road, Unit 12A, Oakville, ON
Telephone: 905-878-9785
Website: https://www.positivespacenetwork.ca/

TransCare BC
Email: transcareteam@phsa.ca
Telephone: 1-866-999-1514
Transgender Health Information Program
Email: transcareteam@phsa.ca
Telephone: 1-866-999-1514/1-800-784-2433
Website: http://transhealth.phsa.ca/

Index

Page numbers followed by *f* indicate figures; those followed by *t* indicate tables.

L. Poretsky and W. C. Hembree (eds.), *Transgender Medicine*, Contemporary Endocrinology, https://doi.org/10.1007/978-3-030-05683-4

D

The manufacturer's authorised representative in the EU is Springer Nature Customer Service Centre GmbH, Europaplatz 3, 69115 Heidelberg, Germany. If you have any concerns regarding our products, please contact ProductSafety@springernature.com

Printed and bound by CPI Group (UK) Ltd, Croydon, CR0 4YY
30/09/2026
02225593-0014